Histopathology Atlas
for the

Sudden Infant Death Syndrome

Findings derived from the National Institute of Child Health and Human Development Cooperative Epidemiological Study of Sudden Infant Death Syndrome (SIDS) Risk Factors

Marie Valdés-Dapena, M.D.
Patricia A. McFeeley, M.D.
Howard J. Hoffman, M.A.
Karla H. Damus, Ph.D.
Ralph R. Franciosi, M.D.
Donna J. Allison, Ph.D.
Marjorie Jones, M.A.
Jehu C. Hunter, B.S.

D1597268

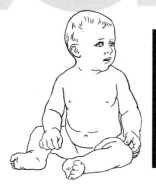

Published by the
Armed Forces Institute of Pathology
in cooperation with the
American Registry of Pathology
and
The National Institute of Child Health and Human Development

Washington, D.C.
1993

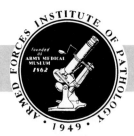 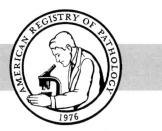

Available from
American Registry of Pathology
Armed Forces Institute of Pathology
Washington, D.C. 20306-6000
ISBN: 1–881041–05–0
1993

Funding of this Atlas was provided in part through Inter-Agency Agreement No. 1-Y01-HD-4-1074 between the National Institute of Child Health and Human Development, NIH, and the Armed Forces Institute of Pathology.

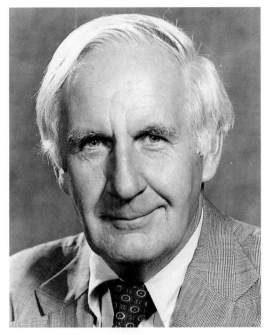

James Weston, M.D.

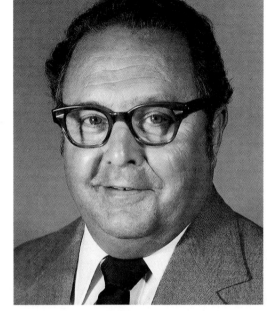

Russell Fisher, M.D.

DEDICATION

The original NICHD Pathology Study Panel, established in 1979 for this project, was comprised of three people: Dr. Russell Fisher, Chief Medical Examiner for the State of Maryland, and Professor, the Johns Hopkins University Medical School; Dr. Marie Valdés-Dapena, Professor of Pathology and Pediatrics, University of Miami School of Medicine; and, Dr. James Weston, Chief Medical Investigator of the State of New Mexico and Professor, University of New Mexico Medical School.

In the course of the five years it took for the panel to complete its work on the study, both Dr. Fisher and Dr. Weston died. They were men of stature in the field of forensic pathology and, despite the heavy burden of their work-related responsibilities, both contributed substantially to the completion of this formidable task. We wish to acknowledge their invaluable effort on behalf of the NICHD Cooperative Epidemiological Study of Sudden Infant Death Syndrome Risk Factors.

With profound gratitude, we dedicate this book to them.

ACKNOWLEDGMENTS

All of the photomicrographs in this book were taken from routine sections prepared for and used in the NICHD SIDS Cooperative Epidemiological Study. The photographer was Mr. John Luscavage, Armed Forces Institute of Pathology, who took these pictures in both black and white and color transparencies for use in a matching study set of kodachromes. We are proud of the quality of these illustrations and express herewith our gratitude to him for the excellence of his work.

J. Thomas Stocker, COL, MC, USA, Deputy Director, Armed Forces Institute of Pathology, was instrumental in facilitating the creation of this Atlas, overseeing its production at the AFIP. Dr. Stocker also provided a liaison with our excellent publications designer, Ms. Fran Card, and managing technical editor, Dena Selby, M.D., who spent many hours organizing the mountains of paperwork required for completing this project.

We thank Duane Alexander, M.D., Director, National Institute of Child Health and Human Development (NICHD), for his support during all phases of this project. Also, we thank Eileen G. Hasselmeyer, Ph.D., R.N., for her leadership from the beginning of the NICHD SIDS Cooperative Epidemiological Study and for reviewing each of the chapters. Ms. Dorothy M. Day provided excellent secretarial assistance throughout the study and typed each of the many drafts of chapters. Heinz W. Berendes, M.D., and Mr. Harvey Shifrin provided managerial and administrative support for this large, multicenter epidemiological and pathological study. We also thank Marian Willinger, Ph.D., for her sustained interest in the Atlas. We appreciate the dedication and perseverence of all our colleagues who have helped to produce this Atlas.

PREFACE

This Atlas has been assembled as a handbook or work manual for practitioners of general and forensic pathology. It was designed for use as a reference by those pathologists who perform autopsies on infants that have died suddenly and unexpectedly. By the nature of their practice many pathologists are more familiar with the pathologic lesions of adults than those of children.

Distinguishing pathologic processes from normal tissues in microscopic sections is not always easy, particularly when the normal histologic features change over time, as they do in infants in the first five years of life. Therefore, following introductory chapters describing the origin of the pathologic material and the study design of the NICHD SIDS Cooperative Epidemiological Study, a chapter is devoted to the normal histology of infants in the first year of postnatal life.

Because there is some confusion about what one expects to see microscopically, in various organs, in the "typical" case of sudden infant death syndrome, another chapter is devoted specifically to illustrations of those minimal lesions.

It is not at all uncommon, in this realm particularly, for a pathologist at autopsy to struggle with a decision as to whether or not a given lesion is sufficiently grave to have caused an infant to die. One chapter, therefore, deals exclusively with these "gray zone" lesions that are so difficult for the practitioner. The aim of the remaining chapters is to present practical guidelines for SIDS through illustrations obtained from the large collection of cases accrued by this national study.

We sincerely hope that this book will be useful to pathologists called upon to diagnose infants who may have died of sudden infant death syndrome.

AUTHOR AFFILIATIONS

Marie Valdés-Dapena, M.D.
Professor of Pathology and Pediatrics
University of Miami School of Medicine
Miami, Florida

Patricia A. McFeeley, M.D.
Chief, Office of Medical Investigation
State of New Mexico, *and*
Associate Professor of Pathology
University of New Mexico School of Medicine
Albuquerque, New Mexico

Howard J. Hoffman, M.A.
Special Assistant for Infant Mortality Research
National Institute of Child Health and Human
    Development, *and presently*
Chief, Epidemiology, Statistics, and Data
    System Branch
National Institute on Deafness and Other
    Communication Disorders
National Institutes of Health
Bethesda, Maryland

Karla H. Damus, Ph.D., R.N.
Assistant Professor, Division of Community
    Health and Epidemiology
Department of Obstetrics and Gynecology
Albert Einstein College of Medicine
Bronx, New York, *and*
Institute for Healthier Babies
March of Dimes Birth Defects Foundation
White Plains, New York

Ralph R. Franciosi, M.D.
Director of Pathology
Children's Hospital of Wisconsin
Milwaukee, Wisconsin

Donna J. Allison, Ph.D.
Project Coordinator, Pathology Coordinating
    Laboratory
Office of the Chief Medical Examiner and
    Coroner
City and County of San Francisco
San Francisco, California

Marjorie Jones, M.A.
Deputy Director, SIDS Data Coordinating
    Center
Department of Biostatistics
School of Public Health and Community
    Medicine
University of Washington
Seattle, Washington

Jehu C. Hunter, B.S.
Consultant and SIDS Study Coordinator
National Institute of Child Health and Human
    Development
National Institutes of Health
Bethesda, Maryland

TABLE OF CONTENTS

◆ *Chapter 1*

Study Design and Protocol for the Pathology Component of the National Institute of Child Health and Human Development Cooperative Epidemiological Study of Sudden Infant Death Syndrome Risk Factors

Introduction 1
Materials and methods 3
    Design of the Epidemiological Study 3
        Study Centers 3
        Ascertainment of SIDS cases and living control infants 4
    Design of the Pathology Component 6
        Necropsy protocol and determination of eligible SIDS cases 6
        Quality control cases 7
        Tissues for microscopic examination 9
        Procedures at the Pathology Coordinating Laboratory (PCL) 9
        Microscopic examination of tissues by the Pathology
            Study Panel (PSP) 10
        Pathology data collection 11
Results 13
    Verification of SIDS cases and explained deaths 13
    Distribution of birth weights and gestational ages 14
    Newborn risk factors 15
    Maternal risk factors 16
    Comparison of selected illnesses/conditions prior to death
        (or interview) 16
Discussion 19
References 20

◆ *Chapter 2*

Death Investigation and Postmortem Examination

Introduction 23
Investigative requirements other than the autopsy 24
    Medical history of the infant 24
    Death and scene investigation 24
The Autopsy 25
    Instruments and materials for the infant autopsy 25
    The autopsy protocol 26

The autopsy method 26
   Preliminary tasks 26
   External examination 26
   Initial incisions 27
   Peritoneal cavity 27
   Thoracic cavity 28
   Opening the normal heart 29
   Removal of the organs en bloc: The Rokitansky Technique 30
   Other pieces of tissue to remove from the body 31
   Spinal cord 31
   Removal of the cranial contents 32
   Dissection of the block of viscera 33
Ancillary studies 36
   Bacterial cultures 36
   Viral cultures 36
   Toxicology 36
   X-ray studies 37
References 37

◆ *Chapter 3*

Normal Histology of the Infant in the Postneonatal Period

Introduction..39
Heart...39
Respiratory tract 41
   Epiglottis 41
   Larynx 42
   Trachea 43
   Bronchus 45
   Bronchiole 46
   Lung 47
   Pleura 52
Spleen 53
Lymph nodes 54
Kidney 56
Ureter 60
Gastrointestinal tract 61
   Esophagus 61
   Cardioesophageal junction 62
   Small bowel 63
Liver 64
Pancreas 66
Ovary 71
Adrenal 73
   Periadrenal adipose tissue 76

Thymus 78
Thyroid 80
Parathyroid 82
Pituitary 86
Skeletal muscle 87
Central nervous system 89
    Wall of lateral ventricle 90
References 92

◆ *Chapter 4*

The Preliminary Diagnosis of SIDS and "Classic" or Typical Gross Findings

Introduction 93
Typical gross findings 94
    External examination 94
        Skin 94
        Mouth and nose 94
    Internal examination 94
        Petechiae 94
        Thymus 95
        Heart's blood 95
        Lungs 95
        Lymphoid tissues 95
        Gastric contents 95
Iatrogenic lesions 95
    Acute 95
    Chronic 95
Requirements for the preliminary diagnosis of SIDS 96
Communication with the family and others 96
References 97

◆ *Chapter 5*

"Classic" or Typical Histologic Findings in SIDS

Introduction 99
Heart 99
    Epicardial petechiae 99
Larynx 100
    Focal fibrinoid necrosis 100
    Laryngitis 101
Trachea 102
    Inflammation 102
Lung 103
    Pleural petechiae 103

Congestion 104
Alveolar hemorrhage 105
Septal hemorrhage/interstitial emphysema 106
Pulmonary edema 107
Alveolar macrophages 108
Atelectasis and emphysema 109
Liver...110
Microvesicular fatty change 110
Thymus...111
Thymic petechiae 111
Brain 112
Perivascular hemorrhage 112
References 113

◆ *Chapter 6*

Explained Sudden Deaths

Introduction 115
Classification of explained sudden deaths 116
Causes for sudden explained deaths determined microscopically 119
Rhabdomyoma of the heart (tuberous sclerosis) 119
Myocarditis 122
Endocardial sclerosis (endocardial fibroelastosis) 124
Acute bronchiolitis 126
Pneumonia 129
Meningitis 134
Boric acid poisoning 138
Encephalitis 140
Cervical cellulitis (Ludwig's angina) 141
Cystic fibrosis of the pancreas (in hot weather) 143
Causes for explained deaths determined at gross autopsy
by historical data and/or by ancillary studies 144
The battered infant 144
Suffocation 144
Congenital heart disease 145
Intracranial arteriovenous malformation 145
Gastroenteritis with dehydration and fluid and electrolyte imbalance.................146
Starvation, neglect, and failure to thrive 148
Massive aspiration of gastric contents 148
References 150

◆ *Chapter 7*

Incidental or Inconsequential Lesions

Introduction 153
Heart 153

Patchy interstitial fibrosis 153
Calcium deposits in a papillary muscle 155
Iatrogenic lesions/needle track marks 156
Epicardial hemorrhage 158
Ischemic necrosis 159
Systemic infections 160
Cytomegalovirus infection 160
Upper airway 164
Epiglottitis 164
Tracheitis 165
Lung 166
Bacterial colonization 166
Patchy overaeration 168
Subpleural emphysema 170
Interstitial pulmonary emphysema 172
Macrophages in alveoli 174
Acute aspiration of gastric content, milk 175
Acute aspiration of solid material 180
Solitary "aspiration granulomas" 182
Bronchiolitis, minimal 186
Bronchopneumonia, minimal 188
Spleen 189
Extramedullary hematopoiesis 189
Kidney 190
Focal subcapsular scars 190
Subcapsular microcysts 191
Focal calcium deposits 192
Nodular renal blastema 194
Gastrointestinal tract 196
Ectopic rests of gastric mucosa in the esophagus 196
Inflammation of the cardioesophageal junction 198
Liver 200
Extramedullary hematopoiesis 200
Fatty Change 202
Hemangioma 203
Pancreas 204
Ectopic splenic tissue in the tail of the pancreas 204
Adrenal 205
Hemorrhage into and calcification of the medulla of the adrenal 205
Cytomegaly 207
Neuroblastoma-in-situ 210
Thymus 211
Extramedullary hematopoiesis 211
Central nervous system 212
Recent subarachnoid hemorrhage 212
Pigment-laden macrophages in the leptomeninges 214

  Residua of old germinal matrix hemorrhages 216
 Blood 218
  Sickling of red cells 218
 References 221

◆ *Chapter 8*

"The Gray Zone"

Introduction 223
 Classification of significant lesions 223
Acute bronchiolitis 226
Pneumonia 232
Macrophages in alveoli in abnormally large numbers
 and extensive distribution 236
Excessive aspiration of amniotic debris 237
Chronic aspiration 242
The "Wilson-Mikity" pattern 248
Sepsis 251
Suffocation with a soft object 251
References 251

◆ *Chapter 9*

Illustrative Cases

Introduction 253
 Case 1: Viral myocarditis 254
 Case 2: *Escherichia coli* sepsis with Waterhouse-Friderichsen syndrome 256
 Case 3: Rhabdomyomas of heart; probable tuberous sclerosis 258
 Case 4: Probable suffocation / compression asphyxia 260
 Case 5: Congenital cardiac anomalies, with large interventricular septal
    defect, a patent ductus arteriosus, right ventricular hypertrophy,
    and congestive heart failure (associated with Down syndrome) 262
 Case 6: Sudden infant death syndrome (status post-resuscitation attempts) 264
 Case 7: Accidental suffocation / asphyxiation by thin plastic sheet 266
 Case 8: Accidental suffocation/bronchopneumonia 268
 Case 9: Suffocation; child abuse 270
 Case 10: Sudden infant death syndrome 274
 Case 11: Bacterial meningitis 276
 References 278

◆ *Chapter 10*

**Summary of Histologic Findings and Implications for Future
SIDS Research**

Introduction 281
Comparability of SIDS and explained deaths 282

      Birth characteristics 282
      Age at death 283
      Causes of explained deaths 284
      Appropriateness of autopsy controls for SIDS cases 286
    Prevalence of histologic lesions 286
    Discussion of selected histologic lesions 292
      Inflammation of the upper airway 292
      Pulmonary congestion 292
      Pulmonary edema 292
      Liver 293
          Extramedullary hematopoiesis 293
          Fatty change 293
      Spleen 293
          Acute splenitis 293
      Adrenal 293
          Presence of periadrenal brown fat 293
      Thymus 293
          Thymic petechiae 293
      Lung..294
          Pleural petechiae 294
          Macrophages in alveoli 294
          Granulomas in lung 294
      Heart 294
          Epi- and/or myocardial petechiae..294
      Intrathoracic 294
          Petechiae 294
      Summary of positive morphological findings 294
    Special studies based on the NICHD histopathology collection 295
    Resources from the NICHD histopathology collection
      for future study and research activities 296
    Conclusion...296
    References 298

Appendix A: Autopsy protocol form 303
Appendix B: Letters 309
Appendix C: Study principal investigators, consultants, & NICHD staff 313
Appendix D: Medical examiners & coroners contributing SIDS cases to
               NICHD Cooperative Epidemiological Study of SIDS Risks Factors 315

Index 319

List of Tables

Table 1–1   Numbers of live births, and infant, neonatal, postneonatal, and SIDS mortality rates by race for the geographical area encompassed by the NICHD SIDS Cooperative Epidemiological Study and for the total United States in 1979. 2

Table 1–2   Number of SIDS cases and selected indices by study center 4

Table 1–3   Distribution of age at death for pathologically defined singleton SIDS cases and age at maternal interview for matched living control infants 5

Table 1–4   Tissues collected at autopsy from potential SIDS and quality control cases 7

Table 1–5   List of major differential diagnoses in sudden, unexpected infant deaths, exclusive of SIDS, based on history, information from gross dissection, microscopic, toxicological, and microbiological studies 8

Table 1–6   Summary of criteria used by the Pathology Study Panel for their impressions after completion of the first review 11

Table 1–7   Critertia used by the Pathology Study Panel for classifying the certainty of the diagnoses of SIDS as the cause of death 12

Table 1–8   Final SIDS pathology classification by plurality of birth of eligible SIDS cases 13

Table 1–9   Distribution of singleton SIDS cases and living control infants by joint birth weight and gestational age categories 14

Table 1–10   Percent and relative risk (odds ratio)of selected newborn factors for SIDS cases compared to living control infants 16

Table 1–11   Percent and relative risk (odds ratio) of selected maternal factors for SIDS cases compared to living control infants 17

Table 1–12   Selected illnesses or conditions of singleton SIDS cases and living control infants as reported by the maternal interview 18

Table 2–1   Summary of recommendations for microscopic sections 35

Table 6–1   Clasification of SIDS cases and explained deaths by source contributing to the NICHD Cooperative Epidemiologic Study 115

Table 6–2	Explained causes of sudden death in infants classified by anatomical site of mortal lesion	117
Table 6–3	Explained causes of sudden death in infants classified by source of information	118
Table 6–4	Diagnoses, cases of explained deaths originally submitted as SIDS	119
Table 8–1	Significant morbid and mortal lesions	224
Table 10–1	Number and percent of singleton SIDS cases and explained deaths by race, sex, gestational age, and birth weight	283
Table 10-2	Age at death distribution of singleton SIDS cases and explained deaths	284
Table 10-3	Specific causes-of-death categories for the explained death infants	285
Table 10–4	Histopathological findings based on the Pathology Study Panel review of microscopic slides for singleton SIDS cases and expained deaths	288
Table 10–5	Percentage of SIDS singleton cases and explained deaths diagnosed as having some degree of pneumonia	292
Table 10–6	Percentage of SIDS singleton cases and explained deaths with macrophages in alveoli	292

CHAPTER *1*

STUDY DESIGN AND PROTOCOL FOR THE PATHOLOGY COMPONENT OF THE NATIONAL INSTITUTE OF CHILD HEALTH AND HUMAN DEVELOPMENT (NICHD) COOPERATIVE EPIDEMIOLOGICAL STUDY OF SUDDEN INFANT DEATH SYNDROME (SIDS) RISK FACTORS

INTRODUCTION

Although several earlier comprehensive studies of the Sudden Infant Death Syndrome involved both epidemiology and pathology findings,[1,3,10,11,15] the NICHD Cooperative Epidemiological Study of SIDS Risk Factors was the first multicenter, population-based, case-control investigation in which, by design, a panel of pathologists played an integral part. The panel, in fact, made the ultimate decisions as to which cases were to be included in the analyses. Another unique feature of the study was the extraordinary care taken to ensure that each of the three-member panel worked independently and conducted his or her review in a "blinded" two-stage process that provided for checks on the consistency and validity of the classification of SIDS versus explained deaths.

The purposes of the review of case material were threefold: 1) to verify the diagnosis of SIDS, (2) to determine whether there were any common pathological findings among the SIDS cases, and (3) to suggest areas in which further research might be profitable. Autopsies were performed on the infant death cases at medical examiner/coroner's offices associated with the six study centers, which were located in the eastern, mid-western, and western regions of the United States. The six centers, with defined geographic boundaries, were: Chicago (Cook County), California (eight counties), New York City (all five boroughs), St. Louis (five county metropolitan area), Seattle (King county), and upstate New York (20 counties). The population of births occurring in the defined geographic areas of the NICHD SIDS Cooperative Epidemiological Study, in 1979, when the study was conducted, represented about 10% of all births in the United States.

Autopsies were performed according to a standard protocol. Selected tissues were obtained and placed in formalin. Those tissues were sent to a central facility, the Pathology Coordinating Laboratory (PCL), located at the San Francisco Medical Examiner/Coroner's Office. At the PCL a standard set of microscopic slides was prepared for subsequent review by the three-member Pathology Study Panel (PSP). That panel included two forensic pathologists, Dr. Russell Fisher and Dr. James Weston, who were, respectively, the Chief Medical Examiner and Chief Medical Investigator for the States of Maryland and New Mexico. Dr. Marie Valdés-Dapena, a pediatric pathologist and Professor of Pathology and Pediatrics at the University of Miami in Florida, was the other original member of the PSP. Drs. Fisher and Weston died after completion of the first tier of the two-tiered review process. After their deaths, Dr. Patricia McFeeley, a forensic pathologist and now the Chief Medical Investigator for the State of New Mexico, and Dr. Ralph Franciosi, a pediatric pathologist,

originally a member of the study's Advisory Committee, who has since become Director of Pathology in the Children's Hospital of Wisconsin in Milwaukee, assumed their roles in completing the second tier of the SIDS pathology review.

In addition to describing the procedures used for the acquisition of the NICHD SIDS pathology collection, this chapter provides an overview of the study design, sample size, and selected characteristics of the cases and control (both living and dead) infants, thereby providing the necessary background for subsequent chapters of this SIDS Histopathology Atlas.

Table 1–1. **Numbers of Live Births, and Infant, Neonatal, Postneonatal, and SIDS Mortality Rates by Race for the Geographical Area Encompassed by the NICHD SIDS Cooperative Epidemiological Study and for the Total United States in 1979***

	Live Births	Infant Mortality Rate*	Neonatal Mortality Rate	Postneonatal Mortality Rate	SIDS Mortality Rate
Black Race					
Cooperative Study	87,371	22.6	14.8	7.8	3.65
United States	577,855	21.8	14.3	7.5	2.82
Non-Black Race					
Cooperative Study	259,909	11.6	8.0	3.5	1.10
United States	2,916,543	11.3	7.8	3.6	1.25
Total Race					
Cooperative Study	347,280	14.3	9.7	4.6	1.75
United States	3,494,398	13.1	8.9	4.2	1.51

* Infant mortality rate equals the number of infant deaths per 1,000 live births. The neonatal, postneonatal and SIDS mortality rates are defined similarly.

MATERIALS AND METHODS

DESIGN OF THE EPIDEMIOLOGICAL STUDY

The NICHD Cooperative Epidemiological Study of SIDS Risk Factors was a multicenter, population-based, case-control study. The study design comprised three distinct but interrelated components: (1) ascertainment of study infants, including the selection of two living control infants for each SIDS infant and the conduct of face-to-face interviews with parents (usually mothers) of both SIDS and control infants, (2) abstraction of all medical records on each infant and his or her biologic mother, and (3) collection and review of autopsies and related pathology materials.

The SIDS cases were ascertained over a span of 15 months from October 1978 through December 1979. The combined population base for the study represented approximately 10% of all live births in the United States during the study period.[5] One-fourth of the live births that occurred in the geographic areas included in the study were black, and the remaining three-fourths were non-black. These data and other selected vital statistics are presented in Table 1–1. The incidence (number of SIDS cases per 1,000 live births) by race is shown in the far right-hand column. The SIDS incidence in the entire United States, as calculated by the National Center for Health Statistics, is compared with the incidence in the study areas. The incidence of SIDS among non-black infants in the NICHD study was 1.10 versus 1.25 for the entire United States, which is 12% lower in the study areas compared to the national incidence.

The SIDS incidence for blacks is higher than for non-blacks. Approximately one-half of the SIDS cases in the NICHD SIDS Cooperative Epidemiological Study were black. In addition, the SIDS incidence among black infants was 29% higher in the NICHD study (3.65 per 1,000 live births versus 2.82 for the entire United States). Although variations in the SIDS incidence between the different study centers occurred among both black and non-black infants, only among black infants was there a marked, overall difference between the NICHD study and the national figures. This difference could not be attributed to the NICHD study areas having higher total infant, neonatal, or postneonatal mortality rates since those rates were virtually the same as the national rates (see Table 1–1). Hence, it may be that black SIDS cases were ascertained better in the NICHD study areas than they were in the United States in general.

Study Centers

The six study centers, together with sample sizes, SIDS incidences, and proportions of all postneonatal deaths due to SIDS, are indicated in Table 1–2. Overall in the NICHD study, 37.9% of all postneonatal deaths were attributed to SIDS.[7] Although the Seattle, Chicago, and California study centers all reported relatively high proportions of postneonatal deaths due to SIDS (48.5%, 46.4%, and 40.6%, respectively), the SIDS incidence rates for Seattle and California were not nearly as high as for Chicago. This difference is explicable, in part, by the racial composition at the three sites, 50.7% of live births in Chicago were black as compared to 9.1% in California and 7.0% in Seattle. As shown in Table 1–1, black infants have a SIDS incidence rate approximately three times higher than white infants in the United States.

With respect to the pathology component, each study center was responsible for developing procedures to ensure cooperation with the local medical examiner/coroner's office(s) in reporting all eligible SIDS cases. The staff also monitored adherence to the standardized necropsy protocol during postmortem examination, and determined that the tissues required for microscopic examination were collected properly and submitted to the Pathology Coordinating Laboratory located at the San Francisco Medical Examiner/Coroner's Office. Materials

Table1–2.   **Number of SIDS Cases and Selected Indices by Study Center***

Study Center	Singleton SIDS Cases (No.)	Multiple Birth SIDS Cases (No.)	SIDS Deaths as Proportion of Postneonatal Deaths (%)	SIDS Rate* (No. per 1,000 Live Births)
Chicago	247	11	46.4	3.48
California	170	9	40.6	1.66
Seattle	46	1	48.5	2.00
New York City	193	10	33.4	1.52
New York State	80	4	26.1	0.86
St. Louis	64	3	33.3	1.29
Totals	800	38	37.9	1.75

*Based on 1979 U.S. vital statistics for resident live births and postneonatal infant deaths within the geographic boundaries of each of the six study centers.

required by the local medical examiner/coroner's offices for those procedures were distributed by the study center staff. The study center staff also obtained informed consent from the parents of the case infants prior to their inclusion in the study. The parents were assured their family's privacy would be protected and confidentiality would be maintained throughout the study.

Ascertainment of SIDS Cases and Living Control Infants

In order to obtain data of the best quality and to avoid introducing bias into the data set, complete ascertainment of eligible SIDS cases during the study period was essential. For that purpose a case notification procedure was established at each study center. According to that procedure, a contact person at the participating medical examiner/coroner's office telephoned the study center on the day of death, or on the next working day after the death, of an eligible SIDS infant. Specific items of information on the case were obtained by the study center personnel during that call. Twice monthly, telephone calls were made by the staff at the study center to the participating medical examiner/coroner's offices to verify the number of eligible SIDS cases reported during the prior two week interval and, also, to obtain information on any potential cases that might have been missed during that period. To establish the completeness of case ascertainment in each study area, death certificates also were screened bimonthly to check that all infants who had died of SIDS, or those listed as "SIDS-pending further study," were accounted for.

An eligible case infant was defined as any infant who died suddenly and unexpectedly, and who met all of the eligibility criteria and none of the exclusion criteria for the study. The eligibility criteria were: (1) death during the specified 15-month time period, (2) death within the geographic limits of a study center (that is, death occurring within the study center's prescribed county or city boundaries), (3) death designated as SIDS or possibly SIDS, following autopsy by a medical examiner or coroner, using the standardized necropsy protocol. Exclusion criteria were: (1) no autopsy performed, (2) major deviations from standardized necropsy protocol during postmortem examination, (3) any death of an infant younger than 14 days or older than 24 months of age, (4) any death of an infant occurring in a hospital if the infant had been in the facility for more than 24 hours immediately prior to death.

Once an eligible case was submitted, the study center initiated control selection procedures which eventually resulted in the identification of two living control infants. The first control (Control A) was randomly selected from a defined pool of birth certificates within the geographic area of the study center and was matched only to the age at death of the SIDS infant. Thus, mothers of living Control A infants were interviewed when their infants were within two weeks of the age at death of the SIDS infant. A comparison of the age at death distribution for the 757 pathologically-validated SIDS cases and the age at interview of the corresponding living control infants is shown in Table 1–3. The second control (Control B) was matched on age in the same way as Control A and, in addition, was matched also by race (dichotomized as black and non-black) and birth weight (categorized as either greater than 2500 grams, or if less than or equal to 2500 grams, then within 250 grams of the birth weight of the SIDS case). For example, a non-black SIDS infant born weighing 1600 grams was matched to a living Control B infant who was of the same age, non-black, and born weighing between 1350-1850 grams.

The mothers of the SIDS infants and living control infants were contacted by the study center staff and invited to participate in the study, which included a detailed home interview. Informed consent was requested for permission to release all medical records concerning the infant

---

Table 1–3. **Distribution of Age at Death for Pathologically Defined Singleton SIDS Cases and Age at Maternal Interview for Matched Living Control Infants***

Age at Death or Maternal Interview	SIDS Cases		Control A		Control B	
	No.	%	No.	%	No.	%
2-5 weeks	118	15.6	98	12.9	94	12.4
6-11 weeks	311	41.1	312	41.2	307	40.6
12-23 weeks	239	31.6	252	33.3	259	34.2
24-51 weeks	73	9.6	78	10.3	80	10.6
52-103 weeks	16	2.1	17	2.2	17	2.2
Totals	757	100.0	757	100.0	757	100.0

*Control A infants were matched on age and Control B infants were matched on age, race (black vs. non-black), and birth weight (to within 250 grams if the SIDS case were less than 2500 grams).

from birth to death (or for control infants until time of the maternal interview), as well as prenatal and delivery records of the mother. Abstraction of medical records was very time consuming, requiring two years following ascertainment of the last case in December 1979. If the SIDS mother agreed to participate, an interview was scheduled for about three weeks after the infant's death and the medical records abstraction process was initiated. About 95% of the mothers of SIDS cases were located and successfully interviewed. Control mothers were selected and interviewed for all of the SIDS cases. If the first chosen control mother did not agree to participate, or could not be located within the allowable period of time (since age of the control infant was a critical matching variable), then an alternate control mother was selected randomly and invited to participate in the study. After written and telephone contact, however, the majority of the first chosen control mothers agreed to participate. About 20% of those initially chosen for the study were *not* interviewed for the following reasons: not home (6%), moved (7%), refused to be interviewed or to release medical records (4%), or other miscellaneous reasons (4%). In all of those instances, alternate control mothers were selected for the study.

DESIGN OF THE PATHOLOGY COMPONENT

Concomitant to the interview and medical records review were the activities of the Pathology Study Panel. The pathology component was designed to assure that each case ultimately included in the data base was deemed to be either definitely or probably SIDS, following a two-tiered review. However, prior to the panel's careful review of all cases, routine postmortem reviews were conducted by the participating medical examiners and coroners who served the regions of the six study centers. That process included prompt notification of the study centers by the medical examiner/coroner's offices when a sudden infant death occurred.

Necropsy Protocol and Determination of Eligible SIDS Cases

A standardized necropsy protocol was followed during the mandatory autopsy. The necropsy protocol was designed to provide a standardized procedure for postmortem examination and collection of tissues for later microscopic examination. For inclusion of a case in the study, the prosector must have followed the necropsy protocol during the postmortem examination.

The prosectors were asked to perform the gross autopsies and dictate the gross autopsy reports in their usual fashion. They were further requested to complete a necropsy checklist which included a short questionnaire about the gross external and internal appearance of the infant at autopsy and to collect the tissue samples listed in Table 1–4. The prosectors then reviewed the autopsy findings, the death investigative reports, and any other materials or available test results (e.g., x-rays, toxicology, etc.), and determined whether the infant death was or was not compatible with the diagnosis of SIDS. A list of differential diagnoses (Table 1– 5) was provided, based on the publication by Jones and Weston,[8] to assist the pathologist in distinguishing a SIDS case from an explained death. If a specific cause of death ("known" cause) was determined, the infant was classified as definitely a *non-SIDS* case and, therefore, not eligible for study enrollment. If the death was not due to a recognized cause, the case was labelled as "eligible for further study" and referred to the study center.

Some of the cases submitted as eligible for further study were later determined to be due to "known" causes of death based on additional investigative information. For example, occasionally the results of laboratory studies, including toxicology, biochemistry, or microbiology, permitted identification of specific causes of death. If the maternal interview had already been completed, those originally "eligible" cases were then designated as "turn arounds" and the information already gathered was used to contribute to a group of *non-living* controls. If the mother had not been interviewed, then those infants were designated as "ineligible" and no further information was gathered from their parents since they no longer met all of the study eligibility criteria.

Quality Control Cases

A small, selected group of 68 infant deaths was submitted by the study centers to the Pathology Coordinating Laboratory. Those infant deaths were control infants chosen deliberately

---

Table 1–4.   **Tissues Collected at Autopsy from Potential SIDS and Quality Control Cases**

I. **Sections from the following tissues:**
Adrenal, one piece through the thickest part of the adrenal, including overlying fat
Brain
　　Basal ganglia, including ependymal surface and the angle of the lateral ventricle
　　Cerebellum, including the dentate nucleus and folia
　　Hippocampus, one randomly selected piece including the leptomeninges
　　Motor cortex, including overlying meninges
　　Temporal bone, one section of the petrous portion of the temporal bone, including
　　　　mucosal lining of the middle ear
Diaphragm, one randomly selected piece
Heart, a section through the walls of both the left and the right ventricles, not
　　including septum, two pieces total (endocardium to epicardium)
Ileum, including a Peyer's patch, the complete unopened ileocecal region, 2 cm above to
　　2 cm below the ileocecal valve
Kidney, one representative section extending from the capsule to the pelvis
Liver, one randomly selected piece
Lungs, a section from **each** lobe, extending from the main bronchus out to the periphery,
　　(five sections in all)
Mesenteric lymph node, one representative section
Spleen, one randomly selected piece
Thymus, one randomly selected piece

II. **Any grossly abnormal tissue(s)**

III. **One costochondral junction, approximately 2 cm in length**

IV. **The following tissue blocks:**
Neck organs, a block to include trachea and thyroid, a mainstem bronchus, and carinal
　　nodes
Larynx, a block of the right half of the larynx, including the epiglottis and 2 cm below the vocal
　　cords
Gastro-esophageal junction, a block including 2 cm of esophagus and 2 cm of stomach
Pancreas, a block to include the head of the pancreas with overlying duodenum
Brain, a longitudinal block to include half of the length of the pons (including the floor of the
　　fourth ventricle and the basis pontis) and medulla (including the olivary bodies)
　　with overlying meninges

Table 1–5.   **List of Major Differential Diagnoses in Sudden, Unexpected Infant Deaths, Exclusive of SIDS, Based on History, Information from Gross Dissection, Microscopic, Toxicological, and Microbiological Studies**

General: Malnutrition
                Poisoning
                Reye's Syndrome
                Sepsis (including meningococcemia)

Blood: Sickle cell anemia with thrombosis

Heart: Congenital heart disease (including aortic stenosis)
                Myocarditis (especially Coxsackie)
                Subendocardial fibroelastosis (endocardial sclerosis)

Lungs and   Bronchiolitis
Airways: Pneumonia
                Idiopathic pulmonary hypertension (pulmonary arteriolar sclerosis)
                Tracheobronchitis

Kidney: Pyelonephritis

G.E. Tract: Enterocolitis (with diarrhea and dehydration)
                Salmonella, Shigella, and pathogenic *E. Coli*

Liver: Hepatitis (including Coxsackie)

Pancreas: Boric acid poisoning
                Cystic fibrosis of the pancreas (sudden death in hot weather)
                Pancreatitis (including Coxsackie)

Adrenal: Congenital adrenal hyperplasia

Brain: Arteriovenous malformation
                Encephalitis
                Meningitis
                Trauma (skull fractures, edema, subdural hemorrhage)

Skeleton: The battered child

as "quality controls" to check on the ability of the pathology review panel to recognize and distinguish explained deaths from SIDS cases. Prior to submission of a quality control case, the study center staff cleared each submission with the principal investigator at the study center and with a pediatric pathologist who, as a member of the study's Advisory Committee, had agreed to screen the potential quality control cases for suitability. Both the Pathology Coordinating Laboratory staff and the Pathology Study Panel members were "blinded" as to which of the submitted infant death cases were believed to be SIDS versus deaths due to known causes.

Tissues for Microscopic Examination

The prosectors were provided with detailed instructions on tissue collection procedures to be followed in those cases which were eligible for further study and in selected quality control cases. They were instructed to place pieces of the tissues listed in Table 1–4 in an 8" X 12" plastic bag containing phosphate buffered formalin and to allow them to fix there for 72 hours. At the end of the fixation period, all but about 2 ml of the formalin was to be decanted from the bag. Excess air was to be expelled and the bag then heat-sealed.

All tissues and corresponding necropsy checklists were packaged and mailed to the Pathology Coordinating Laboratory for microscopic slide preparation. The suspected or assumed cause of death did not appear on any of those forms since PCL staff were to remain "blinded" as to the cause of death. "Unblinding" of the PCL staff occurred at a much later time when copies of the death investigative report, gross and microscopic autopsy reports, and results of additional studies or tests were forwarded to the PCL by the project coordinators at each of the study centers. None of that information was sent until after completion of the first review by the PSP. To assure confidentiality, no identifying data (names, addresses, etc.) appeared on any of the materials sent by the local medical examiner/coroner's offices to the PCL. Cases were identified by the pathology case

number only, which was assigned in ascending numerical order by the PCL staff.

Procedures at the Pathology Coordinating Laboratory (PCL)

At the PCL the fixed wet tissue samples from all submitted cases were oriented and trimmed into standard sections by a forensic pathologist who, like all PCL staff, was blinded as to the cause of death. The condition of each sample was noted, as was the absence of any specifically requested sample. The trimmed tissues were processed, each case separately, in a Technicon processor, using standard techniques. Any remaining tissues were again sealed in a plastic bag with fresh phosphate buffered formalin.

Processed tissues were embedded in paraffin in a standardized orientation using plastic peel-away molds with a paper label, one piece of tissue per block. Sections were cut from the paraffin blocks on a microtome at 5-6 microns, the thickness depending upon the quality of the tissue. Two or more sections from each block were mounted on a microscopic slide. All sections were stained with hematoxylin and eosin. There was an average of 26 slides per case.

Each slide was examined microscopically to determine whether the quality of the tissue and the cutting and staining met acceptable standards. If not, that is, if they varied significantly in quality from a standard slide, then the sections were recut or restained. An average of six recuts per case was required.

When all slides were judged to be of the best possible quality permitted by the condition of the tissues, the slides for each case were arranged in a standard format in anatomical order and numbers were affixed to each slide. The numbers identified both the case and the tissue, each tissue having a specific number. For example, all slides bearing pancreas sections were numbered as 15. A cross-index was maintained of the slide and block numbers for each case.

At that stage, a final determination was made

regarding missing tissues. At least one piece of the following tissues, except where indicated, was essential for a case to be considered adequate: trachea, thymus, lung (at least two pieces required, one central and one peripheral), heart, liver, pancreas, cerebellum, basal ganglia, and hippocampus. A list of cases with any of the above tissues missing was prepared for each study center by the PCL. Those lists were sent to the study centers monthly and served as requests to search for and to submit the missing tissues. Cases that deviated from the standard in a major way, after all available tissues were submitted, were not excluded from the study on that basis alone; as much data as possible was obtained on those cases. The Pathology Study Panel later decided how to categorize the incomplete cases, for example, deciding that some of these cases were "probable" SIDS. Others were labeled as "indeterminate" and excluded from the study, while still others were labeled as "possible" SIDS and excluded from the pathology-validated SIDS cases, which were used in the analysis of SIDS risk factors.

Microscopic Examination of Tissues by the Pathology Study Panel (PSP)

The prepared slides were then sent (six cases to the set) to the PSP as the first part of the two-tiered independent review system. The same slide sets were reviewed by each member of the panel in turn. Each PSP member independently and blindly reviewed the slides on each case, recording all findings on a standard, six page microscopic examination form. The microscopic findings, organ by organ, were noted on that form. After reviewing and documenting their findings the PSP members determined whether the microscopic lesions observed were sufficient to have caused death. The criteria developed at that stage, following the first review of microscopic slides only, are shown in Table 1–6. The only additional information available to PSP members during that initial slide review was the infant's age at death, gestational age, and birth weight.[16]

In order to determine the consistency of the microscopic study among the three PSP pathologists, 30 cases were selected for re-review. Those 30 cases were selected randomly as follows: ten cases that were sent for the original slide review early in the study, ten that had been sent midway during the study, and ten that had been sent towards the end of the study. The slides from each of those cases were renumbered with new pathology case numbers and then were resubmitted to the Pathology Study Panel for a review which should have been identical to the first review. Members of the Pathology Study Panel were unaware of the fact that that consistency check had been built into the study.

In addition to the consistency check, a series of "quality control" cases were also submitted to the panel without their knowing which were presumed to be SIDS or explained deaths. That portion of the first review was meant to assess the precision and accuracy (or validity) of the pathologists' slide review. The outcome of that review will be described in the Results section of this chapter.

Following completion of the first independent review by the panelists, each potential case was sent out for the second stage, or tier, of the review process. For that second review, each member of the Pathology Study Panel re-read his/her own written report of microscopic findings from the first review, supplemented by the local medical examiner/coroner's death investigation and autopsy reports (gross and microscopic) and any other available medical history or special study results. Only after completion of the second-tier of review were joint sessions convened involving all three pathologists to reconsider and resolve every case in which significant discrepancies still existed.

Following the pathology review process (a five year period), all cases were classified as either "SIDS" (further su;bgrouped as "definite," "probable," or "possible" SIDS) or "nonSIDS," that is, an explained cause of death was identified. The basic requirements for the final classification of SIDS deaths is shown in Table 1–7.

Table 1–6.   **Summary of Criteria Used by the Pathology Study Panel for Their Impressions After Completion of the First Review**

A.   Lesion(s) sufficient to cause death

1.   Pneumonia 3+ or 4+ in two or more sections of lung
2.   Myocarditis (any time a good sized focus, 15+ cells, of lymphocytes present in the myocardium)
3.   "Quinsy" in the neck, i.e., severe cellulitis (Ludwig's angina)
4.   Acute inflammation of the leptomeninges
5.   Adrenal hemorrhage 4+, which indicates probable sepsis and Waterhouse-Friderichsen syndrome

B.   Lesions, insufficient to cause death (by themselves)

1.   Inflammation in the upper respiratory tract ≥ 1+ (infants of this age are not subject to fatal epiglottitis)
2.   Patchy pulmonary (alveolar) hemorrhage ≥ 3+
3.   Involution of the thymus, which is evidence of chronic stress
4.   Sickling of blood cells (because infants, especially if less than five months of age, usually do not experience lethal crises)
5.   Modest amounts of iron in macrophages in the lungs (however, if large amounts, it would certainly arouse suspicion about a long-standing and perhaps lethal cardiac lesion or primary pulmonary hemosiderosis)
6.   Aspiration associated with macrophages and polymorphonuclear leukocytes
7.   Apparent pancreatic islet cell hyperplasia
8.   Cholestasis
9.   Triaditis, mild
10.   Extramedullary hematopoiesis, liver and/or spleen
11.   Apparent glomerulonephritis
12.   Cytomegalic inclusion cells
13.   Enteritis, without history of diarrhea or gross findings of fluid contents of the bowel and dehydration or biochemical findings of fluid and electrolyte imbalance
14.   Small, scattered focal hemorrhages in the brain

C.   "Without Lesions" (not considered primary or, of themselves, lethal lesions)

1.   Aspiration, of any degree
2.   Pulmonary edema
3.   "Wilson-Mikity" effect, or alternating patches of atelectasis and emphysema (seen often in babies who have or had bronchopulmonary dysplasia)
4.   Alveolar macrophages, not associated with other lesions

In addition to a decision on the cause of death, each pathologist also indicated the relative usefulness of the materials available in assigning the cause of death. Those reports provided valuable information on which case materials were considered essential in establishing the cause of death.

Pathology Data Collection

All written materials received and generated by the Pathology Coordinating Laboratory were abstracted onto a series of ten forms designed for ease of computer data entry. Those forms consisted of:

1. Comments by Cutter Form
2. Necropsy Checklist Form
3. Death Investigation Report Form
4. Gross Autopsy Report Form
5. Microscopic Autopsy Report Form
6. Special Studies Report Form
7. Terminal Event Cardio-Pulmonary Resuscitation (CPR) Report Form
8. Microscopic Examination Form
9. Second Review Form
10. Cross-Index of Slides, Blocks, and Wet Tissues

When completed and edited, the forms were all submitted to the NICHD SIDS data coordinating center located at the Public Health Computer Center, School of Public Health and Community Medicine, University of Washington in Seattle.

Table 1–7. **Criteria Used by the Pathology Study Panel for Classifying the Certainty of the Diagnosis of SIDS as the Cause of Death**

	Gross Autopsy	Special Studies: Toxicology or Microbiology	Microscopic Review	History and Death Investigation
Definite SIDS (≥ 90% chance)	Negative	Negative or Not Available	No Lesions or Insufficient Lesions	Present and Adequate
Probable SIDS (50-89% chance)	Negative	Negative or Not Available	No Lesions or Insufficient Lesions	Adequate or Inadequate
Possible SIDS (10-49% chance)	Equivocal or Negative	Negative or Not Available	Insufficient Lesions	Adequate or Inadequate
Explained Deaths or Indeterminate (<10% chance)	Positive **OR**	Positive **OR**	Lesions **OR** Sufficient to Cause Death	Positive

RESULTS

VERIFICATION OF SIDS CASES AND EXPLAINED DEATHS

At the conclusion of the pathology review, the panel was unable to distinguish 27 (40%) of the so-called "quality control" cases from SIDS infants. In that regard, it is important to mention that the majority of those 27 quality control cases had been submitted with bronchopneumonia as the presumed cause of death. That issue will be discussed more fully later in the Atlas (especially Chapters 6, 8, and 10). Also, the panel could not decide in three other quality control cases (4%) whether they were SIDS infants or explained deaths because of incompleteness, either of tissues or other materials. However, 38 (56%) of the quality control cases were confirmed by the panel as deaths due to explained causes.[6]

Of the 800 eligible singleton SIDS cases, 757 (94.6%) were ultimately judged by the panel to be either "definite" or "probable" SIDS (Table 1-8). For purposes of the epidemiological analysis of risk factors, and all other reports from the study, those 757 singleton SIDS cases comprise the pathologically-validated SIDS cases. A very similar proportion, 92.1% (35/38), of eligible multiple birth SIDS cases were also deemed to be either "definite" or "probable" SIDS by the Pathology Study Panel, as shown in Table 1-8.

All of the quality control cases in which the panel concurred regarding their having been truly explained deaths were used ultimately in a group designated as "dead" controls. Indeed, all infant deaths, including potential SIDS, "turn-around" cases, or quality control cases, that the Pathology Study Panel labeled as explained deaths were used later in a series of comparisons between SIDS and "dead" control infants. A total of 65 infant deaths from the NICHD SIDS Cooperative Epidemiological Study were considered to have been explained deaths by the panel. The data presented in this Atlas are derived primarily from those two groups: the 65 explained deaths and the 757 singleton SIDS cases. These two groups represent extremes in the spectrum of sudden infant death. The comparison of frequencies of pathologic lesions between these two groups is provided in Chapter 10.

Table 1- 8. **Final SIDS Pathology Classification by Plurality of Birth**

| | Singleton Births | | Multiple Births | |
	No.	%	No.	%
Definite SIDS	627	78.4	29	76.3
Probable SIDS	130	16.3	6	15.8
Possible SIDS	18	2.3	0	0.0
Explained Deaths	14	1.8	1	2.6
Indeterminate Cause	11	1.4	2	5.3
Totals	800	100.0	38	100.0

DISTRIBUTION OF BIRTH WEIGHTS AND GESTATIONAL AGES

The joint classification of SIDS cases and control infants by birth weight and gestational age is shown in Table 1–9. The importance of the second control series, the Control B infants, is evident from the table, since otherwise there would not have been enough very low birth weight and/or preterm infants with which to compare the SIDS cases. One of the main reasons for matching in a case control study is to ensure that there are sufficient numbers of controls for proper comparisons with the cases. The Control B infants perform this function for race and prematurity or low birth weight, which are well-known risk factors for SIDS in the U. S.[2, 9, 11]

Table 1– 9. Distribution of Singleton SIDS Cases and Living Control Infants by Joint Birth Weight and Gestational Age Categories*

	Very Low Birth Weight (800-1499 g)		Moderately Low Birth Weight (1500-2499 g)		Normal Birth Weight (≥ 2500 g)		Totals
	No.	%	No.	%	No.	%	No.
Preterm Gestations (20-36 weeks)							
SIDS Cases	29	21.8	77	57.9	27	20.3	133
Control A	2	5.7	20	57.1	13	37.1	35
Control B	33	26.6	72	58.1	19	15.3	124
Term Gestations (≥ 37 weeks)							
SIDS Cases	1	0.2	68	11.0	550	88.8	619
Control A	0	0.0	26	3.4	696	96.4	722
Control B	1	0.2	72	11.4	560	88.5	633
All Gestations							
SIDS Cases	30	4.0	145	19.3	577	76.7	752
Control A	2	0.3	46	6.1	709	93.7	757
Control B	34	4.5	144	19.0	579	76.5	757

*Either gestational age or birth weight was unknown in five of the SIDS cases.

NEWBORN RISK FACTORS

Relative risks, estimated using odds ratios, for several newborn conditions are shown in Table 1–10. For example, the relative risk of SIDS for low birth weight, or preterm, infants is 4.6 compared to age-matched, living Control A infants. There was no increased relative risk compared to Control B infants since low birth weight (within ± 250 grams) and race were matched. Very low birth weight (< 1500 grams), or very preterm (< 33 weeks), infants had still higher relative risks, 17.8 and 15.6, respectively, as compared to Control A infants. As expected from the pronounced association of SIDS with prematurity, low Apgar scores at both one and five minutes are increased in SIDS compared to Control A infants. This association was not present with respect to Control B infants, however, since Control B infants were matched to the SIDS cases for low birth weight and race. Male infants had approximately a 50% higher risk of dying of SIDS than female infants, regardless of the control series used for the comparison. This is appropriate since sex of the infant was not a matching factor in the study. Black race was associated with an increased risk of two and one half times for SIDS versus Control A infants. Because of matching, race was not a risk factor for comparisons of SIDS versus Control B infants.

Most of the other conditions in the table, those noted by nurses during the newborn nursery stay, were significant with respect to both the Control A and Control B infants. One exception is that jaundice was not associated with SIDS risk. Also, apnea of prematurity was not significantly associated with SIDS risk once low birth weight was properly controlled, namely, by the comparison with Control B infants. Bradycardia was only marginally significant (p<0.05) in the comparison with Control A infants, and was not significant compared to Control B infants. Although the other factors in the table (that is, tachycardia, hypothermia, tachypnea, and fever) were each significantly increased for SIDS infants in comparison to either control group, the differences were not always large. Only "fever" had a relative risk of 2.0 or greater (odds ratio of 2.6 versus Control A infants and 1.9 versus Control B infants). However, the frequency of fever among SIDS cases was only 6.3%. The most common of the conditions was "hypothermia," with 45.9% of the SIDS infants classified as hypothermic at some point during their nursery stay. Yet, the relative risk was only about 1.5 (odds ratio of 1.7 versus Control A infants and 1.3 versus Control B infants). Both tachypnea and tachycardia were reported in about 25% of the SIDS cases, but again the relative risks averaged only 1.5.

MATERNAL RISK FACTORS

Several potential maternal risk factors for SIDS are shown in Table 1–11. These factors have been arrayed in order of increasing strength of association. The majority of maternal factors shown in this table are associated with a relative risk of two or higher. The three most significant factors are: maternal smoking during pregnancy, unmarried mother, and maternal age less than 20 years at the time of first pregnancy (not necessarily the pregnancy of the SIDS infant). On the other hand, factors such as cesarean delivery, toxemia or preeclampsia or hypertension, and alcohol use during pregnancy did not show an increased risk for SIDS. In between these two extremes in relative risk, there were a number of factors which were significantly increased for SIDS: high parity, young maternal age at the birth of the SIDS infant, low weight gain during pregnancy, anemia, late (third trimester) or no prenatal care, less than a high school education, infections (urinary tract or venereal disease), illicit drug use (mostly marijuana use at the time of this study), and mother not breast-feeding her infant.

Many of the maternal risk factors are interrelated. Also, the strongest factors, for example, cigarette smoking and young age at first

Table 1–10. Percent and Relative Risk (Odds Ratio) of Selected Newborn Factors for SIDS Cases Compared to Living Control Infants

	Frequency Among SIDS Infants	SIDS vs. Control A	SIDS vs. Control B
	%	Odds Ratio	Odds Ratio
Low birth weight [< 2500 g]	24.0	4.6[a]	1.0[b]
Very low birth weight [< 1500 g]	4.5	17.8[a]	1.0[b]
Preterm birth [< 37 weeks]	18.2	4.6[a]	1.1
Very preterm birth [< 33 weeks]	5.8	15.6[a]	1.3
Apgar score at 1 min < 7	12.7	2.0[a]	1.0
Apgar score at 5 min < 7	4.1	3.5[a]	0.9
Male sex	59.7	1.4[c]	1.5[c]
Black race	53.6	2.5[a]	1.0[b]
Jaundice of the newborn	39.6	1.1	1.0
Bradycardia	16.7	1.4[e]	1.2
Tachycardia	24.2	1.6[a]	1.5[d]
Hypothermia	45.9	1.7[a]	1.3[e]
Tachypnea	25.6	1.9[a]	1.3[e]
Fever	6.3	2.6[a]	1.9[e]
Apnea of prematurity	5.2	7.2[a]	1.1

[a]Level of significance, p<0.001.

[b]These odds ratios are equal to 1.0 due to the study design, since control B infants were matched to SIDS infants for low birth weight (within ± 250 g) and race.

[c]Level of significance, p<0.005.

[d]Level of significance, p<0.01.

[e]Level of significance, p<0.05.

pregnancy, have been shown repeatedly in epidemiological studies of SIDS.[4, 6, 7, 9, 11, 12, 13, 17] In fact, none of these maternal risk factors are truly new or unique to this study. Instead, the pattern of factors shown suggest a less than optimal *in utero* environment and, also, probably indicate that access to health care after delivery of the infant was impaired due to lifestyle and/or socioeconomic disadvantages.[7]

COMPARISON OF SELECTED ILLNESSES/CONDITIONS PRIOR TO DEATH (OR INTERVIEW)

Selected illnesses or conditions of the SIDS cases and living control infants, as reported during the maternal interview, are shown in Table 1–12. These conditions are listed according to the most recently reported time interval:

Table 1–11. Percent and Relative Risk (Odds Ratio) of Selected Maternal Factors for SIDS Cases Compared to Living Control Infants

	Frequency Among Mothers of SIDS	SIDS vs. Control A	SIDS vs. Control B
	%	Odds Ratio	Odds Ratio
Caesarian section delivery	16.8	1.0	1.2
Toxemia, preeclampsia, hypertension	18.1	1.0	0.9
Alcohol use during pregnancy	61.2	1.1	1.0
Low prepregnancy weight (<110 lbs)	15.8	1.2	1.4[c]
Anemia during pregnancy	20.6	1.4[c]	1.4[c]
Parity ≥ 2	38.1	1.5[a]	1.8[a]
Weight gain < 20 lbs at delivery	35.5	2.0[a]	1.7[a]
Mother's age < 20 years	31.5	2.3[a]	1.6[a]
Urinary tract infection/pregnancy	15.8	2.4[a]	1.8[a]
Late or no prenatal care	22.5	2.5[a]	2.5[a]
Mother's education < 12 years	56.7	2.7[a]	2.6[a]
Venereal disease during pregnancy	4.6	2.9[b]	1.8
Illicit drug use during pregnancy	25.6	2.9[a]	2.0[a]
Mother never breast-fed infant	73.7	3.1[a]	2.3[a]
Cigarette smoking during pregnancy	69.6	3.8[a]	3.4[a]
Mother not married	59.3	3.9[a]	2.5[a]
Mother's age < 20 at 1st pregnancy	75.4	4.4[a]	3.3[a]

[a]Level of significance, p<0.001.

[b]Level of significance, p<0.005.

[c]Level of significance, p<0.05.

less than 24 hours prior to death (or prior to interview in the case of living control infants), within the past two weeks (but not within the last 24 hours), more than two weeks before, or never. Background information on recent illnesses or conditions is provided in the case histories or clinical descriptions of the cases chosen for illustration in the Atlas to assist the reader in interpreting the pathology findings.

Several important findings relating to illnesses or other conditions prior to death, or prior to interview for control infants, emerged from this study. It had been reported previously that a recent history of a cough or a cold was a significant feature of SIDS, although other studies had failed to confirm an association.[4, 14] The data from the NICHD SIDS Cooperative Epidemiological Study indicate that control infants have

Table 1–12. **Selected Illnesses or Conditions of Singleton SIDS Cases and Living Control Infants as Reported by the Maternal Interview**

Illnesses or Conditions	SIDS Cases %	Control A %	Control B %
Cold			
< 24 hours	28.9 } 43.8	25.9 } 35.7[c]	26.2 } 38.8
< 2 weeks, > 24 hours	14.9	9.8	12.6
> 2 weeks	22.9	23.1	24.9
Never	33.2	41.2	36.4
Cough			
< 24 hours	12.7 } 21.0	15.3 } 21.2	16.7 } 26.6[b]
< 2 weeks, > 24 hours	8.3	5.9	9.9
> 2 weeks	14.2	14.5	14.4
Never	64.8	64.2	59.0
Diarrhea			
< 24 hours	6.4	3.7	3.7
< 2 weeks, > 24 hours	12.7 } 19.1	8.5 } 12.2[a]	8.3 } 12.0[a]
> 2 weeks	25.0	17.7	19.9
Never	55.9	70.1	68.7
Vomiting			
< 24 hours	7.9 } 14.6	3.2 } 7.7[a]	4.8 } 9.7[a]
< 2 weeks, > 24 hours	6.7	4.5	4.9
> 2 weeks	14.3	9.5	9.5
Never	71.7	82.8	80.8
Seizure			
< 24 hours	0.6 } 0.7	0.0 } 0.0	0.0 } 0.0
< 2 weeks, > 24 hours	0.1	0.0	0.0
> 2 weeks	1.1	0.1	0.5
Never	98.2	99.9	99.5
Fever			
< 24 hours	5.8 } 13.3	2.9 } 11.8	2.8 } 12.1
< 2 weeks, > 24 hours	7.5	8.9	9.3
> 2 weeks	20.9	17.6	20.8
Never	65.7	70.7	67.1
Listless/Droopy			
< 24 hours	7.8 } 10.5	1.1 } 3.8[a]	0.7 } 2.5[a]
< 2 weeks, > 24 hours	2.7	2.8	1.9
> 2 weeks	4.6	3.7	4.0
Never	84.9	92.5	93.5

[a]Level of significance, p<0.001.　　[b]Level of significance, p<0.01.　　[c]Level of significance, p<0.05.

the same history with respect to coughs and colds as the SIDS cases. However, the study did confirm a significant excess of some illnesses or conditions among the SIDS cases, especially diarrhea and vomiting within the two weeks before death or interview and "listless/droopy" within the last 24 hours.[7] Thus, diarrhea within the last two weeks, including the last 24 hours, was reported in 19.1% of SIDS infants as compared to 12.2% of Control A infants and 12.0% of Control B infants. Similarly, vomiting was reported in 14.6% of SIDS infants compared to 7.7% of Control A infants and 9.7% of Control B infants. Each of these comparisons is significant at the $p<0.001$ level. Combining these two symptoms into a single category, "diarrhea and/or vomiting," increased the rate among SIDS infants to 29.3% versus 17.3% among Control A infants and 18.9% among Control B infants, which were also highly significant differences, $p<0.001$. A listless or droopy condition during the last 24 hours was reported at a much increased rate among SIDS infants, 7.8%, compared to either Control A infants, 1.1%, or Control B infants, 0.7%. Upon further investigation of the infants reported as listless or droopy within the last 24 hours, it was shown that they also displayed other symptoms suggestive of acute infection.[7] Thus, just prior to death a relatively small but significant proportion of SIDS infants manifest symptoms of illness at an increased rate compared to living control infants matched for age and, also, low birth weight and race.

DISCUSSION

A total of 23,729 microscopic slides were prepared from tissues submitted on 971 infant death cases by the Pathology Coordinating Laboratory of the NICHD SIDS Cooperative Epidemiological Study. In addition to assisting in the determination of causes of death in those cases,

the microscopic findings of the Pathology Study Panel provides information on the incidence of specific lesions in cases determined to be SIDS. The findings should be useful in developing guidelines for medical examiner/coroner's offices on the types and degrees of specific findings that are compatible with SIDS as a cause of death. Also, it is hoped that this large collection of microscopic slides, which were prepared in a standardized manner, and their corresponding paraffin blocks and remaining wet tissues will constitute a valuable resource for other SIDS research investigators.

The NICHD SIDS Cooperative Epidemiological Study was designed by a team of public health (biostatisticians, maternal and child health experts, and epidemiologists) and medical (pediatricians and pathologists) professionals to determine the strength of certain associations between SIDS and potential risk factors of both a general nature and, to the extent possible, of a SIDS-specific nature. Thus, the case-control design included both randomly selected age matched living Control A infants, as well as randomly selected age, race, and low birth weight matched living Control B infants. This latter control set was used in distinguishing SIDS risk factors from those that are more generally associated with prematurity or black race. In addition, it was recognized by the study's principal investigators that another, albeit much smaller, control series of infants dying from explained causes would be identified in the course of the study.

The inclusion of a panel of pathologists, especially forensic pathologists, in the initial proposal of a comprehensive study of the sudden infant death syndrome was an innovative and almost visionary approach that reaped benefits, which even the original study designers did not anticipate. This Atlas is one of those benefits that we hope will provide tangible assistance to pathologists at all levels of experience who are faced with the difficult decisions about what is, and what is not, to be considered a SIDS case, often on nearly a daily basis. Those decisions, even under the best of conditions, are not always "black" and "white" and this Atlas reflects the recognized subjectivity in difficult, or "gray" zone, cases.

The criteria developed by the Pathology Study Panel were adopted not so much by negotiation or compromise as by unanimous agreement after each of the panel members had reached nearly identical conclusions independently. Although basic standards were agreed upon prior to starting the pathology review process, this Atlas reflects the modified and expanded experience of more than five years of involvement with the review of nearly a 1,000 cases. The requirements for classification within this system include not only the physical findings of the gross autopsy and microscopic examination but also the investigative and expanded ancillary testing that has become a requirement in modern death investigation. It is not expected that the information included will resolve all perplexing conditions related to the diagnosis of SIDS, but this compilation of experience may help to clarify many of the complex issues involved in arriving at the postmortem diagnosis of SIDS.

REFERENCES

1. Adelson L. Specific studies of infant victims of sudden death. In: Sudden Death in Infants: Proceedings of the Conference on Causes of Sudden Death in Infants, September 1963, Seattle, Washington. Wedgwood RJ, Benditt ER, eds. Washington, D.C.: U.S. Government Printing Office, DHEW, National Institutes of Health, National Institute of Child Health and Human Development, U.S. Public Health Service Publication No. 1412, 1965, pp 11–40.

2. Black L, David RJ, Brouillette RT, Hunt CE. Effects of birth weight and ethnicity on incidence of sudden infant death syndrome. J Pediatr 108:209 214, 1986.

3. Froggatt P, Lynas MA, MacKenzie G. Epidemiology of sudden unexpected death in infants ("cot death") in Northern Ireland. Br J Prevent Soc Med 25:119–134, 1971.

4. Golding J, Limerick S, Macfarlane A. Sudden Infant Death: Patterns, Puzzles and Problems. Seattle: University of Washington Press, 1985, 264 pp.

5. Hoffman HJ, Hunter JC, Damus K, Pakter J, Peterson DR, van Belle G, Hasselmeyer EG. Diptheria-tetanus-pertussis immunization and sudden infant death: Results of the National Institute of Child Health and Human Development Cooperative Epidemiological Study of Sudden Infant Death Syndrome Risk Factors. Pediatrics 79:598-611, 1987.

6. Hoffman HJ, Hunter JC, Ellish NJ, Janerich DT, Goldberg J. Design of the NICHD SIDS Cooperative Epidemiological Study, in Chapter 11: Adverse Reproductive Factors and The Sudden Infant Death Syndrome. In: Sudden Infant Death Syndrome: Risk Factors and Basic Mechanisms. Harper RM, Hoffman HJ, eds. New York: PMA Publishing Corp., 1988, pp 155–64.

7. Hoffman HJ, Damus K, Hillman L, Krongrad E. Risk factors for SIDS: Results of the National Institute of Child Health and Human Development SIDS Cooperative Epidemiological Study. Ann N Y Acad Sci 533:13-30, 1988.

8. Jones AM, Weston JT. The examination of the sudden infant death symdrome infant: Investigative and autopsy protocols. J Forens Sci 21:833–41, 1976.

9. Lewak N, van den Berg BJ, Beckwith JB. Sudden infant death syndrome risk factors. Clin Pediatr 18:404-410, 1979.

10. Marshall TK. The Northern Ireland study: Pathology findings. In: Sudden Infant Death Syndrome: Proceedings of the Second International Conference on Causes of Sudden Death in Infants. Bergman AB, Beckwith JB, Ray CG, eds. Seattle: University of Washington Press, 1970, pp 108-17.

11. Naeye RL, Ladis B, Drage JS. Sudden infant death syndrome: A prospective study. Am J Dis Child 130:1207-10, 1976.

12. Peterson DR. The sudden infant death syndrome — Reassessment of growth retardation in relation to maternal smoking and the hypoxia hypothesis. Am J Epidemiol 113:583-9, 1981.

13. Peterson DR, van Belle G, Chinn NM. Sudden infant death and maternal age. JAMA 247:2250-2, 1982.

14. Stanton AN, Downham MAPS, Oakley JR, Emery JL, Knowelden J. Terminal symptoms in children dying suddenly and unexpectedly at home. Preliminary report of the DHSS multicentre study of postneonatal mortality. Br Med J 2:1249-1251, 1978.

15. Strimer R, Adelson L, Oseasohn R. Epidemiologic features of 1134 sudden, unexpected infant deaths. JAMA 209:1493-7.

16. Valdés-Dapena M. The morphology of the sudden infant death syndrome—An update, 1984. In: Sudden Infant Death Syndrome: Risk Factors and Basic Mechanisms. Harper RM, Hoffman HJ, eds. New York: PMA Publishing Corp., 1988, pp 143-50.

17. Wierenga H. Cot Death in Preterm and Small for Gestational Age Infants in the Netherlands. Pre- and Postnatal Risk Factors. Groningen: Wolters Noordhoff-Grafische Bedrijven [Doctoral Thesis], 1988, 123 pp.

CHAPTER *2*

DEATH INVESTIGATION AND POSTMORTEM EXAMINATION

INTRODUCTION

The autopsy on the body of an apparently healthy infant who has died suddenly and unexpectedly should be at least as thorough as that performed in relation to any other postneonatal death. The principal alternative diagnosis to sudden infant death syndrome (SIDS), and a particularly worrisome one, is child abuse. Other commonly encountered recognized causes are congenital aortic stenosis, viral myocarditis, endocardial fibroelastosis, pneumonia, severe bronchiolitis, dehydration with fluid and electrolyte imbalance, and meningitis. The complex process of establishing or excluding those and other non-SIDS diagnoses became more standardized following an important conference in the mid-1970's.[14]

In 1975 the late Dr. James Weston, Chief Medical Investigator for the State of New Mexico, served as host-coordinator for a conference on the sudden infant death syndrome, held in Santa Fe, New Mexico. The meeting was convened by Dr. Eileen G. Hasselmeyer of the National Institute of Child Health and Human Development (NICHD) and Mrs. Geraldine Norris Funke of the Division of Maternal and Child Health, Health Resources and Services Administration. Approximately 22 pediatric and forensic pathologists and other scientists met to draft recommendations for the conduct of: (1) a practical autopsy protocol to be used by coroners' physicians and medical examiners, and (2) an optimal death investigation in cases of sudden unexpected infant death.

At the beginning of their meeting, the Santa Fe group developed a list of diagnoses to be *excluded* by autopsy. The task of constructing a standard protocol thereafter became much easier; they simply created an autopsy protocol to include all of the procedures required to exclude those other diagnoses. By using the protocol which this group designed, an autopsy pathologist in the field can be confident of having observed, documented, and/or taken permanent microscopic sections of every organ or tissue required to establish or exclude other commonly encountered, alternative diagnoses.

The resulting article[6] and booklet[14] in which these protocols appear are recommended to anyone who is involved in either the death investigation or postmortem examination of any case of sudden unexpected infant death. The autopsy protocol was used by the coroners and medical examiners who collaborated in the NICHD Cooperative Epidemiological Study of Sudden Infant Death Syndrome (SIDS) Risk Factors.

A more detailed and illustrated set of instructions for performing an infant autopsy is available in the 1983 Armed Forces Institute of Pathology publication entitled **Perinatal Autopsy Manual**.[13] Although it contains certain details pertaining almost exclusively to the neonate, on the whole its procedures and protocols are equally applicable to the autopsy on a postneonatal infant.

INVESTIGATIVE REQUIREMENTS OTHER THAN THE AUTOPSY

The autopsy alone does not constitute an adequate investigation of a sudden infant death case.[15] SIDS is a postmortem diagnosis which requires knowledge of the infant's relevant medical history, a careful investigation of the circumstances of death, and, when indicated, ancillary studies (e.g., X-rays, toxicologic, bacteriologic, virologic, fungal, or other special procedures).

MEDICAL HISTORY OF THE INFANT

The postmortem investigation of a sudden and unexpected infant death should include a history of important health related conditions. It should encompass the baby's health since birth, focusing on serious illnesses, as well as all morbidity in the preceding two weeks and, especially, the 24 hours prior to death. A brief review of the baby's birth also should be obtained. The investigator needs to know whether the labor and delivery went smoothly or were complicated and/or difficult. If the infant was one of a multiple birth, the status of the other sibling(s) should be ascertained. When indicated, selected maternal and prenatal factors should be explored including potential substance abuse, trauma, and infections.

Perinatal events not uncommonly involve ischemic insult(s) to the brain, which for the first few months of life may not be apparent, even to skilled observers. Central nervous system lesions (e.g., old subdural hematomas and foci of encephalomalacia) may be recognized for the first time during the performance of an autopsy, and it is of singular importance that they be distinguished, if at all possible, from traumatic lesions indicative of child abuse. For this purpose, hospital records concerning labor and delivery are essential, and the investigator must determine, to the extent possible, the age or ages of any relevant lesions.

Medical records from prolonged hospitalizations after birth and all readmissions should be reviewed to ascertain relevant information.

DEATH AND SCENE INVESTIGATION

It is imperative that the autopsy not be interpreted in a vacuum. Information from the autopsy must be correlated with that obtained from a detailed, ideally on-site, investigation of: (1) the events during the hours and minutes prior to the baby's death and at the very moment of the death, and (2) the physical site and circumstances of the death. The investigator needs to know exactly what happened to the baby, where he/she was, how he/she was, and who was doing what, to, with, or for the infant just prior to the death. Was the baby, for example, sharing a bed with an inebriated mother? Was the baby alert and being fed at the time? Circumstances occurring at the moment of apparent death and in the minutes (and, on occasion, even hours or days) after the death are needed as well. Some infants have been observed to die, or nearly die; then they have been resuscitated and subsequently kept alive, with respirators and other devices, for long periods of time. A variety of pathologic changes occur during protracted life support, and it is sometimes difficult to distinguish them from lesions that precede a sudden, unexpected death.

The investigator is obliged to obtain all of the above information because it is essential to the ultimate interpretation of autopsy findings. Photographs of the death scene and recording of the environmental and infant's temperature soon after death may provide additional valuable information for the interpretation of autopsy findings.[3,8]

THE AUTOPSY

INSTRUMENTS AND MATERIALS FOR THE INFANT AUTOPSY

The infant's total body weight is one of the most important determinations to make in the infant autopsy thus a **weighing scale** is necessary. Body weight is critical to the autopsy diagnosis of: (1) failure to thrive or starvation, and (2) dehydration with fluid and electrolyte imbalance. There seem to be two reasons why this feature is so often neglected: (1) the general pathologist is often not aware of its singular importance in these cases, and (2) autopsy rooms designed and maintained primarily for adult cases are seldom equipped with accurate scales to determine infant body weight to the nearest gram.

Also critical is the balance for weighing infant organs, up to 500 grams. Well adjusted, **small scales**, accurate to the tenth of a gram, are ideal.

Other Instruments (items in italics are considered essential):

1 —*Scalpel with fresh #22 blades*
1 —Durham knife with fresh blades
1 —Brain cutting knife
1 —*Medium forceps with teeth*
1 —Medium forceps without teeth
1 —Small forceps with teeth
2 —Mosquito hemostats
1 —*50 cm ruler*
1 —*Pair of stout scissors for cutting bone*
1 —Pair of coronary artery scissors
1 —*Pair of Metzenbaum scissors*
1 —Pair of small scissors with sharp points
1 —Fine probe with rounded ends
1 —Brick-shaped, moist sponge (roughly 8 x 4 x 2.5 cm) (to serve as a movable "work-bench" for dissection of organs)
2 —Smaller soft sponges (to keep the body and working area clean)
1 —Means of magnification (such as a dentist's lens or dissecting microscope)
1 —Set of gauze squares (2 x 2 in) (to keep the field of dissection clear and dry)
2 —Types of string (1 spool of thin, waxed string and 1 spool of moderately stout thread)
1 —Dissection board (wood or plastic)
1 —Graduated cylinder for measuring volumes of fluid up to 100 ml
1 —Small ladle or large syringe (for removing fluid from body cavities)
2 —Sets of sterile and non-sterile disposable syringes and needles
1 —Plastic bag for tissues to be returned to the body
1 —Stool of adjustable height
1 —Small box in which to store the set of instruments for infant autopsies (to keep them separate from those used in adult autopsies)

Materials for Bacteriologic Cultures:

6 — Sterile #22 blades
3 — Test tubes of liquid culture medium (e.g., thioglycolate broth)
1 — Sterile #22 needle
1 — Sterile 10 ml syringe
1 — Aerobic blood culture bottle
1 — Anaerobic blood culture bottle

Materials for Virologic, Fungal, or other Cultures:

6 — Sterile #22 blades
3 — Sterile containers (e.g., petri dishes) for tissue with appropriate media

Materials for Toxicologic Analysis:

3 — Pairs of screw-top toxicology tubes (1 plain, 1 with preservative, e.g., sodium fluoride)

THE AUTOPSY PROTOCOL

The autopsy protocol recommended is detailed in the Armed Forces Institute of Pathology publication **Perinatal Autopsy Manual**;[13] a blank copy of the form appears in Appendix A. It was developed by Dr. James B. Arey of St. Christopher's Hospital for Children in Philadelphia and is, in general, as useful in cases of sudden and unexpected infant death as it is in instances of perinatal death. A blank copy can be kept at the autopsy table and used not only for note-taking (e.g., for the weight of the body and weights of individual organs) but also to itemize routine procedures which might otherwise be forgotten, such as measuring the height of the diaphragm on each side and counting the numbers of ribs.

All subsequent methods described herein reflect adaptations from Dr. Arey's protocol.

THE AUTOPSY METHOD

Preliminary Tasks

Before beginning the autopsy it is important to document carefully the following information: name of the patient, age, sex, race and/or ethnicity, date and time of death (or when the infant was last seen alive), date and time of autopsy, and the name(s) of the autopsy pathologist and of any other pathologists in attendance.

External Examination

Weigh the body and determine crown-to-rump and rump-to-heel lengths, as well as the circumferences of the head (occipito-frontal), chest (at the level of the nipples), and abdomen (at the level of the umbilicus).[9,16]

Each tube in the body should remain in place (if necessary, secured there) until the exact position and state of the distal tip is noted during the course of the autopsy. Hospital personnel should be instructed not to remove tubes when they prepare the body for transportation to the morgue.

One of the most important, recognizable (and, unfortunately, often unrecognized) causes for sudden infant death is diarrhea with consequent dehydration and fluid and electrolyte imbalance, to which infants under one year of age are extremely susceptible. Babies succumb to this combination of fluid and biochemical derangements much more readily than do adults. The history of diarrhea may not have been called to the attention of the investigators or of the examining pathologist, but certain features of the external examination will alert him or her to that possibility; principal among them are skin turgor and the state of the eyes. If skin turgor is poor, as it is apt to be in dehydration, it will remain "tented" when pinched even though the body is warm. In dehydration the eyes appear sunken. However, if these two features are not looked for specifically they may not be noticed and/or noted in the protocol. If in doubt about dehydration, the pathologist should take a sample of the vitreous humor for determination of electrolytes and urea nitrogen. In some forensic offices, this is done routinely.

Retinal hemorrhages in the eyes may also alert the pathologist to the possibility of child abuse. Retinal hemorrhages, subdural and/or subarachnoid hemorrhages with minimal or absent signs of external trauma may or may not be indicative of the shaken baby syndrome.[4] This clinicopathologic entity may be demonstrable at autopsy, and is not consistent with SIDS.[11]

Rigor mortis is checked in the jaw and in all four extremities.

Jaundice, particularly in infants in whom the skin is deeply pigmented, is best ascertained in the sclerae and, ideally, in daylight.

Cyanosis is checked in the vermillion border and the finger- and toenail beds.

Edema, especially pitting edema, should be looked for, particularly over the dorsal surfaces of the feet, the anterior aspects of the tibiae, and over the back.

The size, shape, regularity, and equality of the *pupils* can be determined only prior to the time that the corneae become cloudy, some hours after death.

The *external ears* should be examined with reference to the shape of the pinna on each side, as well as the patency of the external auditory canal.

In inspecting the *oral cavity*, the color and moisture of the lining mucosa should be examined first.

Needle puncture marks and other evidence

of resuscitative endeavors should be noted as to number and site.

Initial Incisions

Make the incision in the skin across the chest and abdomen in the usual Y-shape, with each upward segment of the Y extended to the very top of the shoulder. The midline abdominal segment, extending from the xiphoid process to the symphysis pubis, deviates slightly in a small arc around the left side of, rather than through, the umbilicus.

Carefully lay bare the clavicles, ribs, and sternum when reflecting the three skin flaps (resulting from the above incisions) away from the chest wall and sever the attachments of muscles and peritoneum to the costal margins bilaterally.

Then, lift the umbilical vein and explore it for patency; if patent, it should be double-tied and transected between the ties. Identify the two (obliterated) umbilical arteries and transect them at a level cranial to the urinary bladder and deep in the pelvis so that they can be removed subsequently together with the urinary bladder.

Peritoneal Cavity

If a splenic culture is to be taken as a double-check on the blood cultures, that should be done before any other procedure involving the contents of the peritoneal cavity is undertaken. The method is the same as that employed for taking lung cultures (see p. 29). Thereafter, measure the height of the liver diaphragm on each side by inserting the index finger of the right hand up to the dome from below and then counting down, on the anterior aspect of the thorax, to the corresponding rib or interspace with the left forefinger.

Measure the extent to which the lower border of the liver projects below the cleared costal margin vertically in three planes: the anterior axillary line, the mid-clavicular line, and the midline (from the base of the xiphoid process down); for the fourth determination, measure the horizontal breadth of the exposed left lobe of the liver from the midline to the point where the lower border disappears behind the costal margin. These particular measurements are arbitrary but they serve to document possible enlargement of the liver.

Inspect the stomach and small and large intestines externally to determine the nature and color of the serous surface as well as the average diameter of each.

To inspect the mesenteric lymph nodes (for number, size, and color) sweep the loops of the small bowel to the right. While holding them there, observe both the mesenteric lymph nodes and the attachment of the mesenteric root. Normally the attachment extends obliquely across the posterior wall of the abdomen from the left upper quadrant (ligament of Treitz) to the right lower quadrant, near the lower pole of the right kidney. If it is abnormally short, as it is in malrotation of the gut, it is confined to the immediate vicinity of the origin of the superior mesenteric artery.

At this stage, it is advisable to cleanse the body, table, and instruments once more; cleanliness, and particularly the absence of blood or dried blood in the field, is an absolute necessity for the performance of a good infant autopsy.

Thoracic Cavity

The easiest method to determine the presence or absence of a pneumothorax is to insert a sterile needle into each hemithorax, between the ribs anteriorly and supero-laterally for a distance of about 4 mm; the attached syringe is filled beforehand with sterile saline. If a pneumothorax is present and under pressure, air bubbles will rise spontaneously in the saline as soon as the tip of the needle enters the pocket of air immediately beneath the chest wall.

To open the chest easily and obtain the best possible view of the thoracic contents, use a #22 scalpel blade to separate the manubrium sternum from each clavicle. Then, with the tip of the forefinger resting 2-3 mm from the tip of the blade, simply run the blade tip rapidly and smoothly down through all of the cartilaginous portions of the ribs, just medial to the costochondral junctions on each side. Each incision flares laterally as it proceeds caudally providing wide exposure inferiorly. No bone is severed so that all skeletal cut edges are smooth and nontraumatic and will not tear rubber gloves or cut the prosector's hands. After these incisions are made, it is easy to elevate the plastron, lifting it with the left hand while cutting away any loose connective tissue attachments posteriorly with either scissors or a scalpel blade.

In young infants it is advisable, at this time, to scrape away the loose tissues from the front and back of the removed plastron, to transilluminate it, and visualize the centers of ossification in the manubrium and in each of the four sternebrae. As the baby grows, these centers become larger and eventually fuse to form one large, elongate center for the sternum. Examination of this bone will assist the prosector in assessing the adequacy of the infant's growth and development.

Inspection of the thoracic contents, at this juncture, should reveal, in the midline, from above down: (1) a sheet of skeletal muscle superiorly, overlying the cervical poles of the thymus, (2) caudal to that, the thymus, overlying the great vessels and upper part of the heart, and (3) the heart. Using Metzenbaum scissors and working from below upward, employ the "separating technique" to lift the sheet of skeletal muscle away from deeper structures. It is necessary to have the skin flap loose enough so that, reflected, it will allow for exposure of the neck organs up to the level of the thyroid. Once the sheet of muscle has been removed the thyroid will be visible above with the cervical extensions of the thymus immediately caudal to it.

Using the same separating technique, lift the thymus, from below upward. In so doing it is essential to watch carefully for the brachiocephalic vein, which courses across the "back" of the thymus and is sometimes a bit embedded in it. If at all possible, it should not be incised because it bleeds freely and creates a bloody field in which it is difficult to work.

The anterior wall of the pericardial sac is then removed by cutting it superiorly as close to the great vessels as possible, and laterally and inferiorly, as completely as possible. Before the heart is touched, blood cultures should be taken from the convexity of the right atrium with a sterile #22 needle and 10-ml syringe. If the required 2-3 ml cannot be obtained readily, lift the head for a few moments, and/or the feet, to drain more liquid blood into the heart; 1 or 2 ml each are injected into aerobic and anaerobic blood culture bottles. The remainder can be saved for other studies, or the serum can be frozen and saved.

Take cultures of the lung next. First, clamp a medium-sized hemostat on the acute angle of the anterior portion of the base of the right lung. Then, lift the lung from the thoracic cavity by pulling on the hemostat, assiduously avoiding contamination of the serous surface to be cultured. The lung can easily be held steady, outside of the cavity, using only the weight of a large hemostat hanging freely, draped over the opposite side of the chest, or it can be maintained in that position by an assistant. With both hands free the prosector can then use two fresh, sterile #22 blades to remove a little wedge of lung tissue (about 3 mm in greatest diameter) from an exposed sharp edge of the right lower lobe; one blade is used to stabilize the tissue and/or cut against, while the other is used to cut with. The same procedure is used on the left side. Each tiny sample is dropped into a separate sterile tube of thioglycolate, or other sterile medium, and labeled. Samples should also be taken from any portion of lung that seems to be consolidated, although such foci are very difficult to ascertain in infants of this age. The same techniques can be used in taking cultures of lung or other tissues in search of mycobacterial, fungal, or viral agents. Appropriate media are employed in each instance.

At this juncture, divide the brachiocephalic vein, if that has not already been accomplished; tie it on both sides of the midline and cut between the ties. This procedure will expose the origins of the great arteries and their branches. Using the spreading technique again, and working from below upward, expose completely the three major branches of the aortic arch and explore the division of the brachiocephalic on the right to be certain that it does divide into a subclavian and common carotid; if it does not, the subclavian will be found to arise from the posterior aspect of the descending thoracic aorta just beyond the entrance of the ductus arteriosus. The complete thoracic aorta is best seen by lifting the heart and left lung and pushing them, together, to the right, incising the sheet of posterior pleura overlying the aorta most carefully, and then using the "spreading-scissors-technique" to clear that vessel from below upward.

If there should be a coarctation present, it will come into view at this point in dissection and appear as a sharp indentation or cleft in the lateral convexity of the arch directly opposite the entrance of the ductus arteriosus. Each of the three great vessels can now be tied, about 1 cm above its origin from the aorta.

In cases of congenital heart disease, one may wish to perfuse the heart-lung preparation for better visualization and demonstration. In that instance, it is better to double-tie each vessel and transect the vessel between the ties. Leave the upper tie long for the funeral director, and cut the lower one short. Also, transect the aorta just above the diaphragm to leave the attached aortic segment as long as possible.

Opening the Normal Heart

In the great majority of autopsies on infants who die suddenly and unexpectedly, at home, there is no reason to expect to encounter any congenital abnormality of the heart. If there is no history suggestive of that and the heart appears grossly normal externally, it is probably best to open the heart in situ. The procedure is simple and involves only two matching sets of three cuts; there are three on the right and three on the left, and all but one are straight.

In each cut, it is imperative that the rounded

end of the small straight scissors be put into place first, like a probe, and then the cut be made as one continuous incision rather than in a series of little nicks.

The first cut is made *from above down*, along the right anterolateral aspect of the right atrium, from the entrance of the superior vena cava to the entrance of the inferior vena cava. If it is done from below upward, the scissors is apt to damage the upper edge of the foramen ovale.

The second cut extends from the middle of the first, down more or less the middle of the back of the heart, immediately to the right of and parallel to the posterior descending coronary artery or about 3 mm from the interventricular septum. This cut proceeds to the apex of the heart and thus exposes the entire "inflow tract" of the right heart.

At this time, assess the state of the foramen ovale. (This is one of the principal merits of the in situ procedure, because it preserves intact the interatrial septum without any distortion of the foramen ovale.) While looking at the foramen, press gently on the interatrial septum forcing the blood still within the left atrium to press upon the valve for closure of the foramen ovale. This maneuver will cause the membrane to bulge to the right; if it is functionally adequate, the residual foramen will not leak. Then one can easily probe the antero-superiorly placed natural opening and determine whether or not it is anatomically patent.

The third cut is made by proceeding from the apex up across the front of the heart to and through the pulmonic valve, again along and immediately adjacent to the septum. This step exposes the "outflow tract" of the right ventricle and completes the examination of the right side of the heart.

Cuts four, five, and six are the left-sided equivalents of those on the right.

To expose the convexity of the left atrium, transect the inferior vena cava and lift the apex of the heart in a cranial direction as far as it will go. The left atrium can now be incised with a straight cut extending from a pulmonary vein on one side to one on the other.

The fifth cut extends from the middle of the fourth, "down" the posterior aspect of the heart immediately adjacent to the septum (this time on the left side), to the apex. This exposes the "inflow tract" of the left ventricle.

The sixth and last cut is the only one not made perfectly straight. Begin at the apex and extend the cut up the anterior aspect of the left ventricle, adjacent to the septum. Be careful, in doing this, to peek inside occasionally to avoid nicking the aortic leaflet of the mitral valve. At the level of the pulmonic valve direct the cut horizontally to your left to transect the pulmonary artery about 5 mm above the pulmonic valve; then abruptly continue the cut cranially again, opening the aortic valve and the root of the aorta.

This final S-shaped incision requires more care than any of the others but, like them, should be performed with a cut as close to a continuum as possible.

Detailed examination of the interior of the heart is made after removal of all of the organs en bloc according to the Rokitansky technique and separation of the heart from the lungs. At that time, the circumference of each valve is measured by placing a straight ruler over the valve, laid out flat. In the atrioventricular valves, the measurement is made from one cut end of the annulus fibrosis to the other. In the two three-cusped valves, the aortic and the pulmonic, the measurement is taken along the upper free edges of the cusps. The thickness of the wall of each ventricle is measured, from endo- to epicardium, just below the atrioventricular valve.

Removal of the Organs en bloc:
The Rokitansky Technique

Using the spreading-scissors-separating technique and working from below upward, lift the skin of the neck up and away from underlying anatomic structures of the neck. To remove the tongue it is probably easiest to work with the tip of a scalpel blade, dividing the muscular base of the tongue from its attachment to the inner aspect of the mandible. Once the tongue has been cut loose, slide your right index finger up into the mouth from below, curve it around the tongue, and pull the tongue down into the neck. Extend the incision, encircling the tongue around the sides and the back so that both tonsils, the posterior wall of the pharynx, and the soft palate with the uvula remain attached to the tongue. When the tongue "is delivered" caudally, into the chest, all of those structures will accompany it.

Deliver the tongue and neck organs downward by severing the attachments between the posterior pharyngeal and esophageal walls and the cervical vertebral column, keeping the knife blade close to the vertebral bodies. The two lateral incisions should be made immediately medial to the common carotid arteries, which will remain in the body, tied as described previously.

Continue delivering the block of organs by cutting them away from the anterior aspects of the vertebral bodies, proceeding caudally toward the pelvis. At the thoracic inlet, the right innominate vein, some nerves, and loose connective tissue of the lateral superior mediastinum must be sectioned. The attachments of the diaphragm to the lateral chest wall and posterior body wall are best cut with Metzenbaum scissors. This incision should extend completely around the posterior circumference, including the attachments of the crurae of the diaphragm to the vertebral column.

When the level of the lower poles of the kidneys is passed, the block may be replaced in the body while the aorta is tied, directly above the bifurcation, and transected above the tie.

With the organs lying loosely in what was roughly their original anatomic position, it is convenient to detach the pelvic structures from the bony pelvis. This is done by inserting a scalpel blade, from above down, between the anterior aspect of the bladder/prostate and the posterior aspect of the pubis, transecting the urethra distal to the prostate and then the anus, as close to the pelvic floor as possible. In the

female infant, the scalpel is inserted along the posterior aspect of the pelvis, severing the distal vagina and anus as close to the pelvis as possible. Then, with a circling motion, all of the pelvic organs can be cut away from their attachments and delivered upward. As they are lifted, transect the two internal iliac arteries and separate the block of organs from the vertebral bodies posteriorly. In continuing that procedure in an upward direction, the earlier plane of dissection will be encountered. Lift the entire block out of the body, in one unit, from the tongue to the anorectal junction; the umbilical arteries, bladder, urachal remnant, and umbilicus are included.

Other Pieces of Tissue to Remove from the Body

Once all of the organs have been removed from the body, count the number of ribs on each side and remove two costochondral junctions, each segment to a length of about 1 cm. Place them in formalin. This is also an appropriate time to resect a portion of psoas muscle, as a representative sample of skeletal muscle. Portions of nerve, skin, and testis can be removed at this time.

Spinal Cord

The spinal cord can now be removed by the anterior approach. Cut through one of the lower lumbar intervertebral discs with a scalpel. Insert the rounded end of a stout, durable scissors into the space between the dura and the vertebral bodies and cut the bony column through the left pedicles from the lower lumbar to the upper cervical region. Repeat this cut on the right. Lift the column of vertebral bodies away from the dura, separating the dura from the bone by blunt dissection so that the cord remains completely surrounded by dura. Two vertebral bodies are separated from this column; these are bisected longitudinally for fixation in formalin.

With a fine scissors incise the dura anteriorly, from below upward, and then, having exposed it, carefully remove the spinal cord together with the posteriorly attached dura. Handle it by lifting it on the opened dura upon which it is lying.

Removal of the Cranial Contents

Make one long incision in the scalp beginning on either side, directly behind the pinna. Bring the incision up over the vertex, well behind the anterior fontanelle, and down the other side. With a little help from the scalpel, it now will be easy to reflect the scalp away from the cranium, first anteriorly to about the level of the eyebrows, and then, posteriorly to a point just below the occiput.

Measure the length and breadth of the anterior fontanelle and note whether the edges of the posterior fontanelle are approximated or not.

With the tip of the scalpel blade, make a sagittally-oriented nick in the lateral extension of the anterior fontanelle on each side. Into one of these insert the tip of the same stout scissors used previously on the vertebrae. Then, create a large, oval lateral flap of bone on that side by cutting forward first, parallel to the sagittal suture, about 8 mm lateral to it, then curving laterally around the anterior extension above the eyebrow, downward and around posteriorly to finish at a point just above the pinna on that side. Re-insert the scissors blade at the fontanelle on the same side and continue the incision posteriorly, curving around laterally and downward in the occipital region; then direct the cut anteriorly once more; terminate this cut about 2 cm from the extremity of the anterior-inferior extension to create a bony hinge for the flap, directly above the ear.

Drape this first bony flap in wet paper towel (or its equivalent) so that the sharp edges of the bone will not damage the delicate leptomeninges or your gloves or hands. Let the flap fall back naturally into its original position.

Create the same sort of bony flap on the opposite side and wrap it in a wet paper towel as above.

Inspect the falx cerebri from above, lifting the cerebral hemisphere gently away from it with a moistened scalpel handle. Transect the midline residual bony bridge (and the underlying sagittal sinus) at its anterior and posterior extremities. Remove this bony bridge and open the sagittal sinus.

Holding the head in the left hand, tilt the cerebrum forward and, again using the wet scalpel handle, lift and tilt the occipital lobes gently up (off of the tentorium on each side) to inspect the tentorium for tears at the junction of the falx and tentorium. Look below the tentorium for any accumulation of blood. With the tip of the scalpel blade, or a small scissors, cut the attachment of the tentorium all around its peripheral edge. Lay the head down on the table top, occiput down, allowing the soft brain to tilt and slide backward a bit. Beginning with the first cranial nerves, remove the cerebral hemispheres and attached portions of the cranial nerves, working from the anterior to the posterior aspect of the head. Throughout all of this, the gloved hands of the prosector must be wet so as not to damage the delicate leptomeninges. Allowing the brain to "fall" backward gradually, while the head rests on the tabletop, permits gravity to work for the prosector and frees up his two hands for dissection. When the brain is almost out of the base of the skull, the undersurface of the brain stem and the cervical spinal cord can be visualized well. Transect the cervical cord as far down as possible. The brain will slide out on to the moist table top. Inspect the brain, weigh it, and place it in a large container of formalin. Allow it to fix for approximately seven to ten days before cutting it.

The confluence of the *dural sinuses*, the transverse sinus, and the sigmoid sinuses are then opened in situ.

The *pituitary* is removed next by cutting the attachment of its tentorium to the anterior and lateral walls of the sella leaving it attached posteriorly. The posterior clinoid processes are severed from the remainder of the sella using a scalpel. Finally, the tentorium is picked up with small, toothed forceps, and the pituitary (*with* attached posterior clinoids) is gently teased from its bony nest.

The *middle ears* are now examined. The petrous portions of the temporal bones are removed by making two cuts in each using heavy bone scissors. The first cut is made along the lateral junction of the petrous portion with the rest of the temporal bone, transecting that junction downward and anteromedially. The bone scissors should be kept flat against the adjacent squamous portion of the temporal bone. The second cut is made along its medial border beginning near the sella and cutting downward and laterally to meet the first cut. The wedge-shaped petrous portion can now be lifted out. The middle ear cavity, the ear drum, and the ossicles are thus exposed. Cultures should be taken of any unusually thick or purulent material found in the middle ear.

Dissection of the Block of Viscera

It is easiest to work with the block of viscera if it is placed on a moist sponge roughly the size and shape of an ordinary brick. Initially they should be upside down, i.e., with the anterior surface of the organs down, against the sponge.

At the outset, the block of viscera should be oriented with the tongue towards the prosector and the caudal end away. Holding the tongue in the left hand and a round-tipped small scissors in the right, open the *esophagus*, from above down, to the level of the diaphragm.

Inspect the esophageal mucosa searching for ectopic gastric mucosa at the level of the larynx (if present, it will appear as a small, elevated, sharply demarcated, pale pink, ovoid patch adjacent to the larynx) or any other defect including an ostium of an unsuspected tracheoesophageal fistula. Then, working from the top downward, reflect the esophagus caudally; use a small scissors to cut the esophagus away from the larynx, trachea, and posterior pericardial sac, all of which lie anterior to it. Lay the freed-up esophagus, still in continuity with the stomach, down over the abdominal organs.

Open the *larynx and trachea* longitudinally and posteriorly with a small scissors, inspecting the lumen and mucosa of each and looking at whatever material each may contain. Transect the trachea just below the level of the lower poles of the thyroid and fix the tongue, pharynx, tonsils, larynx, thyroid, trachea, and parathyroids in one block in a container of formalin for trimming later.

Since the heart has already been opened in situ, and it has been ascertained that the arterial and venous connections between the heart and lungs are normal, the two lungs may now be removed from the heart and from the major bronchi. Multiple sections should be made through each lobe of each lung, and all cut surfaces should be inspected. One or two thin slices from each lobe should be saved in formalin. The trachea and bronchi can be saved in formalin, as they are. Remove the heart and fix it, in its entirety, in formalin.

Following this procedure, dissection of the *abdominal organs* may begin. First, open the aorta posteriorly, from above down. Inspect the celiac and superior mesenteric artery ostia and those of the two renal arteries. Open the renal arteries.

On the top of the diaphragm, next to the aorta is the cut upper end of the inferior vena cava. Open it from above down. Open the renal veins from the lumen of the vena cava laterally and inspect them for thrombi. Turn the sponge around 180° so that the caudal end of the block is directed toward the prosector. Begin lifting the *diaphragm* away from the posterior aspects of the kidneys and adrenals. With toothed forceps, lift one leaf at a time and clip away loose connecting tissues with small scissors. After each leaf has been freed and elevated, cut the entire diaphragm away from the block. Retain a 1 cm square section of that muscle in formalin.

After the leaves of the diaphragm have been detached from the block, separate the *adrenals* most carefully from the kidneys. Hold each adrenal by grasping the loose connective tissue immediately about the gland rather than the friable gland itself. Separation from the kidney is best accomplished a bit at a time, with small scissors. After the adrenals have been removed and weighed together, they can be hemisected in the sagittal plane, from above down, through the thickest part of the gland and then fixed, to be sectioned serially following fixation. On the left side it may be well to detach the *spleen* at this time, cutting across the splenic artery and vein at the hilus and separating the organ from the tail of the pancreas to which it is sometimes tightly adherent. Weigh the spleen, section it serially, and fix representative sections. Hemisect each kidney in the coronal plane before severing its attachments and vessels at the hilus, so that the organ can be anchored there and held securely while the coronal cut is made.

Each half of the *kidney* is then stripped of its capsule, down to the hilus, and the remnants of the capsule are cut away. The color and character of the external surfaces are noted. The pelvis is laid open and the ureter opened with a small round-ended scissors from the ureteropelvic junction down to the *urinary bladder*. If no lesions are found in the kidney, and there is no contraindication to it, each kidney is detached. The kidneys are weighed; if they are similar to each other, they may be weighed together. The bladder is then opened from below, using a small round-tipped scissors. In the male this cut is made through the anterior wall of the prostatic urethra and the entire length of the anterior wall of the urinary bladder. Particular attention is paid to the fundus (in search of urachal remnants) and to the ureteral ostia. The bladder and prostate can be fixed in continuity with the umbilicus for sectioning later. In the female, the bladder is opened in the same manner and then separated from the internal genitalia posterior to it. After the bladder is removed, the vagina, cervix, and body of the uterus can be opened from below in the same manner as the bladder. The internal genitalia can be fixed as a whole after the fallopian tubes and ovaries are inspected.

At this time, turn over the entire block of remaining organs so that the anterior aspect is up. Sweeping the loops of small bowel caudally and to the right and lifting the transverse colon cranially, exposes the area where the duodenum emerges from behind the peritoneum at the ligament of Treitz. Transect the duodenum there and begin to remove by cutting it away from its attachment to the mesentery. This can be done with either a sharp scissors or a #22 scalpel blade; the cut must be made close to the bowel wall or the detached bowel will curl on itself like an apple peel and, as a consequence, be very difficult to open. The entire small and large bowel is removed in continuity; the length of each is determined. To obtain ideal histologic preparations, it is best to remove an intact, unopened, 1 cm segment of small bowel and large bowel at this time, putting both immediately into formalin for trimming later.

The remaining segments of *small and large intestine* are then opened with a round-tipped small scissors. The character and color of the mucosa in each are noted, as are the color and consistency of the contents of each. Appropriate samples of the bowel are fixed in formalin. A 1.0 cm length of each will fix nicely if pressed, serosa down, onto a piece of dry paper towel.

Next, the *liver* is reoriented with its caudal surface upward to expose the attached stomach, esophagus, duodenum, biliary tract, and pancreas. The esophagus is reentered with the rounded end of a small scissors and the incision made there earlier, continued down through the cardioesophageal junction, along the greater curvature of the *stomach* and out through the cut end of the duodenum.

All of the mucosal lining of that specimen is examined and described as to color and the presence of any lesions. The content of every segment is duly noted with regard to character, sheen, color, volume, and consistency.

The block is then reoriented to provide easy access to the ampulla of Vater. The *gallbladder* is inspected and carefully pressed upon to determine whether or not the bile in it can be expressed readily through the ampulla. Sometimes it is difficult to force the bile out, and it is necessary to free the gallbladder from its bed in the liver and to squeeze it firmly between two fingers to achieve that end.

Without too much difficulty the *common bile duct* can be opened from below with the rounded end of a very small scissors. However, if the bile has emerged from the ampulla, there is really no necessity for that maneuver. The gallbladder can be removed and put into formalin in its entirety. Separate the liver from the block containing the stomach, duodenum, pancreas, and mesentery by severing the lesser omentum and other attachments. The esophagus, stomach, duodenum, and pancreas can be fixed as a unit, or appropriate portions can be fixed, e.g., the cardioesophageal junction, pyloric region, mesentery, and pancreas. The remainder can be discarded. In its same upside-down position, the liver is arranged so that the cut end of the umbilical vein is directed toward the prosector. The umbilical vein is opened to its confluence with the sinus intermedius, and this incision is continued along the length of the sinus intermedius. The orifice of the ductus venosus is located in the cephalic wall of the sinus intermedius, directly opposite the orifice of the

---

Table 2–1.   **Summary of Recommendations for Microscopic Sections**

• Strongly Recommended:

Heart (left ventricle and right ventricle)	Adrenal
Lungs (left 2 lobes, right 3 lobes)	Spleen
Trachea	Thymus
Larynx	Mesenteric lymph nodes
Kidney (left and right)	Liver
Pancreas	

• Recommended:

Esophagus	Psoas
Cardioesophageal junction	Rib
Stomach	Vertebral body
Ileum	Tongue
Colon	Diaphragm
Anus	

• Recommended When Indicated:

Submaxillary gland	Peripheral nerve
Urinary bladder	Fallopian tube and ovary
Breast	Testis
Umbilicus	Prostate
Uterus-cervix-vagina	
Skin	

umbilical vein. The vessel, if it is still patent, should be opened from its orifice to its confluence with the hepatic veins and the inferior vena cava. (The orifice of the ductus venosus closes within a few days of birth.) Examine the *liver* and weigh and serially section it. Note any lesions and save them, along with a number of thin sections representative of the two lobes.

ANCILLARY STUDIES

Bacterial Cultures

The only routine cultures recommended in the study of the sudden and unexpected death of an apparently healthy infant are for bacteria.

Equipment and materials:

- Sterile 10 ml disposable plastic syringes and 18 gauge needles

- Blood culture media, aerobic and anaerobic

- Sterile tubes of thioglycolate broth (or any similar medium)

- Sterile swabs and routine bacterial transport media

- 4 sterile #22 scalpel blades

When no inflammatory process is apparent, a single culture of each lower lobe of lung and one of the heart's blood (right atrium) should be taken. One of the spleen also may be taken as a double check for the blood culture. Hence, if only one pathogen is isolated from the blood culture and it is also found in the spleen, you can be assured that the agent was in the blood stream at death and may well have been responsible for sepsis; with nothing more than the presence of one agent in the heart's blood there may be some doubt as to the validity of the finding.

If there is an obvious inflammatory proc-

ess present anywhere, such as pneumonia or meningitis, appropriate cultures should be taken from the affected tissues or sites.

At least two scientific surveys[1,7] have demonstrated that systematic cultures for *Clostridium botulinum* will apparently be positive for the bacteria (and toxins can be demonstrated) in only 4-5 percent of SIDS autopsies. Therefore, most forensic offices do not perform them on a routine basis. Even when, in a given case, the bacteria are isolated and the toxin demonstrated, there remains some uncertainty about how those findings are to be interpreted. No one knows whether this combination necessarily means that the particular infant died of infant botulism.

Viral Cultures

Experience has shown[2,10] that in many suspected SIDS cases routine cultures for viruses will demonstrate the presence of a wide spectrum of viral agents, reflecting any of those present in the community at the time. Those assorted viruses also will be found in various organs, which will almost always show no histologic evidence of inflammation. Viral cultures are, therefore, not warranted as part of the routine postmortem, but may be useful in selected cases.

Viral pneumonia has never been shown to be responsible for any significant fraction of sudden unexpected infant deaths. While viral myocarditis is implicated in a small percentage of these sudden unexpected deaths (see pp. 122 and 254), it is impossible to diagnose grossly.

Although an infant who dies from AIDS (acquired immune deficiency syndrome) is not likely to be mistaken for one who has succumbed to SIDS, HIV testing may be considered for babies at risk, e.g., the infant of a mother who is a drug abuser, or known to be HIV positive and/or diagnosed as having AIDS.

Toxicology

Two samples each of blood, urine, gastric contents, and vitreous humor should be set aside routinely in every case of sudden infant death, one saved in a tube with preservative, and the other in either the fresh refrigerated or frozen state. When indicated, these stored materials can be used for toxicologic analysis.

Some forensic centers conduct a general, qualitative "drug screen" for alcohol, aspirin, and acetaminophen in all cases even though toxic levels of these agents are seldom found.[5,12] Analysis for drugs of abuse (e.g., narcotics, cocaine, barbiturates, etc.) is warranted, especially when parents or caretakers are suspeof being drug abusers.[11]

X-Ray Studies

It is recommended that x-rays of the entire body be taken before the autopsy is begun. If, in any instance, child abuse becomes an issue, x-rays may be crucial to establishing the ultimate diagnosis.

REFERENCES

1. Arnon SS, Midura TF, Damus K, Wood RM, Chin J. Intestinal infection and toxin production by *Clostridium botulinum* as one cause of sudden infant death syndrome. Lancet I:1273-7, 1978.

2. Brandt C, Patrick JR, Chandra R, Parrott RH. Infectious agents from cases of SIDS and from members of their community. Clin Proc Child Hosp DC 26:249-60, 1970.

3. Denborough MA, Galloway GJ, Hopkinson KC. Malignant hyperpyrexia and sudden infant death. Lancet II:2068-9, 1982.

4. Duhaime AC, Gennarelli TA, Thibault LE, Bruce DA, Margulies SS, Wiser R. The shaken baby syndrome. A clinical, pathological, and biomechanical study. J Neurosurg 66:409-15, 1987.

5 Finkle BS, McClosky KL, Kopjak L, Carroll JM. Toxological analyses in cases of sudden infant death: A national feasibility study. J Forens Sci 24:775-89, 1979.

6. Jones AM, Weston JT. The examination of the sudden infant death syndrome: Investigative and autopsy protocols. J Forens Sci 21:833-41, 1976.

7. Peterson DR, Eklund MW, Chinn NM. The sudden infant death syndrome and infant botulism. Rev Infec Dis 1:630-6, 1979.

8. Peterson DR, Davis N. Malignant hyperthermia diathesis and sudden infant death syndrome (Letter). Anesth Analg 65:209, 1986.

9. Potter EL, Craig JM. Pathology of the Fetus and the Infant, 3rd ed. Chicago: Year Book Medical Publishers, Inc., 1975.

10. Ray CG, Beckwith JB, Hebestreit NM, Bergman AB. Studies of the sudden infant death syndrome in King County, Washington: I. The role of viruses. JAMA 211:619-23, 1970.

11. Smialek JE, Lambros Z. Investigation of sudden infant deaths. Pediatrician 15:191-7, 1988.

12. Valdés-Dapena M. The pathologist and the sudden infant death syndrome. Am J Pathol 106:118-31, 1982.

13. Valdés-Dapena MA, Huff DS. Perinatal Autopsy Manual. Washington, D.C.: Armed Forces Institute of Pathology, 1983, 98 pp.

14. Weston JT, ed. The investigation and postmortem examination of death from the sudden infant death syndrome (SIDS). Proceedings of a conference. Rockville, MD: US DHEW, Office of Maternal and Child Health, PHS (HSA) 76-5150, 1976, 108 pp.

15. Willinger M, James LS, Catz C, et al: Defining the sudden infant death syndrome (SIDS): deliberations of an expert panel convened by the National Institute of Child Health and Human Development. Pediatr Pathol 11:677, 1991.

16. Wigglesworth JS. Perinatal Pathology, Vol 15. In: Major Problems in Pathology. Philadelphia: W.B. Saunders Co., 1984.

CHAPTER *3*

NORMAL HISTOLOGY OF THE INFANT IN THE POSTNEONATAL PERIOD

INTRODUCTION

In general those pathologists who work with autopsy material from adults and children, including infants, are more accustomed to adult histology, i.e., the normal appearance of tissues in the adult, than they are to that of babies.[1] As a result, innumerable, significant mistakes have been made through the years on the basis of misinterpretation of what is really normal histology for the infant. The classic example is the infant lung; normal lung tissue in the baby of two months looks quite different, histologically, from that of a 20 year old man. The walls of the infant alveolus are thicker and more cellular than those of the adult; consequently the normal infant lung has been, and still is, frequently misdiagnosed as representing interstitial pneumonitis. This chapter is devoted to illustrations of normal and near normal histology in the postneonatal period, from 28 days to approximately one year of age.

HEART

The principal difference between the infant heart and that of the adult is the thinner breadth (or diameter) of the myocardial fibers in babies and, therefore, the relatively larger size of the nuclei. Similarly, the endocardium and epicardium are thinner, and there is far less epicardial adipose tissue (Figs. 3–1 through 3–4).[6]

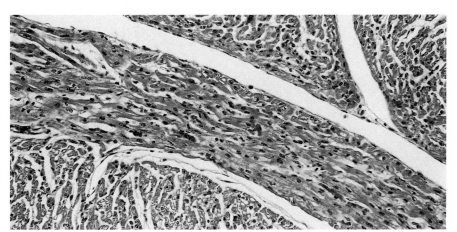

Figure 3–1.
A section of the myocardium taken from the wall of the left ventricle. Myocardial fibers appear here in both cross and longitudinal sections. 160x

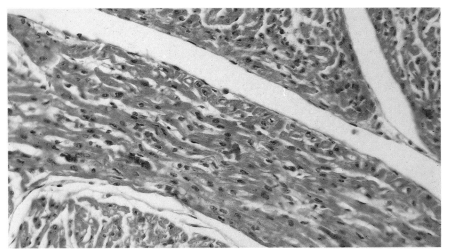

Figure 3–2. The myocardium at higher magnification. Notice the delicate quality of the endocardium lining the space, obliquely oriented, just above the center. 250x

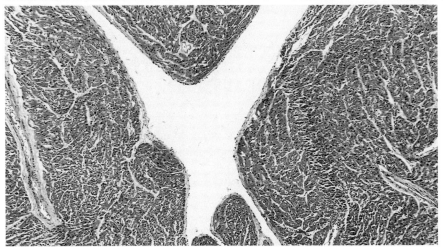

Figure 3–3. The myocardium in the wall of the left ventricle at considerably lower magnification. The endocardium lining the Y-shaped central cleft exhibits an expected variability in thickness and cellularity. 60x

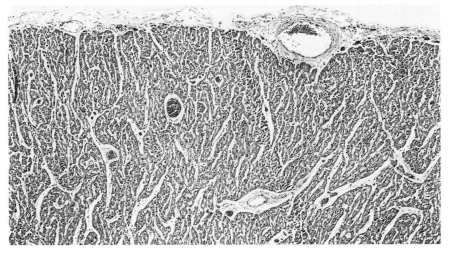

Figure 3–4. The normal epicardium for the same ten-month old infant, at the same magnification, as shown in the preceding photograph. 60x

RESPIRATORY TRACT

Epiglottis

Ideally a midline sagittal section of the epiglottis is taken at every infant autopsy. However, significant epiglottitis is uncommon in the first year of life (Fig. 3–5).

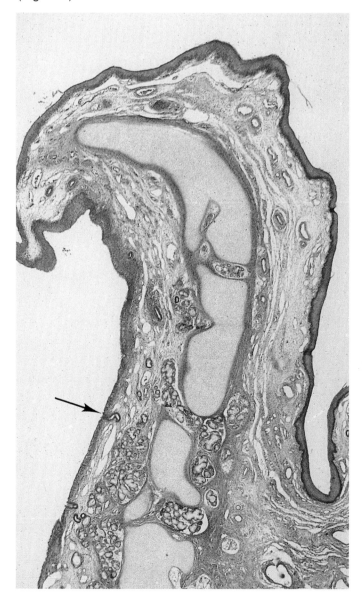

Figure 3–5. A midline, sagittal section of the epiglottis. The tongue is to the right, and the airway to the left. Most of the surface of the epiglottis in this infant is covered with stratified squamous epithelium. Note that there are "defects" in the central bar of cartilage in which can be seen both vessels and mucous glands; the ducts of these glands are directed posteriorly (arrow). 15x

Larynx

It is usually desirable to include in any set of slides from an infant autopsy at least one section of the larynx. Inflammation of the larynx is relatively common among infants in the postneonatal period. A cross section can be taken at or near the laryngeal ventricle; however, many pathologists prefer a longitudinal section, taken anterolaterally, either to the right or to the left of the midline (Fig. 3–6).

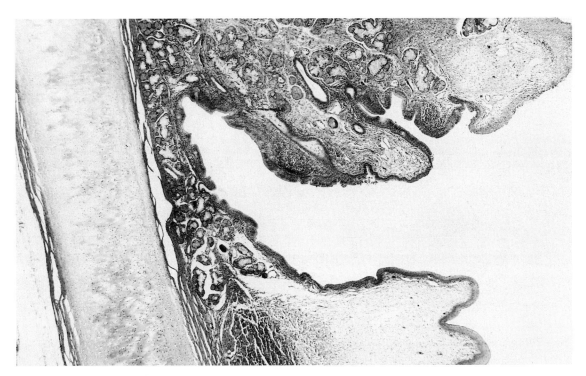

Figure 3–6. A longitudinal section of the larynx, taken to one side of the midline so that the laryngeal ventricle is seen in profile. In this instance most of the ventricle is lined by respiratory epithelium. 25x

Trachea

A cross section of the trachea is taken routinely in most infant autopsies. To maximize the usefulness of that section, pathologists usually elect to take it horizontally, at the level of the thyroid, to include the isthmus, both of the lower poles of the lateral lobes of that organ, and sometimes, one or two parathyroids (Figs. 3–7 and 3–8).

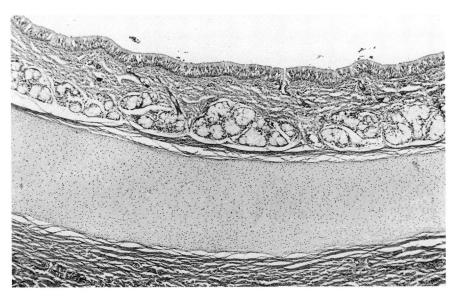

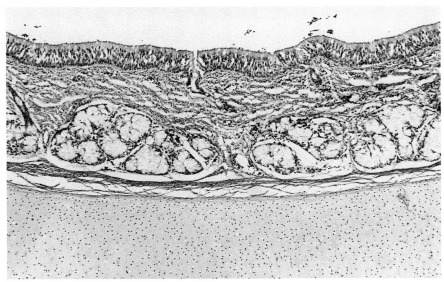

Figure 3–7.
A cross section of the wall of the trachea in an infant.
A (upper): Wall of the trachea, at medium magnification. Immediately superficial to the cartilage ring are numerous mucous glands. 40x
B (lower): Same section at higher magnification. 60x

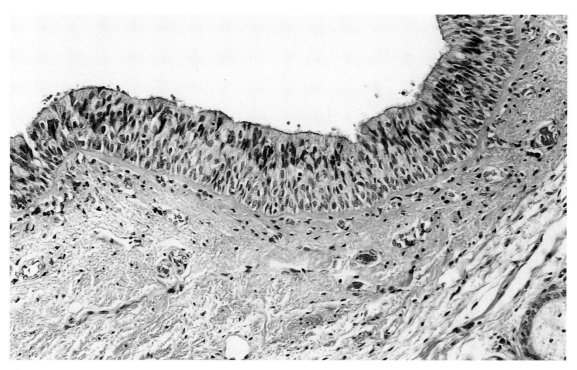

Figure 3–8. The epithelial lining of the infant trachea. The epithelium per se is tall, columnar, pseudostratified, and ciliated. The basement membrane is normally prominent and of uniform thickness. The underlying connective tissue is normally cellular and vascular. 160x

Bronchus

In addition to the routine sections of peripheral lung, it is important to take a section near the hilus to include one or more sections of bronchi (Figs. 3–9 and 3–10).

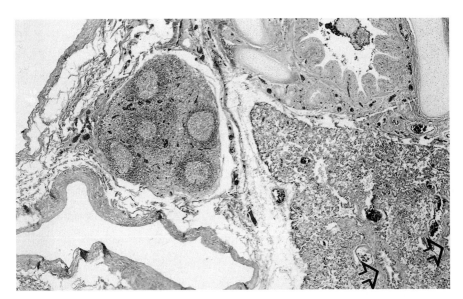

Figure 3-9. Bronchus. A hilar section depicting a bronchus (upper right) cut in cross section, a hilar lymph node, and a vessel (lower left) together with a small portion of lung (lower right corner) bearing two bronchioles (open arrows). Note the markedly convoluted quality of the epithelial lining of the bronchus. 25x.

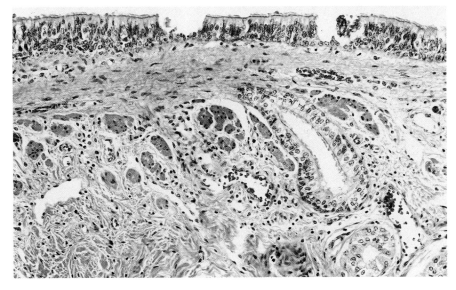

Figure 3-10. The epithelial lining of a normal infant bronchus, at higher magnification. Note the underlying smooth muscle bundles and a portion of a mucous gland and its duct. 160x

Bronchiole

Sections taken from the periphery of the lung usually include adequate numbers of bronchioles for examination (Figs. 3–11 and 3–12).

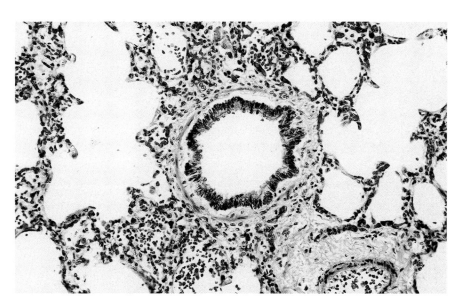

Figure 3–11.
The wall of a bronchiole of an infant. The lining epithelial cells are much shorter than those of the bronchus and their nuclei tend to be basally situated. Note the delicate ring of smooth muscle encircling the structure. Except for a few tiny intra-alveolar hemorrhages, the surrounding lung parenchyma is unremarkable. 160x

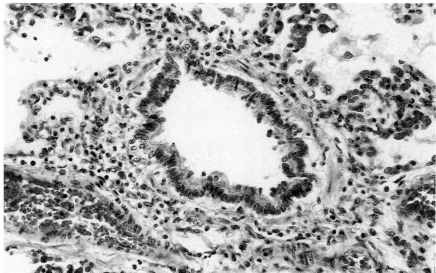

Figure 3–12.
Cross section of another bronchiole, at higher magnification. A bundle of smooth muscle is visible in the wall, particularly in the upper right quadrant. A few small round cells, probably lymphocytes, are scattered within and around the wall. 250x

Lung

A minimum of five sections of the infant lung (one from each lobe) is considered basic for the infant autopsy. Additional sections should be taken of pathologic lesions or worrisome areas (Figs. 3–13 through 3–17).[6]

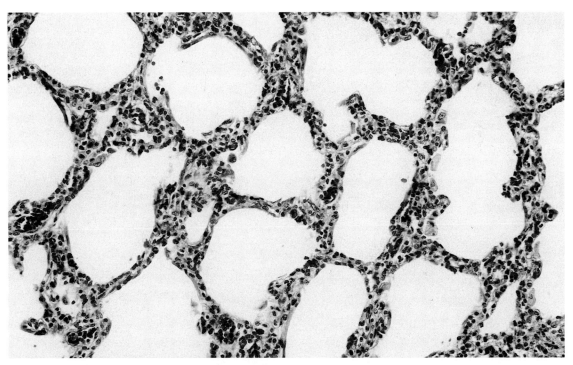

Figure 3–13. Normal alveolar walls in an infant lung. Some of these walls are rather thin, but most are considerably thicker than those of an adult, particularly in relationship to the diameter of the air space. These walls are also more cellular than those of an adult. 160x

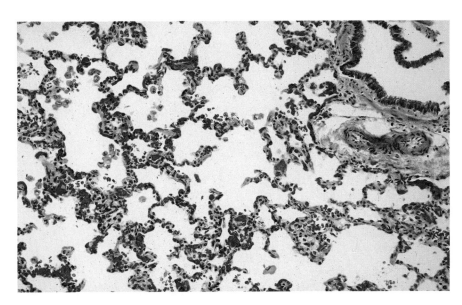

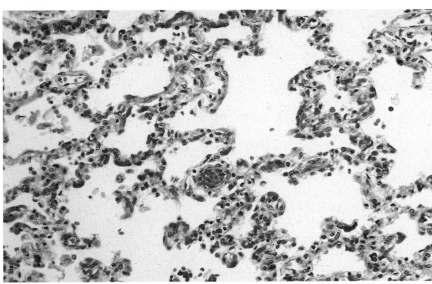

Figure 3–14. Apparent thickening of the walls of air spaces of two different infants, at two magnifications. The apparent thickening shown in these photographs is still within limits of normal for the age. Also, the architecture of the lung in these infants seems not to have been disturbed by artificial respiration at or after the time of death.
A (upper): 160x
B (lower): 250x

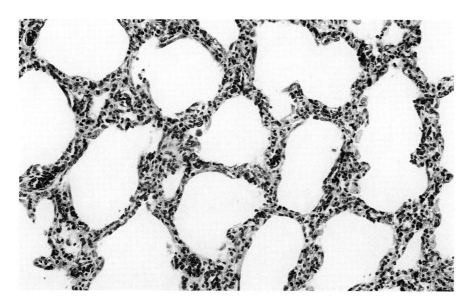

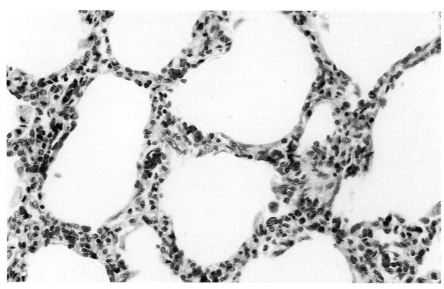

Figure 3–15. Normal lung of an infant, appearing slightly more mature than that in Figures 3–13 and 3–14, at two magnifications. The architecture in this field has not been disturbed by artificial respiration. As in the neonate, these alveolar ducts and alveoli bear some resemblance to crumpled paper bags. In the top picture, it is especially apparent that these inter-alveolar walls are still thicker and more cellular than those of an adult.
A (upper): 160x
B (lower): 250x

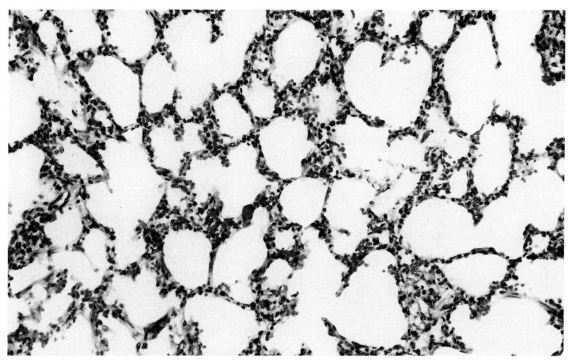

Figure 3–16. Artificial expansion of air spaces produced by assisted pulmonary ventilation at or after the time of death. This is a common artifact in the lungs of infants in whom resuscitation has been attempted. When resuscitation has not been attempted, the configuration of the walls is much more irregular, as shown in Figures 3–14 and 3–15. 160x

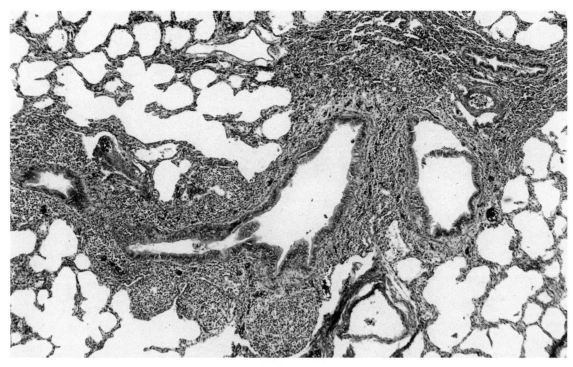

Figure 3–17. Rounded aggregates of lymphocytes, often seen near bronchioles, in an otherwise normal lung. These ought to be considered normal morphologic features of the infant lung in the same way that large tonsils are normal for little children. There are at least three such nodules immediately below and intimately related to a large bronchiole. The distended alveolar ducts and alveoli in the lower left corner suggest that this infant was given assisted ventilation at the time of death. 40x

Pleura

Pleura is usually included in routine sections of infant lung. Although pleural lesions are not common in this age group, secondary changes may correlate with underlying disease (Fig. 3–18).

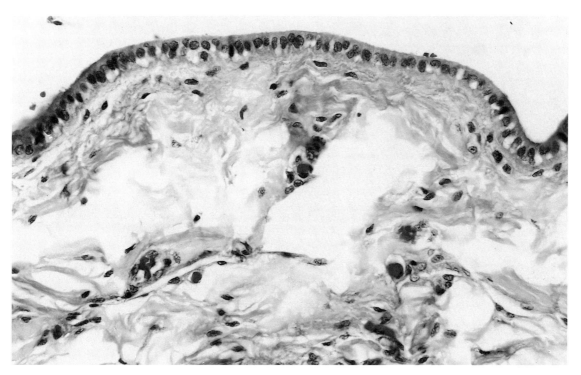

Figure 3–18. The entire thickness of the pleura in an infant. In this illustration there is an unusual, but nevertheless normal, segment of covering mesothelial cells, which here range from cuboidal to columnar. 250x

SPLEEN

A routine section of spleen should be taken for histologic study in the course of every infant atuopsy. By the time of a term delivery, the malpighian corpuscles are fairly large and clearly delineated (Figs. 3–19 and 3–20).

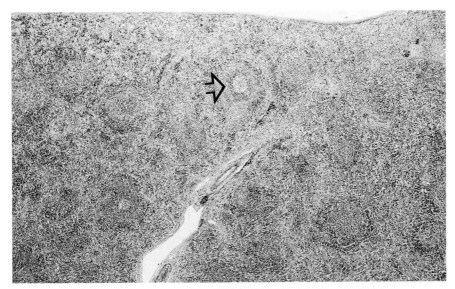

Figure 3–19. The capsule of the spleen (in the upper part of the figure) and five or six malpighian corpuscles (near the middle). One of them (just above the middle) has an active germinal center (open arrow). Several have halos of small, somewhat darker lymphocytes. 25x

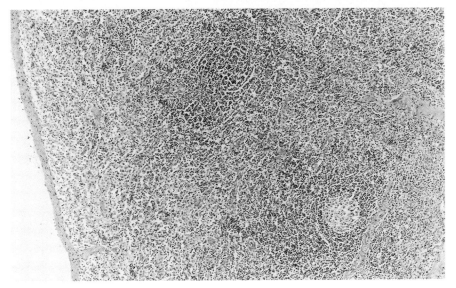

Figure 3–20. The capsule of the spleen, at higher magnification. The malpighian corpuscle in the lower right portion of the picture has a germinal center. 60x

LYMPH NODES

Good sections of lymph nodes can be obtained most easily from a single section of the mesentery. They are normally abundant and generous in size (Figs. 3–21 through 3–23).

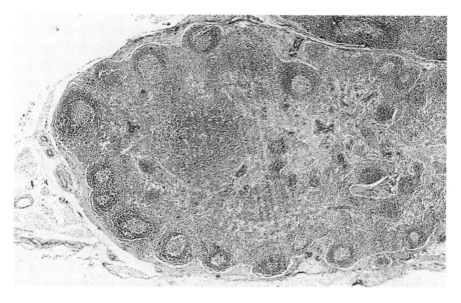

Figure 3–21.
A lymph node with essentially normal architecture. Sixteen lymphoid nodules encircle the node at its periphery; 13 of them have germinal centers. The sinusoids stand out clearly in the right half of the node and the peripheral or subcapsular sinus is clearly delineated around most of the inferior margin. 25x

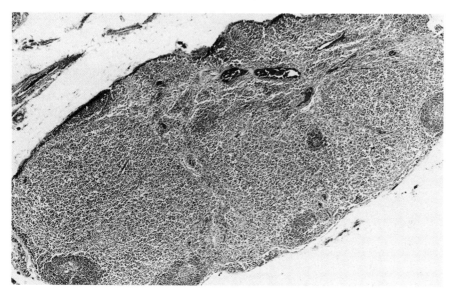

Figure 3–22.
A mesenteric node with only four lymphoid nodules at the perimeter, three with germinal centers. In this particular section the sinuses are not visible; instead there appear to be only monotonous sheets of lymphocytes. 40x

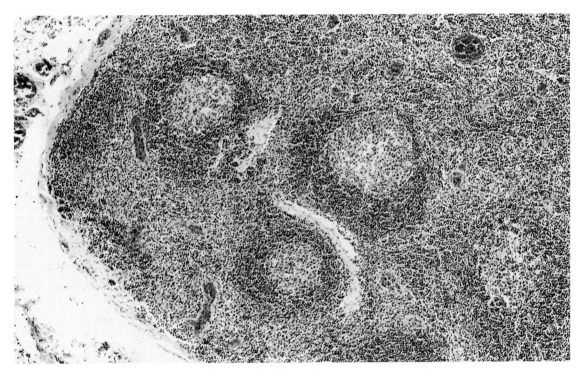

Figure 3–23. Lymph node. Five lymphoid nodules appear here at somewhat higher magnification; four of them have germinal centers. The subcapsular sinus is barely perceptible inferiorly and to the left. 60x

KIDNEY

The histology of the infant kidney varies with the maturity of the infant. In fact, a reasonable estimation of post-conceptual age can be established by an experienced observer based on the features of the glomeruli (Figs. 3–24 through 3–26).[6]

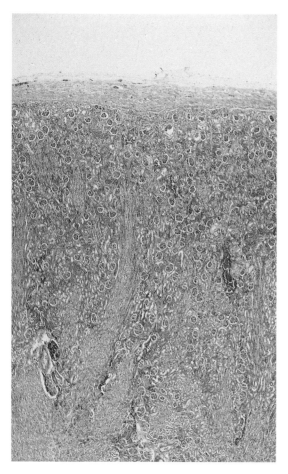 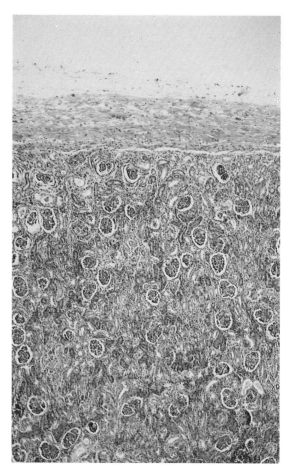

Figure 3–24. Architecture and intimate histology of the renal cortex in infants, at increasing magnification.
A (left): Three medullary rays are seen; the one just to the left of center is the longest. Glomeruli are normally plentiful and all of them seem to be rather mature. The capsule is present and is normally thick. 25x
B (right): The number of layers of glomeruli is adequate and ample numbers of tubules surround glomeruli. 60x

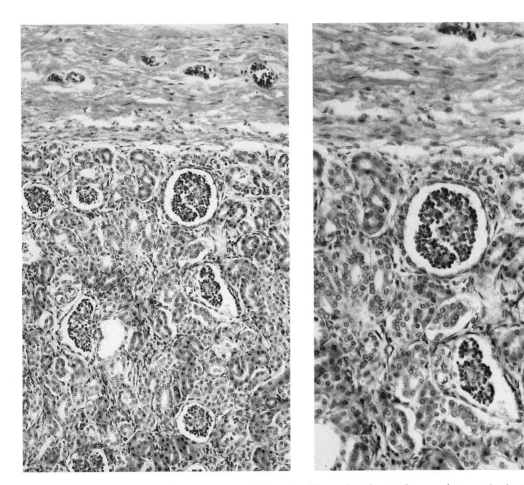

C (left): The glomeruli, at least those most recently formed and hence just deep to the capsule, are not yet mature. The cells at the perimeter of the individual glomerulus provide clear evidence of the fact that this is a section from an infant inasmuch as the rounded nuclei at their edges are very dark and appear tightly packed. Variability of staining among the cells lining tubules is within limits of normal. 160x   D (right): One subcapsular glomerulus with its striking rim of peripheral epithelial cells. Note the prominence also of the epithelial cells lining Bowman's capsule. 250x

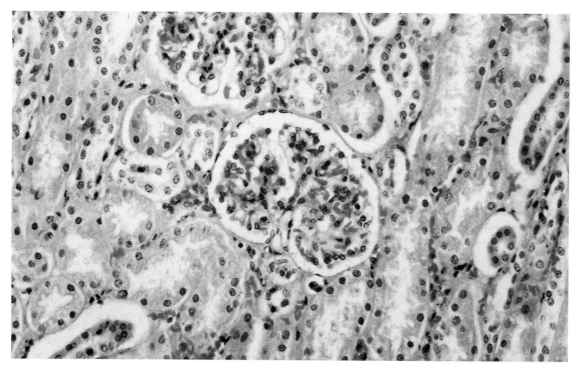

Figure 3–25. A glomerulus from a more mature patient than the one illustrated in Figure 3–24. This glomerulus does not exhibit the striking ring of densely packed, dark nuclei at its periphery. Deeper glomeruli, near the bases of pyramids, are apt to have this more mature appearance in young infants. As babies grow, glomeruli of this type appear higher and higher in the cortex, until eventually all glomeruli are divested of that characteristic rim, even the "youngest" glomeruli located directly beneath the capsule.[6] 250x

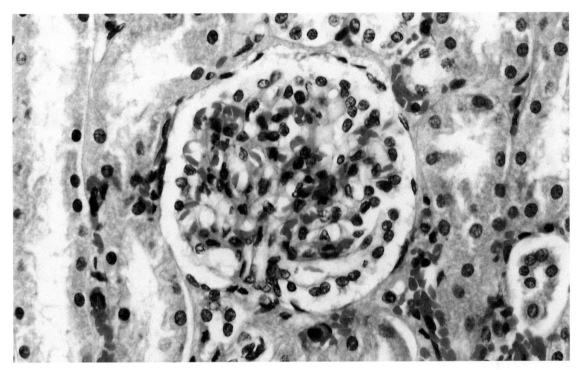

Figure 3–26. A normal infant glomerulus, at high magnification. The cells of this glomerulus are much more plump than those in an adult. Some sickled cells appear in the lumina of the glomerular capillaries. The cells of Bowman's capsule are also slightly more prominent than they are in the adult. The arteriole in the glomerular stalk is normally delicate. The tubular epithelium is well preserved. 400x

URETER

Sections of ureter are not usually included in the set of microscopic sections taken during an infant autopsy. The microscopic architecture of an infant ureter is exactly like that of an adult (Fig. 3–27).

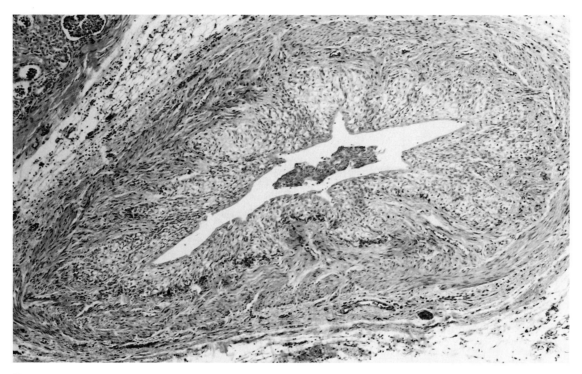

Figure 3–27. A slightly oblique section of a ureter, quite close to the kidney. The transitional epithelial lining is arranged in deep folds. The bundles of smooth muscle in the wall are variously oriented. The entire structure is virtually surrounded by adipose tissue. 60x

GASTROINTESTINAL TRACT

Esophagus

The infant esophagus is much like that of the adult, lined by orderly stratified squamous epithelium. The muscularis mucosae is typically thick in this organ, thicker than in any other part of the gastrointestinal tract (Figs. 3–28 and 3–29).

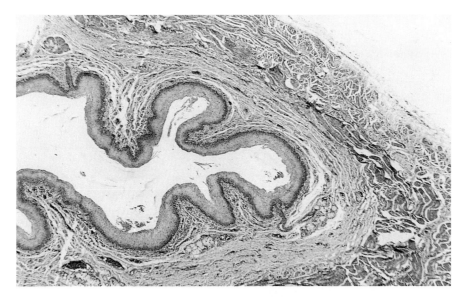

Figure 3–28. A cross section of the esophagus showing the intact lining of stratified squamous epithelium and mucous glands in the submucosa. It is apparent that this section was taken from the middle third of the organ since there is both smooth and skeletal muscle in the wall. 25x

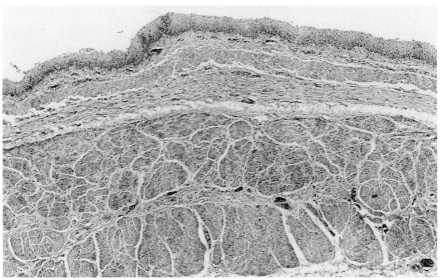

Figure 3–29. A section of esophagus from the inferior portion, taken at slightly higher magnification than the preceding figure. The muscularis propria is made up of smooth muscle exclusively; it is from the lowermost third. 40x

Cardioesophageal Junction

A longitudinal section including esophageal and gastric mucosa is often taken in both adult and infant autopsies (Fig. 3–30).[6]

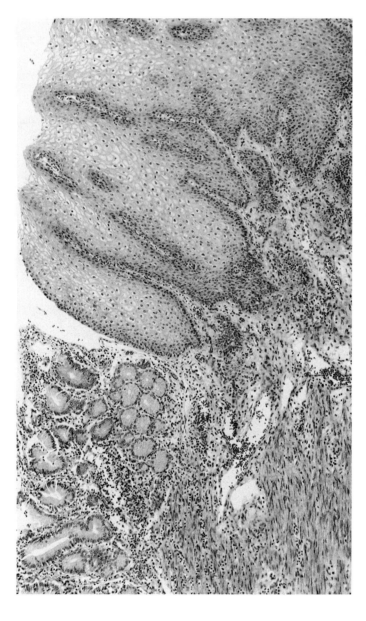

Figure 3–30. Cardioesophageal junction. The stratified squamous epithelium of the esophagus is apparent in the upper half of the photograph and mucous glands of the gastric mucosa in the lower half. A few strands of the muscularis mucosae are apparent along the right edge. 60x

Small Bowel

Sections should be taken from all three segments of the small bowel, i.e., duodenum, jejunum, and ileum. Cross sections of unopened bowel, put immediately into formalin, generally provide good preservation of mucosal histology (Fig. 3–31).[6]

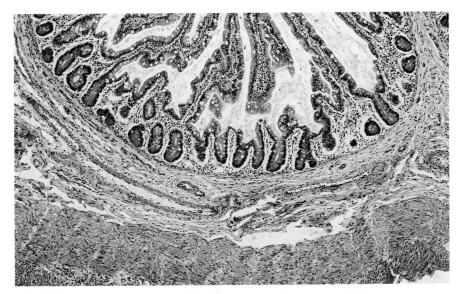

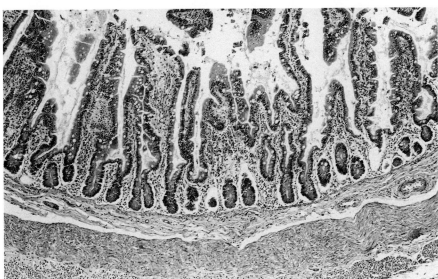

Figure 3–31. Partial cross section of normal ileum, at two magnifications. Both show long, delicate, gracile villi projecting into the lumen, and branching glands.
A (upper): 40x
B (lower): 60x

LIVER

At least one section of liver should be included in every infant autopsy; many pathologists take two, one from the right lobe and one from the left (Figs. 3–32 through 3–35).[6]

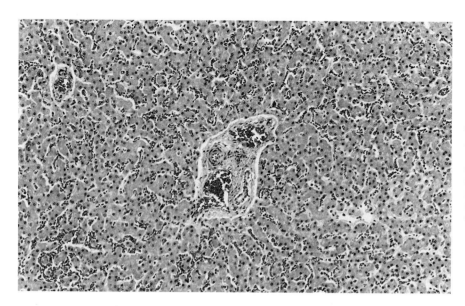

Figure 3–32. General architecture of the liver, at relatively low magnification. Columns of liver cells are delicate and separated from one another by slender sinusoids. In the center of the field is a portal space of medium size with a bile duct on the right side inferiorly, an artery upper left, and two rather large, engorged veins. 100x

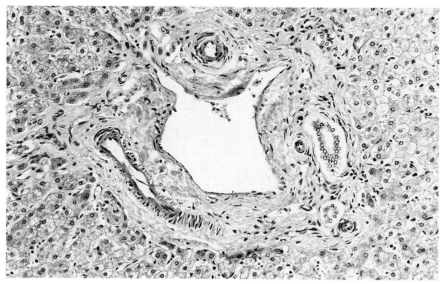

Figure 3–33. Detail of a single portal triad. At the top and to the left are two relatively small arteries. Two ducts appear on the lower right, and a large vein is located in the center of the structure. Many of the hepatocytes are finely vacuolated. 160x

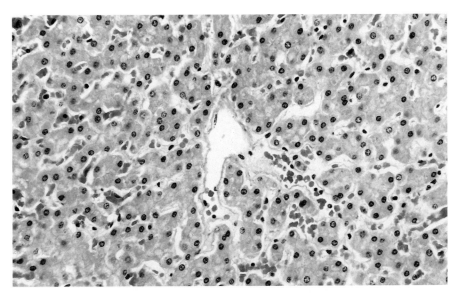

Figure 3–34. A central vein with two sinusoids opening into it, one from below and one from the right. The liver cells are normal. 250x

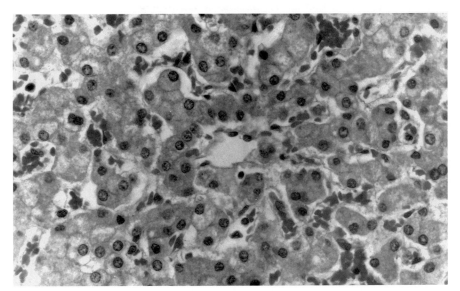

Figure 3–35. A central vein, at higher magnification. Two nuclei of its lining endothelial cells can be seen at the top of the vein. The majority of the hepatocytes in this field exhibit normal, uniformly pale-staining cytoplasm. 400x

PANCREAS

Sections of pancreas should be taken from the head and tail. Interpretation of the number and size of the islets of Langerhans may be especially difficult for those unaccustomed to normal infant histology (Figs. 3–36 through 3–40).[2,3,7]

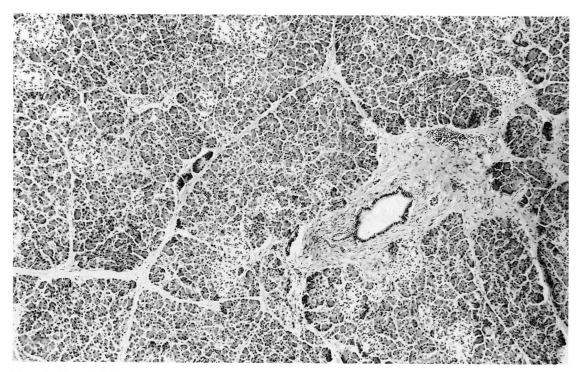

Figure 3–36. The infant pancreas. A large duct is just below and to the right of center. Individual lobules of the pancreas are clearly separated from one another by delicate septa of connective tissue. Acini, back-to-back, make up the bulk of each lobule; scattered among them are round, pale islets, moderately cellular, and of expected size and number. 60x

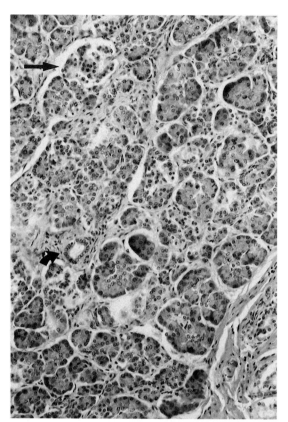

Figure 3–37. Detail of the pancreas.
A (upper): The central portion is occupied by an obliquely oriented band of crowded acini. Acini show central cytoplasm and peripheral nuclei. On the left (curved arrow) is an intralobular duct; in the lower right are several interlobular ducts lined by tall columnar epithelium. In the left upper corner (straight arrow) is a single very small islet. 160x

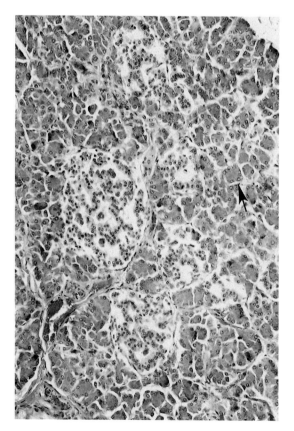

B (lower): A cluster of three islets. Each of these exhibits the characteristic twirled ribbon pattern. The acini (one is marked with an arrow), have typical, solid-appearing central zones and peripheral nuclei. 160x

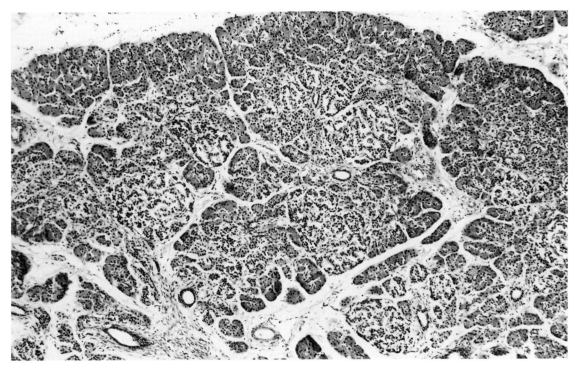

Figure 3–38. Apparent islet cell hyperplasia. This field illustrates crowding of several islets, each of generous proportions. This appearance has led some investigators to suspect hyperplasia of islets and potentially fatal hyperinsulinemia in some cases of sudden infant death syndrome. Subsequent investigations using immuno-histochemistry and/or computerized image analysis have demonstrated that this appearance does not represent real hyperplasia.[2-3,7] 60x

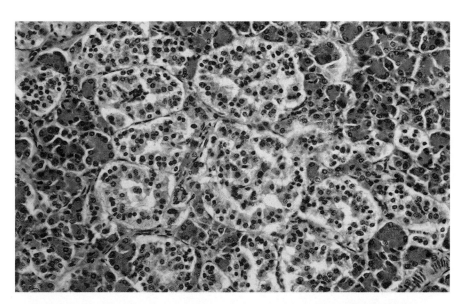

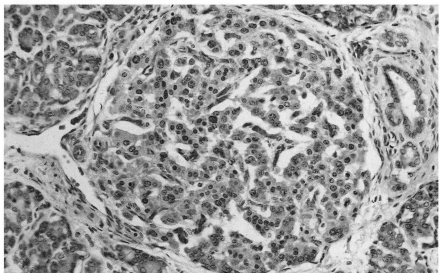

Figure 3–39.
Apparent islet cell hyperplasia.
A (upper): A cluster of islets of normal size fills the middle of the picture. 250x
B (lower): A single islet, at the same magnification. Compare the size of the acini in the two pictures. An occasional large islet, such as this, especially without hypertrophy of individual cells, has no apparent functional significance. 250x

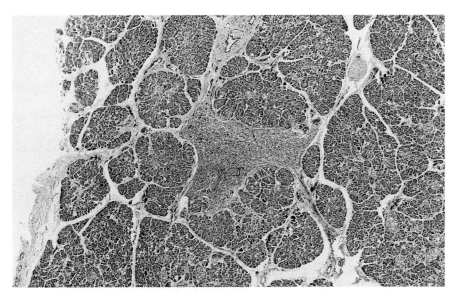

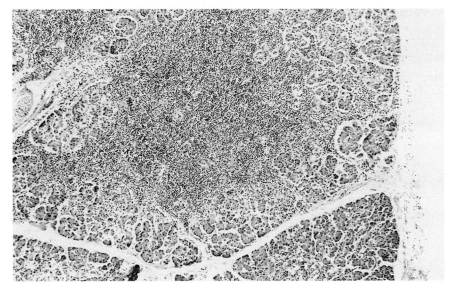

Figure 3–40.
Lymphoid tissue within the pancreas.
A (upper): One large aggregate of lymphocytes, larger than one of the surrounding lobules, appears in the center of the field; it is discrete and has no nodules within it. This type of aggregate is common in infants in the first year of life and seems to have no functional significance. 25x
B (lower): A less well-defined aggregate, similarly monotonous, in which a few acini and intralobular ducts appear stranded. 60x

OVARY

The infant ovary is tiny, thin, flat, and lingulate. The pathologist may submit one entire organ for histologic sections, in which case, the microscopic section will be an elongate oval. Very often, however, the section selected is taken in the sagital plane to include the attached mesentery and a cross section of fallopian tube. Infant ovaries often contain follicular cysts, some of which are surprisingly large (Figs. 3–41 and 3–42).[5,6]

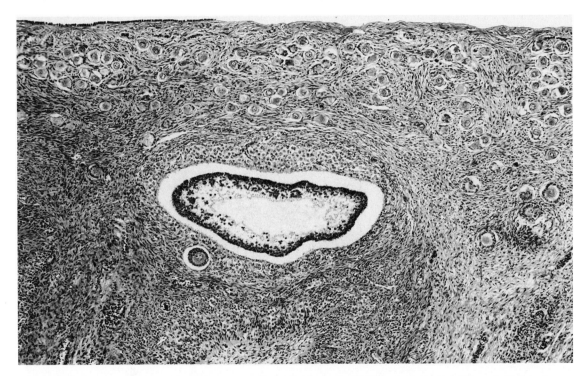

Figure 3–41. The normal cortex of an infant ovary. On part of the surface of the organ (upper left) is a single line of epithelial cells. The others were lost artifactually. Deep to the surface is a band of crowded, primitive follicles, each of which bears a single oocyte. In the center of the field is a secondary follicle lined by granulosa cells which have become detached from the wall artificially. Just above the follicle is a broad band of lutein cells, stouter and paler than granulosa cells. Below and to the left of the secondary follicle is a single primary follicle with a large oocyte in its center. The ovarian stroma is typically tightly woven. 60x

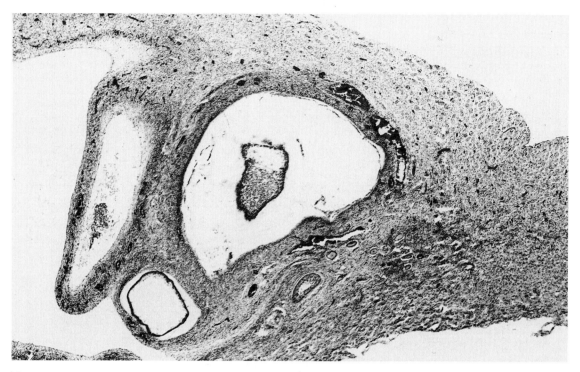

Figure 3–42. Four follicular cysts, normal in ovaries of infants of this age. They are not only numerous but also large, half or more of the diameter of the ovary itself. Only the smallest, at the lower border of the cluster, has a lining of dark, small granulosa cells. 25x

ADRENAL

At least one section of adrenal should be taken in every infant autopsy. That section is usually cut in the sagital plane and through the thickest part of the organ. However, because the organ is friable, one may elect to section it serially *after* fixation and then select one of the central segments for histologic preparation (Figs. 3–43 through 3–47).

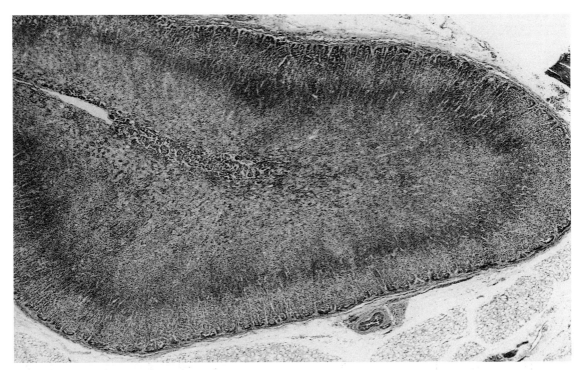

Figure 3–43. The entire breadth of the infant adrenal, at low magnification. There is a slender fibrous capsule about the perimeter and a slender band of medulla in the center. As is normal for this age, the innermost two-thirds of the cortex is still of the fetal type while the peripheral one-third is definitive, or adult, cortex. Even at this magnification it is apparent that much of the periadrenal adipose envelope is brown fat. 25x

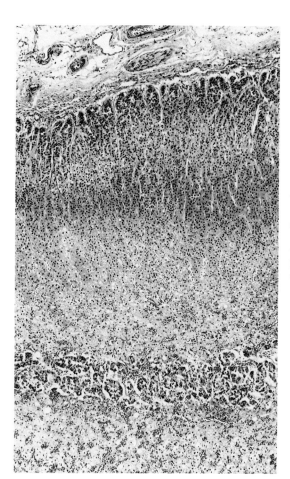

Figure 3–44. Infant adrenal. Cortical cells from the same section as shown in Figure 3–43 are depicted. Near the bottom of the picture is a dark band of medulla. Just above that is a broad band of pale cells constituting the fetal cortex, which, at this age, is diminishing in thickness. The darker cells, making up the outermost band, represent adult cortex, which is gradually becoming the dominant component. 60x

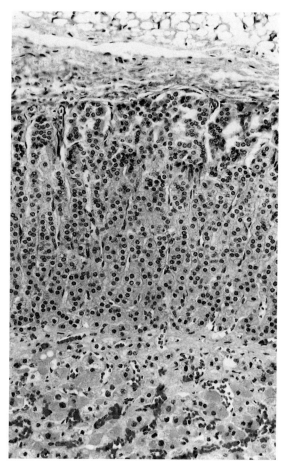

Figure 3–45. Adrenal. This is the fetal cortex, at higher magnification (lowest third of photograph). The adult cortex (upper two-thirds) is arranged in somewhat more regular, slender cords of cells, parallel to one another. 160x

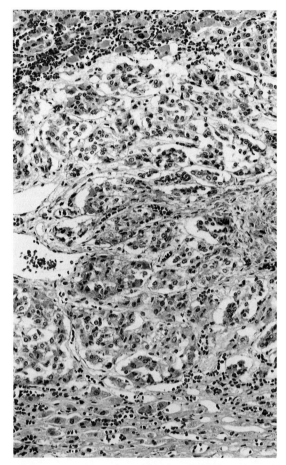

Figure 3–46. Cells of the adrenal medulla. Note the rather haphazard arrangement and pleomorphism. 160x

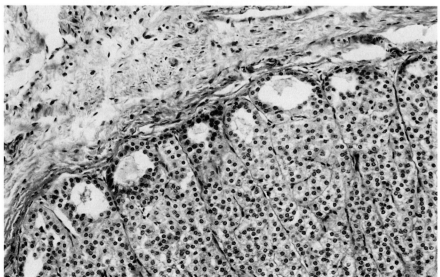

Figure 3–47. Infant adrenal glands with cystic arrangement of cells of the zona glomerulosa. These tiny cysts are of uniform proportions and are always arranged in a ring around the gland just beneath the capsule. Adrenals with this lesion are usually otherwise normal. The significance of these cysts is not known. 160x

Periadrenal Adipose Tissue

The routine section of adrenal taken during an infant autopsy almost inevitably includes periadrenal adipose tissue because this infant organ is extraordinarily delicate and difficult to trim. In the first month of life periadrenal fat is predominantly of the "brown" or multi-vacuolated type. However, during the next seven months of life, progressively more of its cells become univacuolar, or "white", resembling the usual adult adipose tissue cell. Normal newborn babies have about 90% brown fat around their adrenals, while at eight months of age, the normal infant's adrenal is surrounded by adipose tissue, only 40-50% of which is brown fat (Fig. 3–48).[4,8]

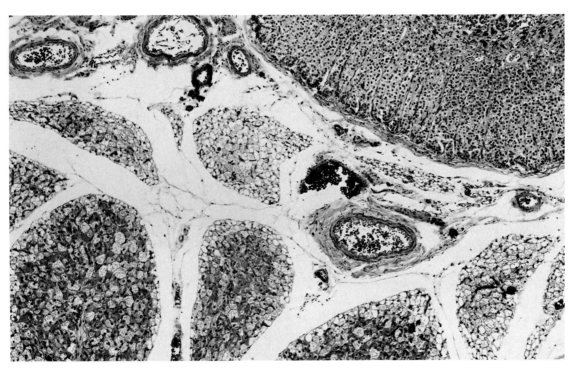

Figure 3–48. Periadrenal adipose tissue comprising both brown and white (mature) fat. A: (above). Islands of adipose tissue surround the gland seen in the upper right corner. Fat cells in proximity to the gland seem to be pale while those at a distance appear more dense. 60x

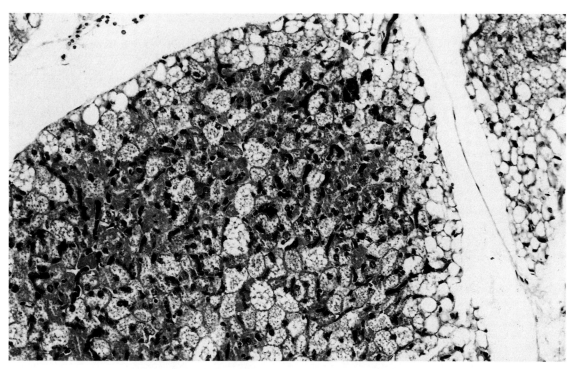

B: A lobule of periadrenal adipose tissue, at higher magnification. The cytoplasm of some of these cells is very dense so that it looks smooth, homogeneous, and grey (brown fat). More peripherally, the cells are diffusely, uniformly, finely vacuolated. At the very perimeter of the lobule is an occasional so-called white fat cell, which is round and bears a single globule of lipid and a peripherally located nucleus. In contrast, the nucleus of a brown fat cell is centrally located. 160x

THYMUS

The thymus is an important component of the routine infant autopsy although little attention is paid to it in the adult. The gross anatomy and histology of this gland are often key factors in interpreting the duration of a disease process in an infant (Figs. 3–49 through 3–51).[6]

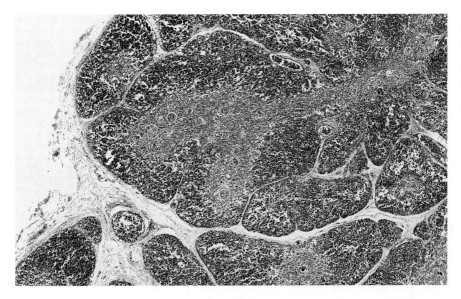

Figure 3–49. Infant thymus, at very low magnification. The clear lobulation reflects the branched architecture of this organ. In the light grey medulla, near the center of the picture, sharply delineated Hassall's corpuscles can be seen. 25x

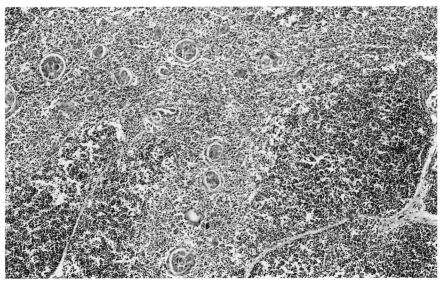

Figure 3–50. The central portion of the thymus illustrated in Figure 3–49, at higher magnification. Approximately 11 Hassall's corpuscles appear in the center of the medulla. 40x

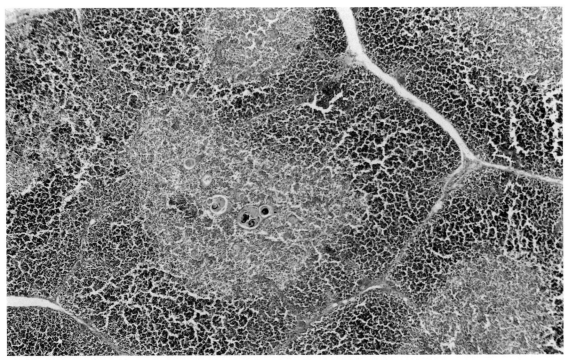

Figure 3–51. A single lobule of the thymus of an older infant. The dark staining material in the Hassall's corpuscles is calcium. Adequate numbers of lymphocytes are present throughout; there has been no appreciable involution. 40x.

THYROID

At least one section of the thyroid is usually included routinely in the set of tissues submitted for microscopic study in any infant autopsy. Ordinarily this section is taken horizontally, through the larynx, to include the lower poles of both lateral lobes and the trachea (Figs. 3–52 through 3–54).

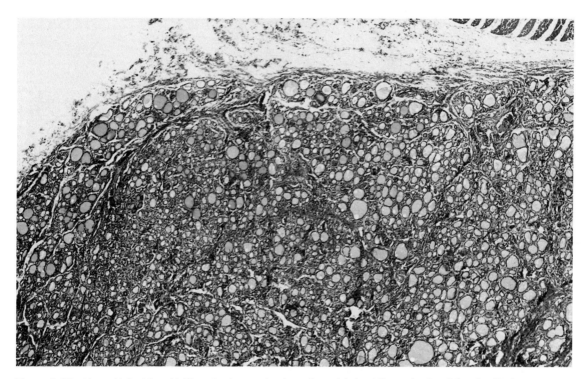

Figure 3–52. Normal infant thyroid. There is always a tendency for acini about the perimeter of the gland to be somewhat larger than those in the center. These acini are filled with colloid and are especially well preserved. 25x

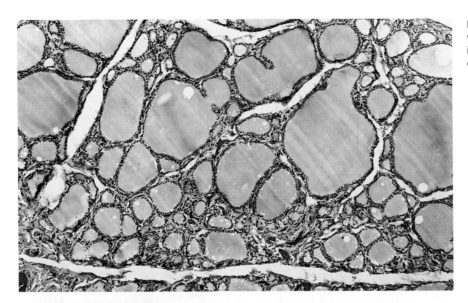

Figure 3–53. Thyroid with normal variability in the size and shape of acini.   60x

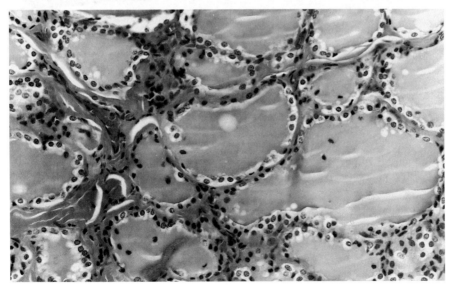

Figure 3–54. Epithelial cells lining thyroid acini. They are cuboidal with central nuclei. The colloid is uniformly stained and not scalloped. 250x

PARATHYROID

The infant parathyroid is not sought deliberately in the routine infant autopsy but appears frequently in the standard section of thyroid and trachea. It contains almost no adipose tissue which is the reason that grossly it has a coral color rather than the somewhat yellow hue of the gland in adults (Figs. 3–55 through 3–58).[6]

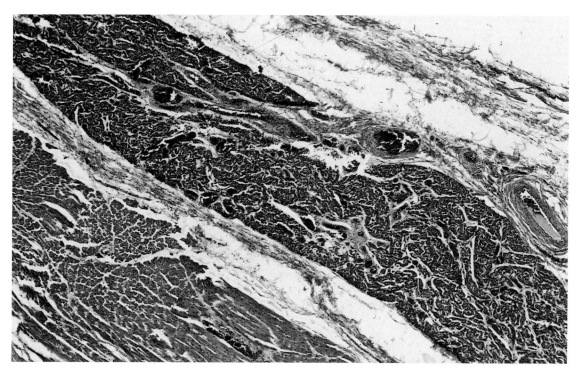

Figure 3–55. A single elongate, slender parathyroid. Even at this low magnification, the typical organoid pattern can be seen. Note the absence of fat cells within the gland. 40x

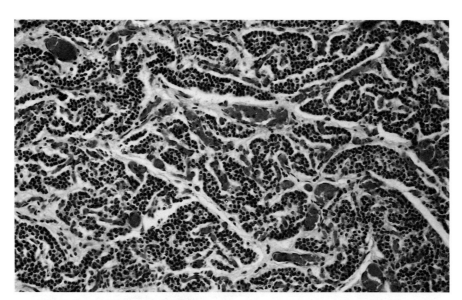

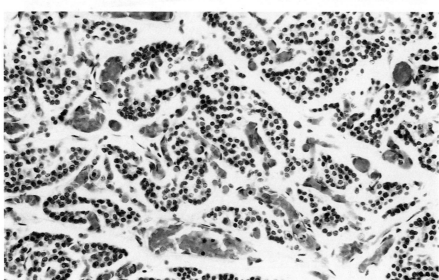

Figure 3–56.
Parathyroid. The same parathyroid as illustrated in Figure 3–55 shown at much higher magnification. These pictures illustrate well the small dark type of epithelial cell native to this organ and the striking vascularity of the gland.
A (upper): 100x
B (lower): 250x

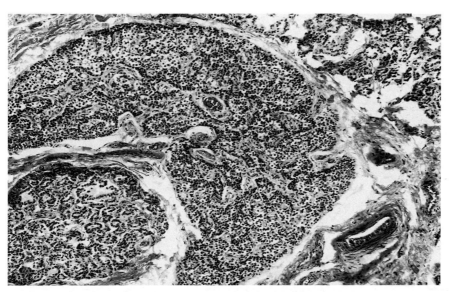

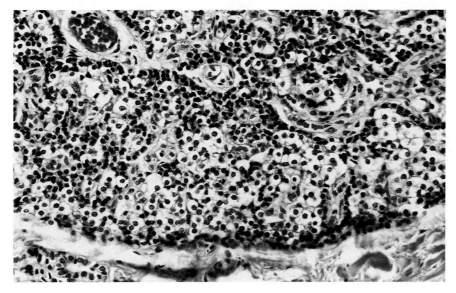

Figure 3–57.
Parathyroid, at two magnifications.
A (upper): Parathyroid gland; note the autolysis that has taken place in the adjacent thyroid (lower left corner). This process proceeds rapidly in infants. 100x
B (lower): There are two types of cells seen in the parathyroid of infants, the small dark ones running like a slender ribbon across the center of this photograph, and the absolutely clear cells (wasserhellen), which are best seen in the lower half centrally. 250x

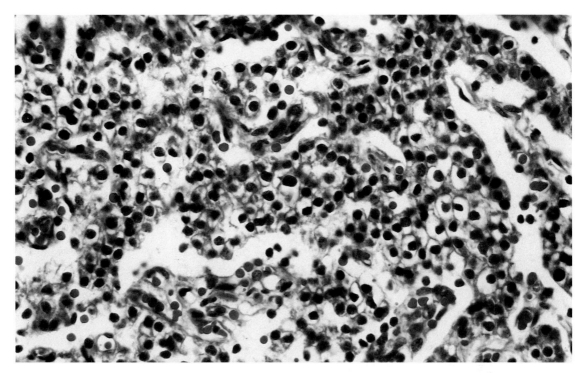

Figure 3–58. "Water-clear" cells in the parathyroid. Most of the nuclei are dense and centrally located and the cell membranes are sharply delineated. 400x

PITUITARY

The infant pituitary histologically has the same three distinct segments as the adult organ, namely the anterior, middle, and posterior portions, all of which are histologically unique (Fig. 3–59).

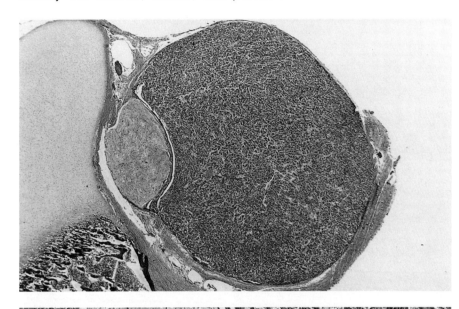

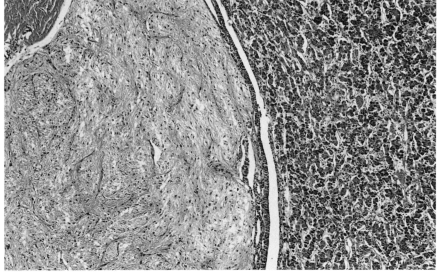

Figure 3–59. The infant pituitary. A (upper): The discrete, large, rounded mass in the center is the anterior pituitary. The small, paler oval mass to its left is the posterior pituitary. On the left above is the cartilaginous portion of the sella turcica, and below that, the bony portion. 15x
B (lower): Epithelial cell cords of the anterior pituitary are on the right. The cleft and cyst-like spaces of the pars intermedia appear in the center and some of the pars nervosa on the left. 60x

SKELETAL MUSCLE

Two sections of skeletal muscle are usually taken in the infant autopsy, one from the diaphragm and one from psoas muscle (Figs. 3–60 and 3–61).

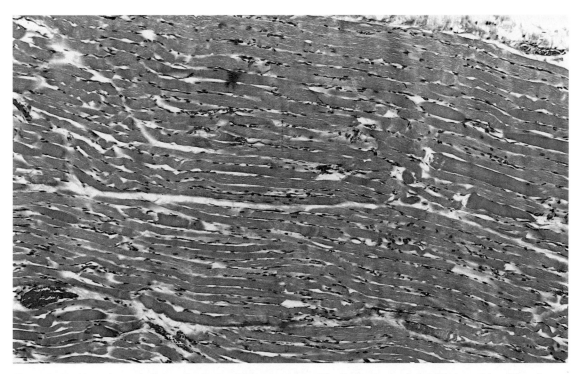

Figure 3–60. Normal muscle fibers of uniform width and staining. The fibers are parallel and their nuclei peripherally oriented. 60x

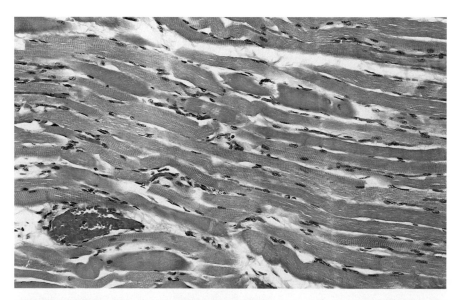

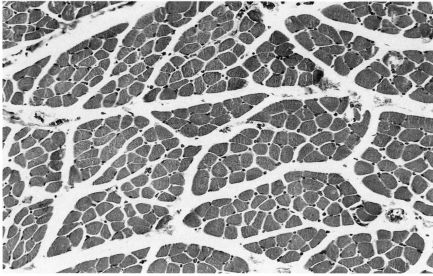

Figure 3–61. Normal skeletal muscle.
A (upper): Cross striations are clearly defined in the center of this longitudinal section. 160x
B (lower): The typical flagstone appearance of a cross section is evident here, as are the peripherally located nuclei. 160x

CENTRAL NERVOUS SYSTEM

Careful gross examination of the central nervous system in the infant seems more difficult than the adult. This is because of the normally soft consistency and less distinctive landmarks of the infant brain. Nevertheless, it is an essential part for a complete autopsy. Evidence of infection (acute or chronic), perinatal hypoxia, and some congenital anomalies, for example, can be detected only by means of thorough gross and microscopic examination. Complete representation of the central nervous system is beyond the scope of this atlas, but is provided elsewhere (Fig. 3–62).[6]

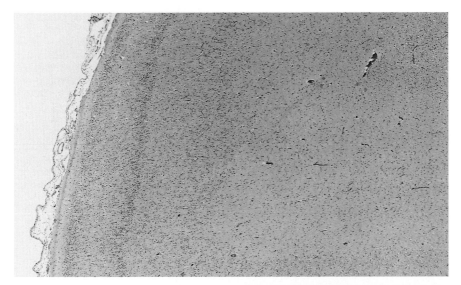

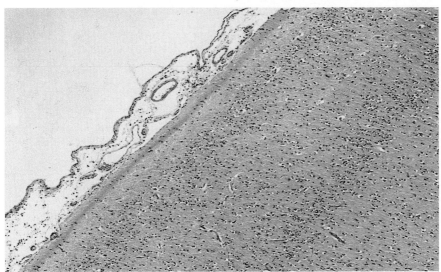

Figure 3–62. The cortex of the cerebral hemisphere. A (upper): The delicate leptomeninges are visible covering the surface; below that is the typical layering of the cerebral cortex. Normal white matter appears in the right side of the photograph. 25x B (lower): A small section of the cortex, at higher magnification. The details of the arachnoid and pia are more readily discerned, as are the layers of the cerebral cortex. 60x

Wall of Lateral Ventricle

The germinal matrix is adjacent to the lateral ventricles. The cells of this densely populated area will later migrate out into the cerebral hemisphere. Sections taken from this location may identify sites where periventricular or subependymal hemorrhages occurred during the neonatal period (Figs. 3–63 through 3–65).

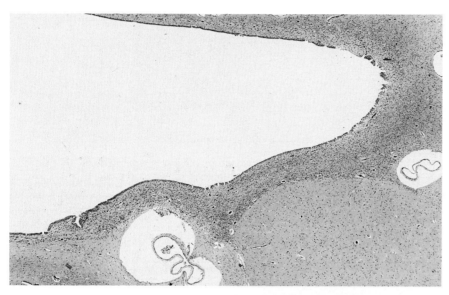
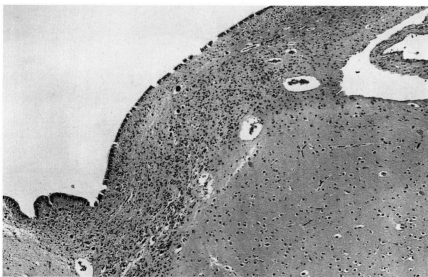

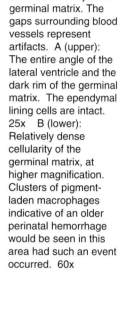

Figure 3–63. The angle of the lateral ventricle and adjacent germinal matrix. The gaps surrounding blood vessels represent artifacts. A (upper): The entire angle of the lateral ventricle and the dark rim of the germinal matrix. The ependymal lining cells are intact. 25x B (lower): Relatively dense cellularity of the germinal matrix, at higher magnification. Clusters of pigment-laden macrophages indicative of an older perinatal hemorrhage would be seen in this area had such an event occurred. 60x

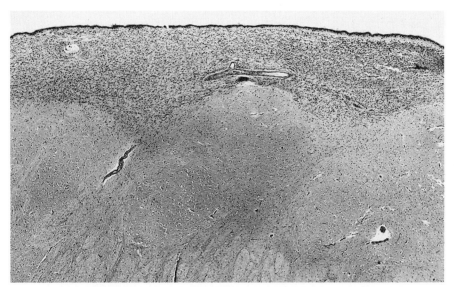

Figure 3–64. A portion of the wall of the lateral ventricle with lining ependymal cells on the left and a portion of the internal capsule on the right. Germinal matrix and somewhat lighter staining white matter separate them. 25x

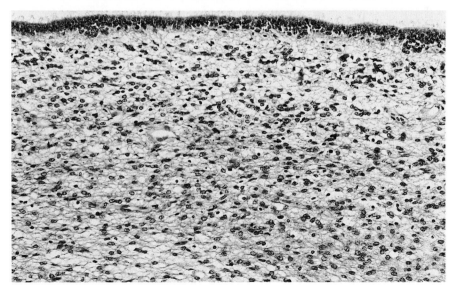

Figure 3–65. Finer details of the ependymal lining cells and of the germinal matrix. Note that the ependymal cells bear countless fine cilia. 160x

REFERENCES

1. Bloom W, Fawcett DW. A Textbook of Histology. Philadelphia: W.B. Saunders Co., 1975.

2. Jaffe R, Hashida Y, Yunis EJ. The endocrine pancreas of the neonate and the infant. Perspect Pediatr Pathol 7:137-65, 1982.

3. Loo SW, Kozakewich HP, Wald RA, Vawter GF. The sudden infant death syndrome and nesidioblastosis: No evidence for pathologic relationship. Lab Investig (Abstract) 46:10, 1982.

4. Naeye RL. Sudden infant death. Sci Am 242:52-58, 1980.

5. Valdés-Dapena MA. The normal ovary of childhood. Ann N Y Acad Sci 142:507-613, 1967.

6. Valdés-Dapena MA. Histology of the Fetus and Newborn. Philadelphia: W.B. Saunders Co., 1979.

7. Valdés-Dapena MA. Insulin-containing islet cells in the pancreas in SIDS. In: Topics in Pediatrics. A Festschrift for Lewis A. Barness. Pomerance HH and Bercu BB, eds. New York: Springer-Verlag: 1990, 99-106.

8. Valdés-Dapena MA, Gillane MM, Catherman R. Brown fat retention in sudden infant death syndrome. Arch Pathol Lab Med 100:547-9, 1976.

CHAPTER **4**

THE PRELIMINARY DIAGNOSIS OF SIDS AND "CLASSIC" OR TYPICAL GROSS FINDINGS

INTRODUCTION

Sudden infant death syndrome (SIDS) is a specific postmortem medical diagnosis. There are no diagnostic tests available to establish the diagnosis; hence, it is a designated, not a definitive, diagnosis. The criteria upon which the SIDS diagnosis is established are included in the official definition, i.e.: the infant's medical history, circumstances of death, and postmortem examination including a complete autopsy. [16, 28]

The diagnosis of SIDS is based upon the inability to identify a probable cause of death in the course of any of the investigative procedures, including the autopsy. Components of an adequate death investigation are discussed in Chapter 2. The autopsy in such a case may be entirely negative, lacking any pathologic lesion whatsoever. In fact, no specific pathologic lesions, either gross or microscopic, are needed to make the diagnosis of SIDS.

Pathologists who perform large numbers of these infant autopsies, however, recognize the fact that certain minor gross lesions are commonly encountered. These lesions have often been referred to as "classic" or typical findings. However, none of them is required for the ultimate diagnosis of the sudden infant death syndrome according to the definition agreed upon at the 1969 International Conference on Causes of Sudden Death in Infants.[1] The definition of SIDS, which emerged from the 1969 meeting is: "The sudden death of any infant or young child, which is unexpected by history, and in which a thorough postmortem examination fails to demonstrate an adequate cause of death."

The definition suggested by Beckwith, plus the recommendations from the New Mexico meeting, remains the standard in the United States. [1, 16] However, some SIDS definitional issues were addressed in 1987 by an expert panel convened by the National Institute of Child Health and Human Development. This panel recommended a rewording of the SIDS definition, especially for use in scientific research studies in the United States, as follows: "The sudden death of an infant under one year of age which remains unexplained after a thorough case investigation, including performance of a complete autopsy, examination of the death scene, and review of the clinical history." [33]

SIDS first became a separate entity for the classification of infant deaths in the United States in 1975.[27] A separate code number (798.0) for SIDS was created in the ninth revision of the International Classification of Diseases, which was introduced in the United States in 1978. More accurate reporting of SIDS in the United States as well as in many foreign countries resulted from these innovations in the classification of infant deaths in official statistics.[13, 17, 32] Based on these data, plus results from a number of SIDS epidemiological studies or surveys, it has been shown that SIDS incidence varies within a fairly narrow range, between 0.6 and 3.0 per 1000 live births, in most population groups.[23]

Furthermore, SIDS is usually the most common cause of postneonatal infant mortality, typically accounting for one-third to one-half of all such deaths.[14, 17]

The great majority of SIDS cases have several "characteristics in common, including death during apparent sleep, a rather narrow age range peaking between two and three months, and a repetitive spectrum of minor morphological lesions at postmortem examination."[2] Epidemiological studies have also indicated a reduced incidence of SIDS in summer months (June, July, August in the northern hemisphere) resulting in rates approximately one half of those reported during the remainder of the year as shown, for example, in the NICHD SIDS Cooperative Epidemiological Study as well as in data from Washington State.[24] Other risk factors, such as, low birth weight and/or premature delivery, have also been documented in several epidemiological studies, including the NICHD study in which 24.0% of the SIDS cases were low birth weight (less than 2500 grams) and 18.2% were born prematurely (less than 37 weeks of gestational age).[14] Based on the initial analysis of the NICHD study, the average birth weight of SIDS infants was 2970 grams compared to 3299 grams among randomly selected living control infants.[31] Differences in birth weight between SIDS cases and living control infants remained after controlling for gestational age differences, which implies that intrauterine growth retardation is also a risk factor for SIDS. These characteristics of low birth weight and prematurity are associated with SIDS, but do not provide an adequate basis for identifying SIDS infants prior to their death. Thus, it is important to recognize that at least three-fourths of SIDS cases in the United States are not low birth weight. In addition, many of the same risk factors that are associated with SIDS are often present in infants who die from explained causes.[14, 18]

The typical microscopic findings seen are dealt with and illustrated in Chapter 5. The most common gross findings are described in this chapter.

TYPICAL GROSS FINDINGS

EXTERNAL EXAMINATION

Skin

The skin of the baby is often mottled in death. Purple blotches in the skin of the face and extremities have frequently been misinterpreted as bruises and led to the mistaken diagnosis of abuse. Patches of purple discoloration of the skin are most striking in dependent portions of the body. Thus, they may appear about the face if the infant was lying in the prone position. Sometimes, in that situation, the tip of the nose is blanched on account of increased pressure at that point.

Mouth and Nose

Frequently the baby is found to have a little blood or mucus, or froth, about the nares and/or mouth. Mucous membranes, the vermillion border, and the finger- and toenail beds are apt to be cyanotic.

INTERNAL EXAMINATION

Petechiae

Showers of petechiae are found commonly in the typical SIDS autopsy; they are most striking in the thymus, particularly in the intra-thoracic portion, but also on occasion and in far less impressive numbers, in the cervical portion.[3] Interestingly, these petechiae are not confined to the external surfaces of the organ, either anteriorly or posteriorly, but are widely distributed throughout the interior as well. They are also present in the visceral and parietal pleura and epicardium. The petechiae in the myocardium are usually so tiny that they can be seen only microscopically. These pinpoint petechiae, so common in the chest, are almost never seen below the diaphragm. Based on the NICHD

SIDS Cooperative Epidemiological Study the prevalence of petechiae on gross examination was 45% for the thymus, 54% for the pleura, and 46% for the epi- and/or myocardium.

Thymus

The thymus in the typical case of sudden infant death syndrome is large, thick, and heavy but still within the range of normal for the age. It becomes thin, flat, and flaccid only in pathologic states, e.g., during the stress of serious infection lasting several days. The discovery that it is less than plump should raise serious questions in the mind of the pathologist about the validity of the diagnosis of SIDS. Involution of the thymus in an infant dictates a search for the cause.

Heart's Blood

Ordinarily the blood within the heart of a SIDS infant is in the liquid state, i.e., not clotted. The reason for this is not known, although laboratory experiments have begun to shed some light on this phenomenon. [26]

Lungs

The lungs, in the typical SIDS infant, are large and slightly heavier than normal. The external surfaces may be a bit purple, darker, and firmer than normal, posteriorly and inferiorly. The cut surfaces superiorly tend to be light pink, spongy, airy, and dry; inferiorly, they are dark red to purple, firm, and rather wet.

In the majority of SIDS cases, two gross diagnoses are made frequently with regard to the lungs, namely, congestion and edema.

It is virtually impossible to rule in or rule out the diagnosis of pneumonia upon gross examination of lungs of this size. All too often even the experienced pediatric pathologist makes the mistaken gross diagnosis of pneumonia when it proves not to be present microscopically or, alternatively, of normalcy grossly when sections reveal the fact that pneumonia is present.

Lymphoid Tissues

Since healthy infants in the first two years of life typically exhibit prominent lymphoid tissues and aggregates throughout their bodies, it is not surprising that at the time of these apparently instantaneous deaths, all lymphoid structures are large. The tonsils are plump as is the large, pallid thymus. Mesenteric lymph nodes are usually pale pink, numerous, and round or ovoid. Pale Peyer's patches stand up strikingly in the ileal mucosa, and even the pinhead-sized, white lymphoid aggregates in colonic mucosa are numerous.

Gastric Contents

The stomach often contains cream-colored, pasty curd (partly digested food), clear, colorless mucus, or dark-brown mucus, presumably stained with old blood as a result of agonal capillary oozing.

IATROGENIC LESIONS

Acute

When resuscitative measures are instituted around the time of an infant's death, a variety of iatrogenic lesions may be induced inadvertently. These include injuries involving the mucosa of the airway (produced by intubation) and acute interstitial pulmonary emphysema. Needle puncture marks may be found in the heart.

Chronic

More difficult to interpret are those lesions that occur (or are induced) between the time of an apparently "aborted" SIDS and the child's eventual removal from life-support systems, occasionally days to weeks later. In prolonged periods of "artificially" sustained life, a certain spectrum of disease states is apt to ensue. Prominent among them is bronchopneumonia, most commonly of bacterial etiology. It may commence within hours after the "rescue" and may persist, or worsen, for days thereafter. If it is determined that these conditions developed after the time of the rescue, they are considered complications of the process. For these cases the original event and determined cause of death remains the sudden infant death syndrome.

A number of other iatrogenic lesions may occur. For example, pressure-induced mucosal ulcers in the airway occur secondary to the use of endotracheal tubes, and pulmonary hyaline membranes as the result of assisted pulmonary ventilation with high levels of oxygen. In most instances, a good history and common sense will permit the pathologist to distinguish such complications from those lesions which could cause or contribute to death.

REQUIREMENTS FOR THE PRELIMINARY DIAGNOSIS OF SIDS

Inasmuch as the diagnosis of SIDS depends, among other things, on the pathologist's inability to explain the child's demise, the autopsy must be reasonably complete and must be, at its conclusion, negative. This means that the autopsy must exclude the presence of any disease process that could logically explain the baby's death. Nothing more, nor less, than this is required.

The presence or absence of one or another of the typical lesions is irrelevant, as is the degree of their intensity when present.[30] Furthermore, the use of morphometry in determining the degree or extent of alleged "tissue markers" of hypoxia or hypoxemia, e.g., brown fat retention[28] is not recommended as routine because there is a wide range of normal values for any of them, at any month of age, within the first year of life.

The final diagnosis of SIDS is based ultimately on a comprehensive and negative scene investigation, coupled with a negative autopsy (including histology) and negative total body x-rays when obtained. All of these procedures cannot be accomplished on the day of the autopsy. In practice, the pathologist is required to make a *preliminary* diagnosis based on an initial investigation, gross autopsy, and what history is

available. It is important to communicate this original determination promptly to law enforcement agencies or social services, when appropriate, and to families and SIDS counselors. In most cases, the preliminary diagnosis of SIDS will be sustained when all studies are completed. Early counseling and parental support can be accomplished in a timely manner only if the pathologist makes this determination upon completion of the gross autopsy.

COMMUNICATION WITH THE FAMILY AND OTHERS

In the early 1970's, when the federally funded SIDS projects were first established, the Office of Maternal and Child Health in the Department of Health, Education, and Welfare required that the family of an infant victim be contacted and provided with at least a provisional diagnosis of SIDS as soon as possible after the performance of the gross autopsy. Many participating pathologists sent letters of condolence and information to parents. Others spoke with parents by phone and a few even visited in families' homes. Of course, some pathologists had been in the practice of communicating with families before the inception of the nationwide program. Such communication should be encouraged as it is of great value to the families of SIDS victims.[4-6, 8-12, 20-22, 25]

On the whole, this practice was well accepted by forensic pathologists at the time and it has continued to be part of the routine procedure in many offices. The custom needs to be encouraged. Communication can be achieved either in person, by phone, or by mail.[29] This type of information sharing can and should be undertaken within 24 hours of completion of the autopsy. In practice, review of microscopic sections and/or culture results only rarely dictates a change in, or an addition to, the original diagnosis of SIDS. When a change does occur, an *additional* contact with the family may be required to explain the new alternative or amended diagnosis and the evidence for it.

For those pathologists who cannot, or prefer not to, communicate with families in person, a series of sample letters that have been, or are being, used by pathologists for that purpose are provided in Appendix B. The first is designed to be sent to the parents immediately after completion of the scene investigation and the gross autopsy; the message it carries is, of course, conditional, but nevertheless helpful. Others are intended to be mailed following completion of the case with or without changes in the diagnosis. For those pathologists who are new to the experience of speaking with parents, perusal of these letters may assist them in finding appropriate words for their own messages to grieving families.

There should be little difficulty in discussing the matter with medical colleagues, whether they are family practitioners or pediatricians, because all of them are aware of SIDS.

Early communication of the diagnosis to the local SIDS center is also one of the primary obligations of the practicing pathologist.[7] The professional staff members of local SIDS centers are eager to be informed and to be of help, once alerted about a potential case.[15, 19] Since SIDS center staff are well educated in the matter, the pathologist should have no difficulty in conveying his diagnosis to them. They know what the diagnosis of sudden infant death syndrome means and what to do in regard to cases pending further study.

In most communities, educational programs for police in training include instruction as to the essential nature of SIDS. This training should facilitate later discussions between pathologists and police who often participate in scene investigation. Statements to law enforcement officials, following scene investigation and the necropsy, should be qualified appropriately. Such qualification is illustrated in the following statement: "Based upon the information we have at this time, the death appears to be consistent with SIDS. In all probability, further studies, including examination of microscopic sections, will not alter that diagnosis. Nevertheless, the diagnosis for the case will not be finalized officially until results from additional procedures have been completed and reviewed."

REFERENCES

1. Beckwith JB. Discussion of terminology and definition of the sudden infant death syndrome. In: Bergman AB, Beckwith JB, Ray CG, eds. Sudden Infant Death Syndrome, Proceedings of the Second International Conference on Causes of Sudden Death in Infants. Seattle: University of Washington Press, 1970, pp 14-22.

2. Beckwith JB. A pathologist's perspective on SIDS diagnosis and the search for predisposing factors. In: Harper RM, Hoffman HJ, eds. Sudden Infant Death Syndrome: Risk Factors and Basic Mechanisms. New York: PMA Publishing Corp., 1988, pp. 507-13.

3. Beckwith JB. Intrathoracic petechial hemorrhages: A clue to the mechanism of death in sudden infant death syndrome? Ann N Y Acad Sci 533:37-47, 1988.

4. Beckwith JB. The value of the pediatric postmortem examination. Pediatr Clin North Am 36:29-36, 1989.

5. Berger L. Requesting the autopsy: a pediatric perspective. Clin Pediatr 17:445-52, 1978.

6. Bergman AB. Psychological aspects of sudden unexpected death in infants and children. Review and commentary. Pediatr Clin North Am 21:115-21, 1974.

7. Booth S. Directory of Sudden Infant Death Syndrome Programs and Resources. McLean, Va:National Sudden Infant Death Syndrome Clearinghouse, 1988, 20 p.

8. Buschbacher VI, Delcampo RL. Parents' response to sudden infant death syndrome. J Pediatr Health Care 1:85-90, 1987.

9. Culbertson JL, Willis DJ. Acute loss and grieving reactions: treatment issues. In: Culbertson JL, Krous HF, Bendell RD, eds. Part II. The Psychological Impact and Management of SIDS, in Sudden Infant Death Syndrome. Medical Aspects and Psychological Management. Baltimore: The Johns Hopkins University Press, 1988, pp. 157-181.

10. DeFrain JD, Ernst L. The psychological effects of sudden infant death syndrome on surviving family members. J Fam Pract 6:985-9, 1978.

11. DeFrain J, Taylor J, Ernst L. Coping with Sudden Infant Death. Toronto: Lexington Books, 1982.

12. Friedman SB. Psychological aspects of sudden unexpected death in infants and children. Pediatr Clin North Am 21:103-11, 1974.

13. Hasselmeyer EG, Hunter JC. A historical perspective on SIDS research. Ann N Y Acad Sci 533:1-5, 1988.

14. Hoffman HJ, Damus K, Hillman L, Krongrad E. Risk factors for SIDS: Results of the National Institute of Child Health and Human Development SIDS Cooperative Epidemiological Study. Ann N Y Acad Sci 533:13-30, 1988.

15. Hunter JC. The federal SIDS support network in perspective. Ann N Y Acad Sci 533:155-7, 1988.

16. Jones AM, Weston JT. The examination of the sudden infant death syndrome infant: Investigative and autopsy protocols. J Forensic Sci 21:833-41, 1976.

17. Khoury MJ, Erickson JD, Adams MJ. Trends in postneonatal mortality in the United States, 1962 through 1978. JAMA 252:367-72, 1984.

18. Lewak N, van den Berg BJ, Beckwith JB. Sudden infant death syndrome risk factors. Prospective data review. Clin Pediatr 18:404-11, 1979.

19. Limerick S. Family and health-professional interactions. Ann N Y Acad Sci 533:145-54, 1988.

20. Mandell F. The family and sudden infant death syndrome. In: Culbertson JL, Krous HF, Bendell RD, eds. Part II. The Psychological Impact and Management of SIDS, in Sudden Infant Death Syndrome. Medical Aspects and Psychological Management. Baltimore: The Johns Hopkins University Press, 1988, pp. 182-97.

21. Mandell F, McClain M. Supporting the SIDS Family. Pediatrician 15:179-82, 1988.

22. McPhee SJ, Bottles K, Lo B, Saika G, Crommie D. To redeem them from death. Reactions of family members to autopsy. Am J Med 80:665-71., 1986.

23. Peterson DR. Evolution of the epidemiology of the sudden infant death syndrome. Epidemiol Rev 2:97-112, 1980.

24. Peterson DR, Sabotta EE, Strickland D. Sudden Infant Death Syndrome in epidemiologic perspective: Etiologic implications of variation with season of the year. Ann N Y Acad Sci 533:6-12, 1988.

25. Stephens BG. Why the autopsy. In: Harper RM, Hoffman HJ, eds. Sudden Infant Death Syndrome: Risk Factors and Basic Mechanisms. New York: PMA Publishing Corp., 1988, pp135-41.

26. Takeichi S., Tokunaga I, Hayakumo K, Naeiwa M. Fluidity of cadaveric blood after sudden death: Part III. Am J Foren Med Path 7:35-8, 1986.

27. U.S. Department of Health, Education and Welfare. Sudden infant death syndrome. In: Nosology Guidelines: Supplement to the Cause-of-Death Coding Manual. Rockville, Md.: National Center for Health Statistics, U.S. Public Health Service, DHEW Publication No. (HRA) 75-1140, 1975, pp 1-4.

28. Valdés-Dapena M. The pathologist and the sudden infant death syndrome. Am J Pathol 106:118-31, 1982.

23. Valdés-Dapena MA. The pathologist's conference with parents following postmortem examination of their child: An application of the Kubler-Ross concept. Perspect Pediatr Pathol 5:263-5, 1979.

30. Valdés-Dapena M. A pathologist's perspective on possible mechanisms in SIDS. Ann N Y Acad Sci 533:31-6, 1988.

31. van Belle G, Hoffman HJ, Peterson DR. Intrauterine growth retardation and the sudden infant death syndrome. In: Harper RM, Hoffman, HJ, eds. Sudden Infant Death Syndrome: Risk Factors and Basic Mechanisms. New York: PMA Publishing Corp., 1988, pp. 203-19.

32. Weiss NS, Green D, Krueger DE. Problems in the use of death certificates to identify sudden infant unexpected deaths. Health Serv Rep 88:555-8, 1973.

33. Willinger M, James LS, Catz C, et al: Defining the sudden infant death syndrome (SIDS): deliberations of an expert panel convened by the National Institute of Child Health and Human Development. Pediatr Pathol 11: 677, 1991.

CHAPTER **5**

"CLASSIC" OR TYPICAL HISTOLOGIC FINDINGS IN SIDS

INTRODUCTION

This chapter presents the typical histologic features of the straightforward or unequivocal case of SIDS. Some are truly classic findings and others are presented because they are commonly encountered (agonal or postmortem changes, or non-lethal processes).[1-3,5,6] As with the typical gross findings discussed in Chapter 4, none of them is *necessary* for the ultimate diagnosis of SIDS. When present, they are reassuring to the pathologist who is often more comfortable with even a few characteristic, objective findings than with none at all.

HEART

Epicardial Petechiae

Just as one typically finds epicardial petechiae grossly (46% of SIDS cases vs 23% in explained deaths in the NICHD study), one can also expect to see them in about 10% of microscopic sections (Fig. 5–1)[7]. They may be numerous and are occasionally confluent. They may also occur within the myocardium. Petechiae are generally smaller than the hemorrhages produced iatrogenically via intracardiac injections during resuscitation, and they are not associated with corresponding hemorrhagic myocardial "tracks" (see Figs. 7–3 and 7–4, Chapter 7).

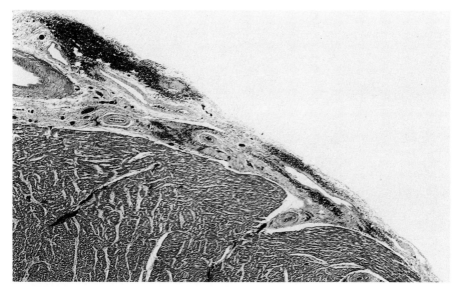

Figure 5–1.
Epicardial petechiae.
25x

LARYNX

Focal Fibrinoid Necrosis

Focal areas of acute fibrinoid necrosis within submucous connective tissue of the larynx are encountered commonly in SIDS cases, but can be worrisome (Fig. 5–2). Although inflammation of the larynx is relatively common in the age group at risk for SIDS, this lesion is not specific for SIDS and is seen in infants who die of other conditions. The etiology of this lesion is unknown.

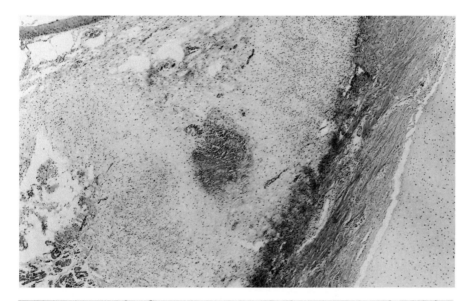

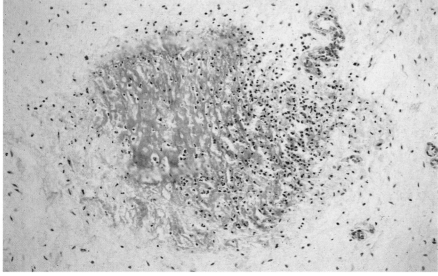

Figure 5–2. Cross section of larynx with focal fibrinoid necrosis. The lesion illustrated here is more advanced than is usual.

A (upper): The laryngeal cartilage is in the lower right corner, and the stratified squamous epithelial lining of the laryngeal ventricle is in the upper left. 40x

B (lower). The lesion is seen here at a higher magnification. 160x

Laryngitis

A relatively common finding in this series of autopsies was mild to moderate (acute or "chronic") inflammation in the larynx (Fig. 5–3). This was often associated historically with mild upper respiratory symptoms. Unless marked and associated with an appropriate clinical history, it would not be expected to cause death.

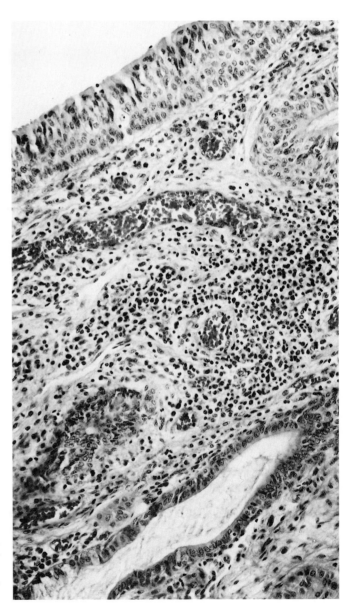

Figure 5–3. Laryngitis. A section of the larynx, showing a moderate mononuclear inflammatory cell infiltrate (lymphocytes, histiocytes, and few plasma cells) in the submucosa. 160x

TRACHEA

Inflammation

Inflammation of the trachea must be evaluated in the context of the entire autopsy and, especially, respiratory tract findings (Fig. 5–4). Many babies who die of SIDS have clinical histories of mild upper respiratory tract infection. In fact, 29% of parents of SIDS infants in the NICHD study reported that their babies had upper respiratory infections within 24 hours of death. The incidence of reported upper respiratory infection increases to 44% when the entire last two weeks of life are considered.[4] The degree and extent of the involvement is critical, however. Mild, or even moderate, focal inflammation that would not be expected to cause significant respiratory distress should not alter final designation of SIDS as the cause of death.

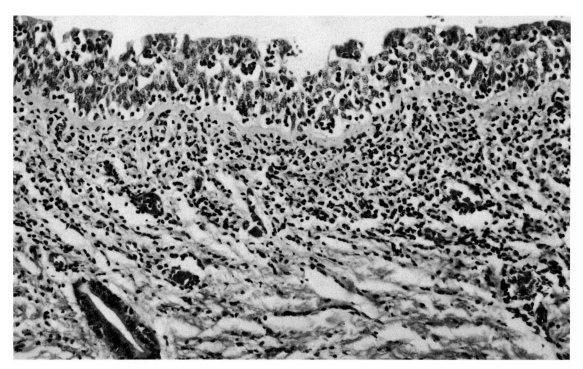

Figure 5–4. Tracheitis may be reflected by an infiltrate of acute or chronic inflammatory cells in the mucosa and/or submucosa. The inflammation in this case was not thought to represent an adequate cause of death; the death was classified as SIDS. 160x

LUNG

Pleural Petechiae

Petechiae are encountered commonly in the pleura in both gross and microscopic examination in cases of sudden infant death (Fig. 5–5). They probably represent agonal events and can be expected in 38% of microscopic sections of lung in SIDS cases.[7] The gross prevalence of petechiae was 54% in the NICHD study. In contrast, petechiae were encountered in 16% of microscopic sections of lung in the explained deaths. The gross prevalence was 35% in the explained deaths. These petechiae are often associated with petechiae in the heart (Fig. 5–1) and thymus (Fig. 5–13). Altogether pleural petechiae were noted, either in the gross autopsy, or microscopically, in 63% of SIDS cases and 38% of explained deaths.

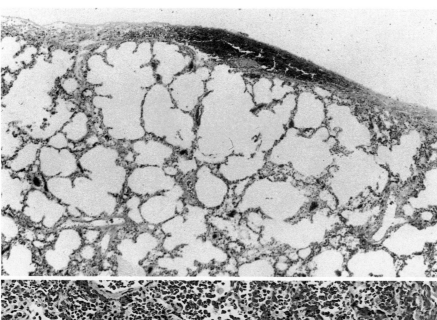

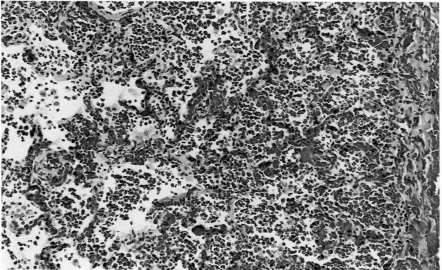

Figure 5–5
A (upper): Focal hemorrhage (petechiae) in the pleura. 100x
B (lower): Focal hemorrhages (petechiae) into and beneath the visceral pleura. 160x

Congestion

Pulmonary congestion is often impressive in the autopsy of an infant who has died of SIDS. Grossly, the deep red color and firm consistency of the lungs may be misdiagnosed as pneumonia. Microscopically, engorgement of dilated capillaries is often striking; normally thick and cellular alveolar walls seem even thicker than usual and the pathologist may interpret them as being abnormal even though no inflammatory exudate is apparent (Fig. 5–6). It should be expected in most instances as it was present in 89% of the SIDS cases in the NICHD study. However, it is not a specific finding for SIDS since it was also observed in the vast majority (80%) of infants in the study who had died of recognized causes.[7]

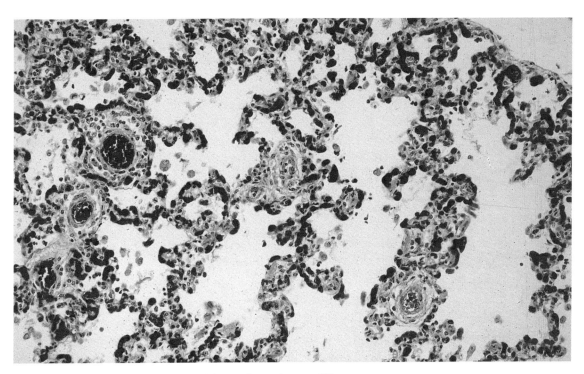

Figure 5–6. Pulmonary congestion of a mild to moderate degree. 160x

Alveolar Hemorrhage

When pulmonary congestion is moderate to marked, some degree of alveolar hemorrhage is almost always present (Fig. 5–7). This should not suggest a coagulation defect, a primary pulmonary lesion, or a cardiac abnormality. It is common in sudden infant death syndrome, especially in dependent parts of the lung, and is probably an agonal or postmortem event. In the NICHD study the incidence of intra-alveolar hemorrhage was 66% for the SIDS cases and 54% for the explained deaths.[7]

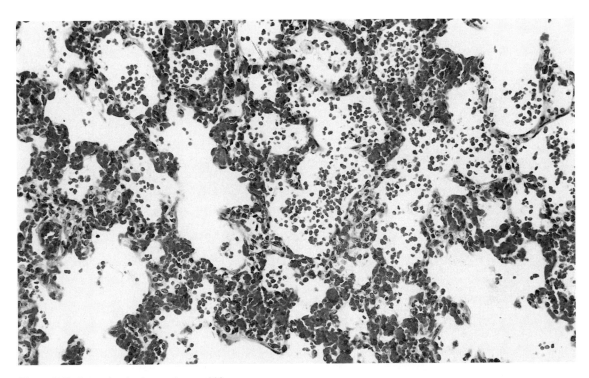

Figure 5–7. Intra-alveolar hemorrhage. 160x

Septal Hemorrhage/Interstitial Emphysema

Just as alveolar hemorrhage often accompanies moderate to severe congestion, so can septal hemorrhage, and in much the same distribution. Septal interstitial emphysema is another common finding, but one secondary to artificial pulmonary ventilation (Fig. 5–8). When extensive or advanced it may lead to an even more confusing post-resuscitation picture, that of pneumothorax.

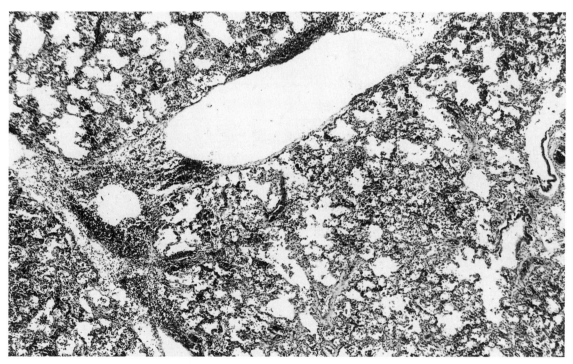

Figure 5–8. Septal hemorrhage and interstitial emphysema. The constellation of findings displayed here is one very commonly encountered in infants in whom vigorous resuscitation has been attempted, as in this infant. 40x

Pulmonary Edema

One of the classic findings in the lungs in the sudden infant death syndrome is mild to marked intra-alveolar edema (Fig. 5–9). It is interpreted as an agonal event rather than a true premortem condition. It may reflect hypoxemic damage to alveolar capillaries in the agonal period or it may be a postmortem artifact. As with congestion, it is an extremely common finding in both SIDS cases and in infants dying of explained causes of death, with the percentages for the NICHD study being 63% and 51%, respectively.[7]

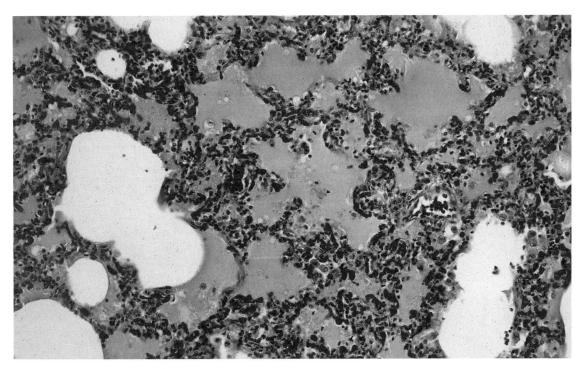

Figure 5–9. Pulmonary edema, moderate to marked. 160x

Alveolar Macrophages

Macrophages are sometimes abundant in alveoli in the sudden infant death syndrome (Fig. 5–10). Their presence is another histologic finding that many pathologists, more accustomed to dealing with adult tissues, are perhaps too quick to consider abnormal. Although the reason(s) for their presence (frequently in large numbers) are not well understood, they are commonly encountered and should not be interpreted as representing pneumonia. Moderate numbers of alveolar macrophages were found in 15% of the SIDS cases and in 18% of the explained deaths in the NICHD study.[7]

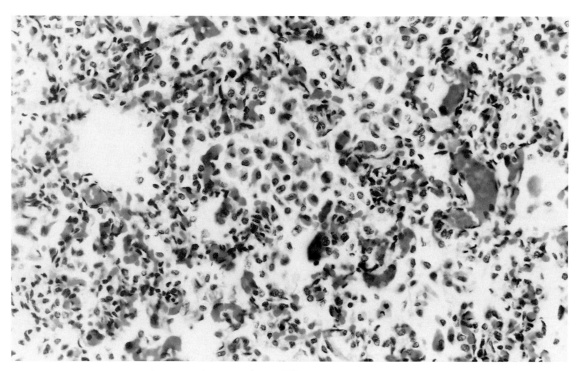

Figure 5–10. Alveolar macrophages, moderate numbers. 250x

Atelectasis and Emphysema

Atelectasis and emphysema often appear together, usually the result of attempted resuscitation (Fig. 5–11). Because such mechanical maneuvers involve blowing air forcibly into the lungs and forcing it out with compression of the chest, the result is uneven aeration. Patchy atelectasis must not be confused with consolidation or pneumonia. Infant alveolar septa are naturally thicker than those of adults and, when collapsed, side-by-side, with no intervening air spaces, may give a false impression of increased cellularity.

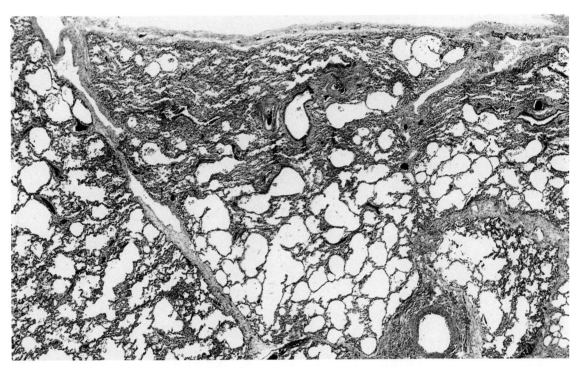

Figure 5–11. Atelectasis and emphysema secondary to resuscitative attempts. Collapse of air spaces in one area (center, above) and overdistention in an adjacent area (below). 25x

LIVER

Microvesicular Fatty Change

Although infant liver cells are normally vacuolated because of their glycogen content, fine microvesicular fatty change is much less common. In fact, fatty change in the liver is uncommon, appearing in only 8% of the SIDS cases in the NICHD study.[7] Among the explained deaths, however, the frequency was significantly more common, occurring in 19%. Mild or even moderate accumulations are probably of little significance (Fig. 5–12). If fatty change were marked, one would need to investigate the possibility of malnutrition or a toxic insult. In true lipid storage disease, the liver is markedly enlarged at autopsy and the histologic picture is much more uniformly abnormal, involving all hepatocytes.

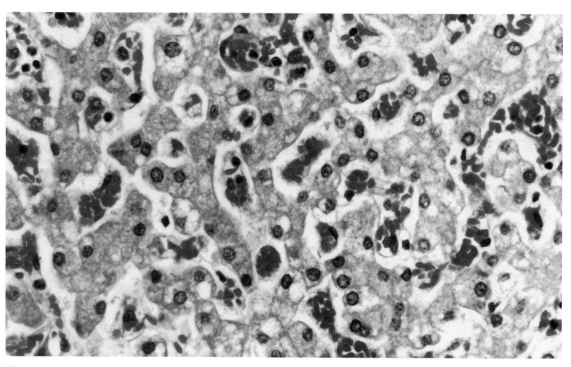

Figure 5–12. A section of liver with mild to moderate fine vacuolization of the hepatocytes and congestion. 400x

THYMUS

Thymic Petechiae

Although not always present, thymic petechiae are a recognized hallmark of SIDS. They are seen frequently at the autopsy table and in histologic sections of the gland (Fig. 5–13). Although characteristic, they are not diagnostic for SIDS and are often found in other types of deaths such as asphyxia. The gross prevalence of petechiae in the thymus was 45% in SIDS cases and 22% in explained deaths. Based on histologic review only, however, the prevalence of thymic petechiae in SIDS cases was 44%, and in explained deaths, 23%. Altogether, thymic petechiae were noted, either in the gross autopsy or microscopically, in 69% of SIDS cases and 38% of explained deaths.

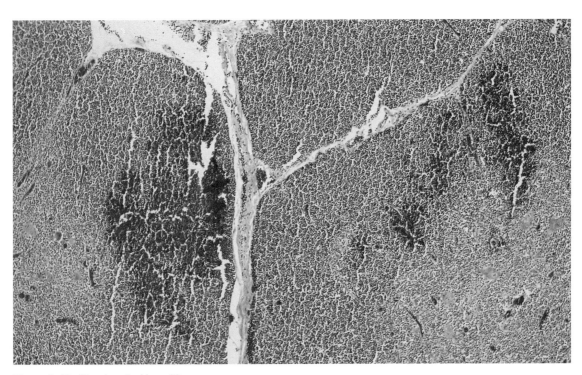

Figure 5–13. Thymic petechiae. 60x

BRAIN

Perivascular Hemorrhage

Small foci of hemorrhage appear grossly and microscopically in organs other than the thymus in typical SIDS cases, and that list includes the brain. Perivascular hemorrhage is observed routinely in otherwise completely unremarkable sections of brain (Fig. 5–14). For example, it was noted in 17% of the SIDS cases and 16% of the explained deaths in the NICHD study.[7] It is not a primary pathologic lesion, but seems rather to be agonal. It should not be confused with other, larger areas of clearly antemortem hemorrhage.

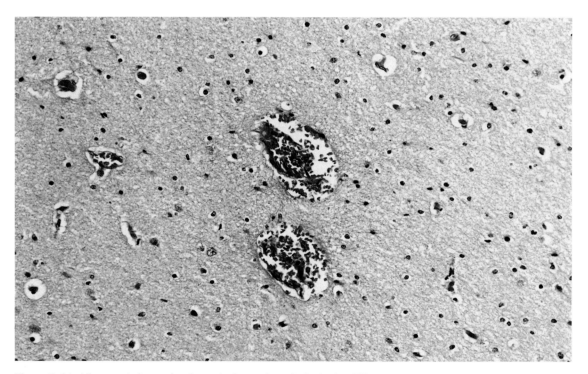

Figure 5–14. Microscopic focus of perivascular hemorrhage in the brain. 160x

REFERENCES

1. Adelson L, Kinney ER. Sudden and unexpected death in infancy and childhood. Pediatrics 17:663-99, 1956.

2. Adelson L. Specific studies of infant victims of sudden death. In: Wedgwood RJ, Benditt EP, ed. Sudden Death in Infants, Proceedings of the Conference on Causes of Sudden Death in Infants, September 1963, Seattle, Washington. Washington, D.C.: U.S. Government Printing Office, US DHEW, National Institutes of Health, National Institute of Child Health and Human Development, Public Health Service Publication No. 1412.

3. Beckwith JB. Observations on the pathological anatomy of sudden infant death syndrome. In: Bergman AB, Beckwith JB, Ray CG, eds. Sudden Infant Death Syndrome, Proceedings of the Second International Conference on Causes of Sudden Death in Infants. Seattle: University of Washington Press, pp. 83-107, 1970.

4. Hoffman HJ, Damus K, Hillman L, Krongrad E. Risk factors for SIDS: Results of the National Institute of Child Health and Human Development SIDS cooperative epidemiological study. Ann N Y Acad Sci 533:13-30, 1988.

5. Marshall TK. The Northern Ireland study: Pathology findings. In: Bergman AB, Beckwith JB, Ray CG, eds. Sudden Infant Death Syndrome, Proceedings of the Second International Conference on Causes of Sudden Death in Infants. Seattle: University of Washington Press, pp. 108-17, 1970.

6. Valdés-Dapena M. The pathologist and the sudden infant death syndrome. Am J Pathol 106:118-31, 1982.

7. Valdés-Dapena M, McFeeley P, Hoffman HJ, Damus K, Franciosi RR, Allison DJ, Jones M, Hunter JC. Chapter 10: Summary of histologic findings and implications for future SIDS research. In: Histopathology Atlas for the Sudden Infant Death Syndrome: Histopathologic Autopsy Findings derived from the National Institute of Child Health and Human Development Cooperative Epidemiological Study of Sudden Infant Death Syndrome (SIDS) Risk Factors. Washington, D.C.: Armed Forces Institute of Pathology, this volume.

Sudden Infant Death Syndrome

CHAPTER **6**

EXPLAINED SUDDEN DEATHS

INTRODUCTION

Recognizable causes of death can be identified for some infants who have been purportedly well and who die suddenly and unexpectedly. For example, in the NICHD Cooperative Epidemiological Study of SIDS Risk Factors, a group of 65 infants were identified whose deaths were attributed to recognizable causes other than SIDS.

Infants included in the pathology component of the NICHD study came from two sources:

(1) those submitted from the field as SIDS or pending further study (N=912), and (2) those submitted as autopsy controls (N=68). Table 6–1 indicates the number and percentage of SIDS cases (definite or probable), indeterminate or possible SIDS cases, and explained deaths derived from these two sources.

Table 6–1. **Classification of SIDS Cases and Explained Deaths by Source Contributing to the NICHD Cooperative Epidemiologic Study**

Determined by Panel	Submitted as SIDS or Pending Further Study No.	%	Submitted as Autopsy Controls No.	%
SIDS - Definite or Probable	845	92.7	27	39.7
Indeterminate or Possible SIDS	40	4.4	3	4.4
Explained Deaths	27	3.0	38	55.9
Total Infants	912		68	

Of the 68 infants submitted as autopsy controls, 56% (N=38) were classified as explained deaths by the panel. Conversely, 40% (N=27) of the infants submitted as autopsy controls were classified by the panel as SIDS cases. Many of these infants were signed out locally as bronchopneumonia deaths. The indeterminate or possible SIDS cases were incompletely documented deaths. The lack of information in these instances precluded their classification into either the SIDS or explained death categories. From each source, 4.4% were left in the indeterminate or possible SIDS category.

Of the 912 infants submitted as SIDS or pending further study, only 3% (N=27) were classified by the Pathology Study Panel as having died of explained causes. Further analysis of this group indicates that out of the 74 infants submitted as pending further study, there were 12 which were ultimately classified as explained deaths by both the local medical examiner/pathologist and the Pathology Study Panel. In addition, of the remaining 838 eligible SIDS cases, 15 were eventually classified as explained deaths by the Pathology Study Panel following their rigorous two-tiered review. In ten of those 15 deaths, the specific lesions considered to be fatal, were identified by the panel during the first review of microscopic sections only. The remaining five were explained during the second review, after consideration of the gross autopsy findings, the death investigative report, the history, and results of laboratory studies. This underscores the need to perform a thorough microscopic review in conjunction with a detailed assessment of circumstances surrounding the death, historical information, and data from any ancillary tests performed.

The 65 infants whose deaths were ultimately designated as explained represent a group of infants in whom a cause of death other than SIDS became apparent either from the identification of a mortal histologic lesion or from additional sources of information about the case. Thus, a classification system for explained causes of sudden deaths in infants has been developed based on: (1) anatomical site of the mortal lesion (e.g., the heart, the brain, etc.), and (2) source of information (e.g., gross autopsy, study of microscopic sections, death investigation, toxicologic analysis, etc.).

CLASSIFICATION OF EXPLAINED SUDDEN INFANT DEATHS

Examples of sudden explained infant deaths classified by anatomical site of the mortal lesion are provided in Table 6–2. The cardiovascular, respiratory, gastrointestinal, pancreas, central nervous system, and systemic categories provide a reasonable anatomic grouping for causes of sudden infant death other than SIDS.

Table 6–2.   **Explained Causes of Sudden Death in Infants Classified by Anatomical Site of Mortal Lesion**

- **Cardiovascular**
  Myocarditis (usually viral)
  Congenital heart disease
  > -Congenital aortic valvular stenosis
  > -Endocardial fibroelastosis
  > -Anomalous origin of the left coronary artery
  Cardiomyopathy
  Rhabdomyoma (especially in tuberous sclerosis)
  Coronary arteritis (Kawasaki's disease)

- **Respiratory**
  Upper airway obstruction
  Bronchopneumonia
  Bronchiolitis, severe

- **Gastrointestinal Tract**
  Cystic remnant of thyroglossal duct in the base of the tongue (causing obstruction to the airway)
  Enterocolitis with diarrhea, dehydration and/or fluid and electrolyte imbalance

- **Pancreas**
  Cystic fibrosis of the pancreas (with overheating)

- **Endocrine**
  Congenital adrenal hypo- or hyperplasia

- **Central Nervous System**
  Trauma
  > -Cerebral edema secondary to trauma
  > -Subdural hematoma
  Meningitis
  Encephalitis
  Arteriovenous malformation

- **Systemic**
  Dehydration
  Cervical cellulitis (Ludwig's angina)
  Poisoning (carbon monoxide)
  Overheating (especially in infants with cystic fibrosis)

In Table 6–3, recognized causes of sudden infant deaths are grouped by the source of information from which the cause of death was ascertained. Clearly for most sudden deaths complete information needs to be obtained from several different sources; missing information can lead to erroneous designation of the ultimate cause of death.

Table 6–3.   Explained Causes of Sudden Death in Infants Classified by Source of Information

- **Death Investigation**
    - Suffocation with a soft object (e.g., accidental with thin, soft plastic sheet adherent to infant's face, or deliberate)
    - Carbon monoxide poisoning (with gross autopsy findings and toxicologic analysis)
    - Drowning
    - Interrogation of caretaker or others
- **Gross Postmortem Examination**
    - Dehydration (with chemical analysis of vitreous humor)
    - Trauma (including child abuse with x-rays)
    - Congenital heart disease
        - 1) Endocardial fibroelastosis
        - 2) Aortic valvular stenosis
    - Rhabdomyomas of the heart in tuberous sclerosis
    - Cardiomyopathy
    - Congenital adrenal hypo- or hyperplasia
    - Bacterial meningitis (with microscopy and microbiologic studies)
    - Intracranial arteriovenous malformation
    - Cystic lingual remnant of thyroglossal duct remnant
- **Histologic Examination**
    - Myocarditis, viral
    - Bronchopneumonia
    - Bronchiolitis
    - Viral hepatitis (Coxsackie)
    - Cystic fibrosis of the pancreas (apparent hyperthermia)
    - Viral pancreatitis (Coxsackie)
    - Myocardial rhabdomyoma in tuberous sclerosis (occasionally these first become apparent in microscopic sections)
    - Boric acid poisoning
    - Viral encephalitis
- **Whole Body X-Rays**
    - Skull fractures
    - Battered child
- **Microbiology**
    - Blood culture (if positive for single pathogenic agent found in both heart blood and the spleen)
- **Toxicology**
    - Poisoning

In the NICHD Cooperative Epidemiological Study of SIDS Risk Factors both classification systems (i.e., the anatomical site, and the source(s) and completeness of information) were useful in determining explained causes of death. This approach, reflected in the two-tiered pathology review (see Chapter 1), identified a small but important number of explained deaths. The ultimate causes of death for these 15 infants are given in Table 6–4.

Table 6–4. **Diagnoses, Cases of Explained Deaths Originally Submitted as SIDS**

Diagnosis	No. of Cases
Bronchopneumonia*	3
Bronchopneumonia* (with dehydration)	1
Bronchopneumonia with bronchiolitis*	1
Dehydration alone	2
Viral myocarditis*	1
Meningitis*	1
Ludwig's angina* (i.e., cervical cellulitis)	1
Tuberous sclerosis*	1
Polysplenia-asplenia syndrome (Ivemark's syndrome)	1
Sickle cell disease* (child of 16 months)	1
Microcephaly and cerebral atrophy	1
Multiple congenital anomalies	1
Total	15

*Mortal lesions identified microscopically on first review by the Pathology Study Panel. Ten of the 15 explained deaths were identified by this microscopic review.

CAUSES FOR SUDDEN EXPLAINED DEATHS, DETERMINED MICROSCOPICALLY

Rhabdomyoma of the Heart

Rhabdomyomas of the heart occasionally cause sudden and unexpected death in infants.[7] Of children recognized to have these lesions, 75% are one year of age or less. Although this lesion may occur independently, it is often only one manifestation of *tuberous sclerosis* (Bourneville's disease), a phakomatosis transmitted as a an autosomal dominant trait.[32,43,50] About one-third of those persons with cardiac rhabdomyomas are ultimately diagnosed as having tuberous sclerosis. About 50% of those with tuberous sclerosis appear to represent new mutations. Since some of the morphological evidences of the generalized disorder are subtle, the disease may be more prevalent than is reflected by the presence of cardiac rhabdomyomas.

The cardiac rhabdomyoma itself may be the cause of sudden death, presumably because of interference with cardiac conduction.[69]

At autopsy, the heart of the affected patient may be enlarged. Occasionally the lesions are overlooked during the performance of a necropsy. They are sometimes first perceived when the tissues are trimmed for the preparation of microscopic sections. To the naked eye, they appear on cut surfaces of heart muscle to be discrete, solid masses of pale tissue of the same consistency as the myocardium itself. Frequently, however, they are detected only in examination of histologic sections.

Microscopically, cardiac rhabdomyomas are circumscribed but not encapsulated. Individual tumor cells are large, and their content of glycogen is best demonstrated in relatively fresh, frozen sections or following non-aqueous fixation and staining with periodic acid-Schiff technique or Best's carmine stain. In sections fixed in formalin, the tumor cells are large, ovoid, vacuolated structures with islands or strands of cytoplasm compressed against the cell membrane or, less frequently, in the center of the cell. Some of the typical cells are referred to as "spider cells" because they have strands within the cytoplasmic mass bearing the nucleus. Some of these strands and, on occasion, some of the cell membranes have cross striations.

Case History

This white male infant was born at term, at 40 weeks of gestation, with a weight of 3630 grams. He died at the age of 26 days. He seemed to be normal at birth and continued in apparent good health until the day he died, suddenly and unexpectedly.

At the time the necropsy was performed, no findings were identified that could have accounted for the infant's death. According to the initial autopsy protocol the heart was normal grossly except for the presence of petechiae. This case was submitted as a typical, unexplained sudden death. Review of the two microscopic sections of the heart revealed the presence of rhabdomyomas in both (Figs. 6–1 and 6–2). It is likely that this infant had tuberous sclerosis and that the other findings that might have confirmed this disorder were so subtle as to have been overlooked, both clinically and pathologically.

Figure 6–1. (Upper, facing page) Subendocardial rhabdomyoma. Myocardium of the wall of the left ventricle and mitral valve. The single lesion is discrete, sharply demarcated, and pale staining. This appearance is typical of rhabdomyomas of the heart in infants with tuberous sclerosis. 25x

Figure 6–2. (Lower, facing page) Rhabdomyoma of the heart. Individual tumor cells on the right are in striking contrast to those of the normal myocardium on the left. A spider cell is marked with an arrow. 160x

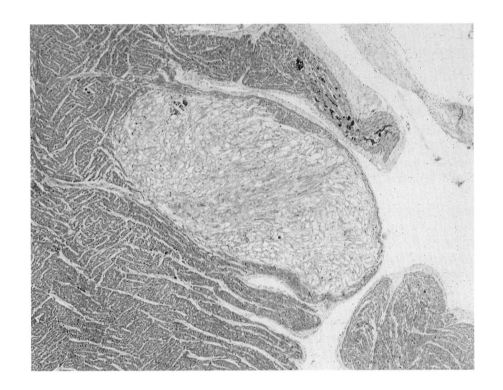

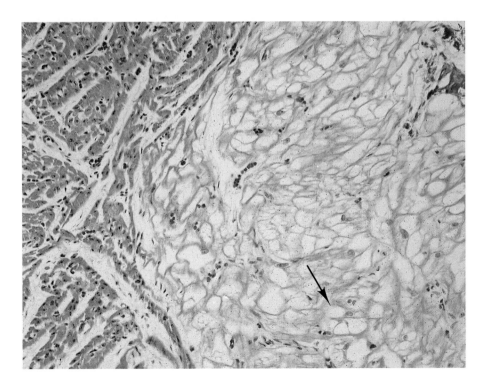

Myocarditis

Inflammation of the myocardium has been described in infants and children in association with a variety of infectious diseases: bacterial, viral, and fungal.[6, 51] In the first year of life, the most common cause of myocarditis in apparently healthy infants is Coxsackie virus, especially group B.[24,34,70] Most of the reported cases have involved babies in the neonatal period; the only other form that occurs with any frequency at this age is that caused by *Toxoplasma gondii*.

Coxsackie B myocarditis in infants is most prevalent in the summer and early autumn. The disease is usually acquired either during or shortly after birth. Clinical manifestations become apparent during the first or second week of life. The onset is sudden with lethargy, anorexia, tachycardia, respiratory distress, and cyanosis. The infant's temperature is usually elevated but may be subnormal. One-third of affected babies have hepatosplenomegaly; some are icteric.

The clinical spectrum of Coxsackie myocarditis is variable. Some children recover completely. Some Coxsackie infections are mild and even inapparent, but others are rapidly fatal. The latter group may be considered initially to be potential SIDS cases.

At autopsy the heart may be enlarged and heavy. There may be scattered petechiae in the epi- and myocardium, a common finding in typical SIDS cases. However, a completely normal heart in gross examination does not exclude the diagnosis.

Histologically, there are variable numbers of necrotic myocardial fibers and an exudate consisting predominantly of lymphocytes, histiocytes, and plasma cells. In some instances necrosis is the predominant lesion; in others, there is a heavy cellular infiltrate with little necrosis (Fig. 6–3).

Lesions in organs other than the heart are common; these organs include the liver, lung, kidney, and central nervous system. Meningoencephalitis is present in slightly more than half of the infants who die. It is characterized by mild, focal, or diffuse infiltrates resembling those described in the heart. Within the brain, lesions are most often present in the pons, medulla, cerebellum, and spinal cord. There may be clusters of neutrophils in the choroid plexus.

Case History

This black female infant was born at term and weighed 4086 grams. She was eight and a half months old when she died. She had experienced one prior illness diagnosed as pneumonia, which was accompanied by difficulty in breathing. Just before her death, she had a slight cold. She was found dead in her crib; her death was totally unexpected.

The case was submitted with the diagnosis of bronchopneumonia. After histologic review by the Pathology Study Panel, the case was reclassified as an explained death due to myocarditis (Fig. 6–3).

Figure 6–3. Myocarditis, probably viral.
A (upper, facing page): The myocardium bears an infiltrate of many lymphocytes, concentrated in the center of the field but also diffusely scattered. The heart muscle fibers are intact. There is no necrosis. 160x
B (lower): Higher magnification. The inflammatory cells are clearly lymphocytes. 250x

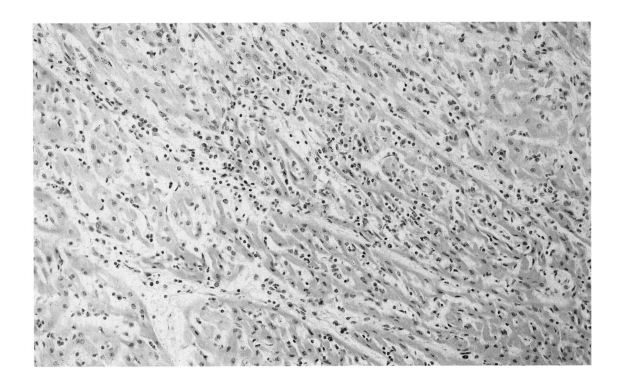

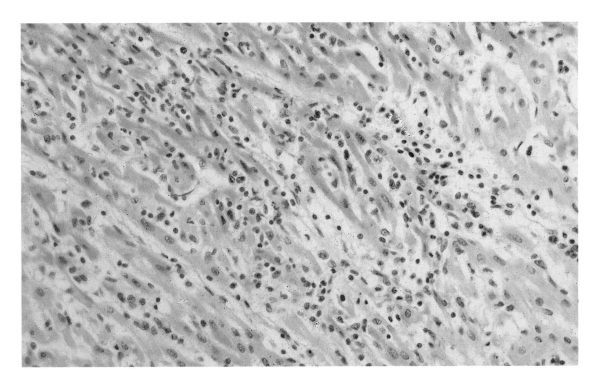

Endocardial Sclerosis (Endocardial Fibroelastosis)

Endocardial sclerosis is gross thickening of the endocardium, the result of an increase in numbers of collagen and elastic fibers. There are two forms of the disease, primary or idiopathic, for which there is no known cause, and secondary, which may be produced by an abnormality in blood flow as the consequence of an associated cardiac anomaly. The best known example of the latter is endocardial sclerosis of the left ventricle in cases of congenital aortic valvular stenosis.[5]

The idiopathic type causes sudden and unexpected death in infants usually in the first few weeks or months of life. These are the cases which, at least clinically, may mimic SIDS. At autopsy, the endocardium of the left atrium and the characteristically globular, dilated left ventricle has endocardium which is thickened, white, and opaque. Often it is the external aspect of the heart, however, that first catches the attention of the pathologist because of its unique spherical shape. Grossly the heart is clearly enlarged, and that enlargement is attributable to a combination of dilatation and hypertrophy.[12,37,44]

The striking endocardial thickening envelops the papillary muscles (Fig. 6–4). When thickening of the endocardium of the left ventricle is not very marked and the diagnosis seems equivocal to the pathologist, it is sometimes helpful to compare the endocardium of the two ventricles because that of the right is usually normal. The endocardium on the right ordinarily remains quite thin, translucent, and pink; only in contrasting it with the relative opacity and white color of the endocardium of the left ventricle does it become clear that the latter is abnormal. In this situation the pathologist has a "built-in" control.

Microscopically, it becomes apparent that long, slender, finger-like extensions of fibroelastic tissue project down into the underlying myocardium and may unite with one another to isolate bundles of myocardium. Sinusoid-like spaces lined by thickened endocardium also stretch out into the myocardium beneath.

There are usually no other associated anomalies in these cases. However, coarctation of the aorta is observed in about 10%.

The etiology of the disease is unknown. Most cases are sporadic; a few are familial. At the present time it is thought that a primary myocardial defect, possibly metabolic, which may be familial, leads to myocardial weakness and "secondary" endocardial thickening. However, this lesion is extremely rare in either stillborn fetuses or newborns.

Case History

This white female infant was born at term with a birth weight of 3629 grams. She seemed well until she died suddenly at 26 days of age. On that day she was a passenger in the car with her parents when suddenly she appeared to them to become cyanotic. The baby's color change was accompanied by what her parents reported as "difficulty in breathing." The infant died suddenly and unexpectedly.

An autopsy was performed, and the infant's death was ascribed to congestive heart failure due to congenital endocardial fibroelastosis (Fig. 6–4, compare with normal endocardium in Fig. 6–5). The case was submitted as one of the quality control cases with an explained cause of death, and the Pathology Study Panel concurred in the diagnosis of congenital endocardial fibroelastosis.

Figure 6–4. Endocardial fibroelastosis. A (upper, facing page): The endocardium is strikingly thickened in this section of the inner portion of the wall of the left ventricle. 25x   B (middle, facing page): A section of the inner portion of the wall of the left ventricle is shown at somewhat higher magnification than in the preceding photograph. 60x

Figure 6–5 (Lower, facing page). Section of the inner portion of the wall of a normal left ventricle with myocardium and endocardium. Contrast the thickness of this endocardium with that in Figure 6–4B. 60x

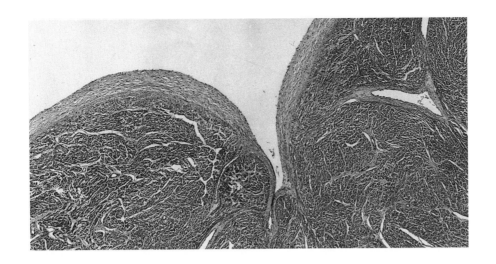

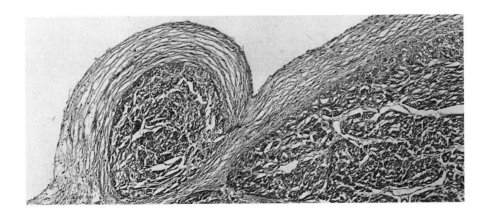

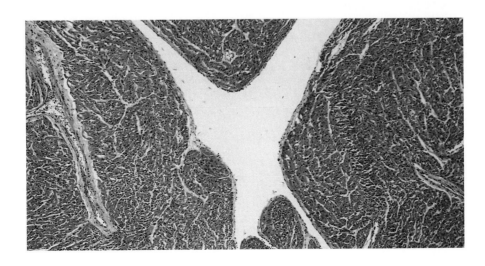

Acute Bronchiolitis

Acute bronchiolitis is common in infants in the first two years of life; its peak incidence occurs at approximately six months. Like SIDS it is most prevalent in the winter and early spring.

Bronchiolitis is a viral disease. In more than half of the cases the respiratory syncytial virus is the causative agent; other agents include para-influenza 3 virus, mycoplasma, and some adenoviruses. Babies with the disease are first noted to have mild symptoms of upper respiratory tract infection with a serous nasal discharge and sneezing. Those symptoms generally last for several days and are followed by fever and diminished appetite. Respiratory distress may develop with a wheezy cough, dyspnea, and irritability.[59]

Histopathologically, the disease is characterized by thickening of the bronchiolar walls produced by edema and inflammatory cell infiltration; mucus and cellular debris fill their lumens. Particularly in the slender airways of small children, even minor thickening of the wall may have a profound effect on airflow. Nevertheless, the case fatality is below 1%.[2]

The role of bronchiolitis should not be exaggerated in any consideration of the possible causes of sudden death in infants. Undoubtedly, a few apparent SIDS cases are due to bronchiolitis. But the determination, in each instance, is the pathologist's to make. If, in any given case, many bronchioles, in many sections, from different parts of the two lungs are affected then the diagnosis of death from bronchiolitis is warranted, and the sudden infant death syndrome is excluded from consideration. However, if only a few bronchioles in any of the sections are affected then, the designation should be one of SIDS with mild bronchiolitis.

In regard to morphology, lymphoid nodules in the immediate vicinity of small airways are probably normal for the age and part of the general wealth of lymphoid tissue that infants exhibit in so many places, e.g., Peyer's patches, tonsils, and mesenteric lymph nodes. They are commonly encountered at autopsy in cases of possible SIDS as well as in infants who have died in accidents or of acute disease processes. They do not encircle the bronchiolar wall nor do they narrow the lumen.

Case History

This 2 month old black male infant was born apparently at term with a birth weight of 3090 grams. He was hospitalized and seen by physicians intermittently for diarrhea and upper respiratory infections up to 10 days prior to his death. The circumstances surrounding the death were not noted.

The case was submitted as an acute dehydration with a history of chronic gastroenteritis. There was no note of a microscopic examination being done.

On initial review, all three members of the Pathology Study Panel agreed that the amount of bronchiolitis seen microscopically was sufficient to cause death (Fig. 6–6). The diagnosis was maintained after the second review which included medical, investigative and autopsy reports. It was felt that the physical findings and vitreous electrolytes did not reveal dehydration significant enough to be fatal.

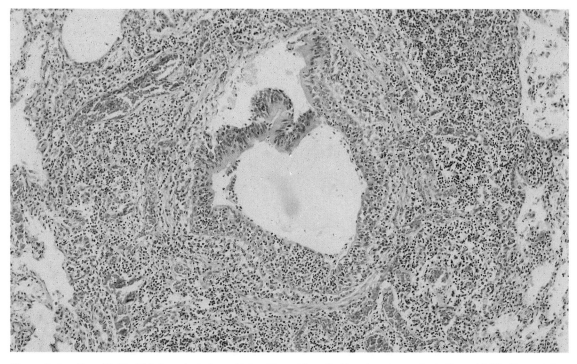

Figure 6–6. Bronchiolitis. This is a single bronchiole with a wide cuff of lymphocytes, typical of bronchiolitis. Essentially all the bronchioles of all five lung sections sampled showed a similar histologic picture.   75x

Case History

This black male infant reportedly had been in good health following an uncomplicated pregnancy and delivery. A check up at 2 weeks of age was "fine." He was found dead in his bed several hours after he had been seen sleeping normally. He was 2 months old.

The gross autopsy was unremarkable except for multiple petechial hemorrhages involving the thymus, lungs and heart and moderate pulmonary congestion. Microscopic examination revealed pneumonia and bronchiolitis (Figs. 6–7 and 6–8). The Pathology Study Panel occurred.

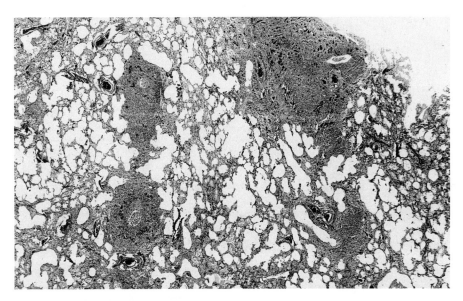

Figure 6–7.
Bronchiolitis and bronchopneumonia. A low power photomicrograph demonstrates numerous airways surrounded by a heavy lymphocytic infiltrate. 15x

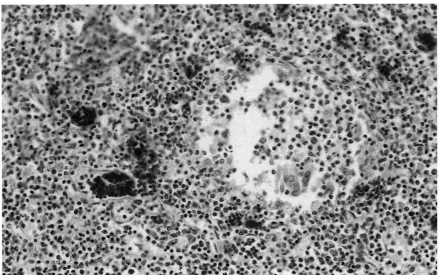

Figure 6–8.
Bronchiolitis and bronchopneumonia. The mucosa of the bronchiole is denuded, and the wide cuff of lymphocytes is evident on higher magnification (arrows). Approximately half of the bronchioles in the five lung sections sampled showed this extent of inflammation. The remaining bronchioles showed minimal to moderate inflammation. Elsewhere, focal bronchopneumonia was evident (not shown). 150x

Pneumonia

For practical purposes, the only morphological type of pneumonia seen in infants who die suddenly at home is bronchopneumonia. Lobar pneumonia does not occur in this age group. In addition, virtually all of these cases are attributable to bacterial infection, and the most common organisms are *Streptococcus pneumoniae, Staphylococcus aureus,* or *Hemophilus influenzae, type b.* [60]

Interstitial pneumonia, presumably viral, does occur, on occasion, in infants of this age, but death as a consequence of it is rare. In one published series of SIDS deaths, no instances were observed histologically in 109 consecutive autopsies in which the investigators were focusing their attention on attempts to isolate viruses from the lungs and other organs.[65] The sections of lung in these cases and others showed occasional examples of apparently thick cellular alveolar walls. This is the feature that has given rise to so many errors in the microscopic interpretation of sections of infant lung (see Chapter 3). Under normal circumstances, alveolar walls in infants are thick and cellular compared with those of adults.

In the NICHD SIDS Cooperative Epidemiological Study, less than 1% (only 3/800) of the cases submitted as potential SIDS were eventually designated by the Pathology Study Panel as attributable to bronchopneumonia. The number is clearly not large. Among the 65 explained deaths, there were 18 deaths classified as due to bronchopneumonia (see Chapter 10). None of the non-SIDS deaths were attributed to viral pneumonia. In fact, no large series, complete with detailed clinical information, histology, and reliable microbiologic investigation of sudden infant deaths due to pneumonia has yet been published.

Pneumonia in infants, like SIDS, occurs most commonly in late winter and early spring when respiratory infections are at their peak. In many instances, pneumonia is preceded by a viral upper respiratory infection. Males are more often affected than females.

The classic history of pneumococcal pneumonia in adults, with shaking chills followed by high fever, cough, and chest pain, is rarely observed in infants. The clinical features are much more variable in babies. Usually, a mild upper respiratory tract infection with a stuffy nose, fretfulness, and a diminished appetite for several days precedes the onset of pneumonia. The illness proper is characterized by an abrupt onset of fever, apprehension, and respiratory distress. Cough is unusual. Physical examination of the chest is seldom helpful.

Pneumonia in the infant lung may be difficult or even impossible to diagnose at the autopsy table. Frequently, nothing is suspected even after careful gross inspection of the lung in cases in which histologic examination reveals full-blown pneumonia. The reverse also occurs, in that the pathologist suspects pneumonic consolidation grossly, only to discover, on examination of microscopic sections, that the lungs are clear.

Fibrinous or fibrinopurulent pleuritis is almost never included in the gross pathologic picture in the cases of sudden death due to fulminant pneumonia.

When the diagnosis is clear microscopically, numerous, fairly large patches of consolidation are apparent in the histologic sections; in these areas, individual air spaces contain countless polymorphonuclear leukocytes. Postmortem bacterial colonization in affected air spaces is considered an incidental finding.

If in studying routine sections from all five lobes one has the impression that the disease was sufficiently severe and extensive to have caused the infant's death (the judgment of which is unfortunately wholly subjective), then the designation of death due to pneumonia removes the case from the ranks of SIDS. The problem is, however, that frequently the pathologist has difficulty deciding, in a given instance, whether it is or is not sufficient (see also Chapter 7).

Case History

This white female infant was born at term with a birth weight of 2384 grams. She was seven and one half months old when she died. The baby had been left alone all night and found dead in the morning.

This case was submitted as an explained death due to bronchopneumonia (Fig. 6–9). The Pathology Study Panel concurred.

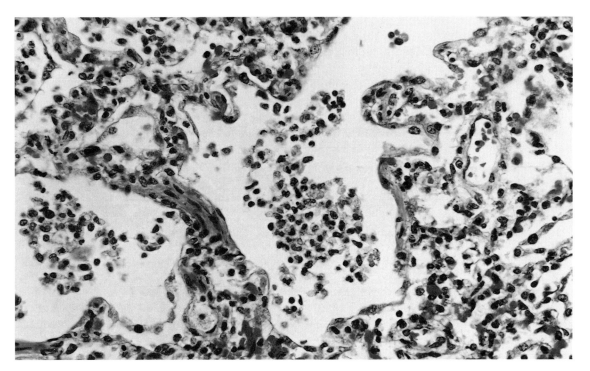

Figure 6–9. Bronchopneumonia. There is a single air space in the middle of the field containing polymorphonuclear leukocytes. An alveolus in the lower left corner also contains pus. Bronchopneumonia was florid in three of the lobes sampled; the remaining two lobes had mild bronchopneumonia. 250x

Case History

This black male was one of twins. He was small at birth but had been healthy and had received all of his immunizations. He was found unresponsive in bed 30 minutes after being fed. He was resuscitated but had severe cerebral anoxia and was pronounced dead approximately 12 hours later. He was 85 days old.

Although there was discussion as to whether this represented a "delayed SIDS," the Pathology Study Panel felt that the extent of the pneumonia was more than would be expected to have developed entirely during the short period of hospitalization and respiratory support. This case was designated as an explained death, due to bronchopneumonia (Fig. 6–10).

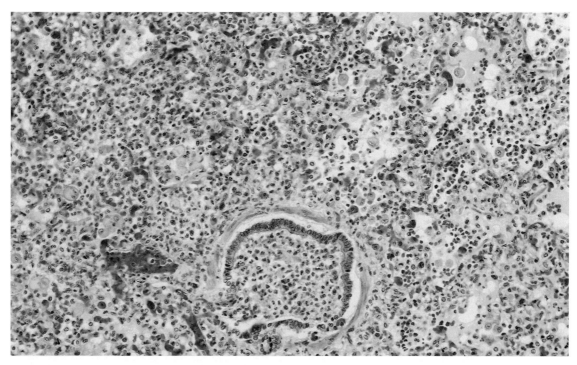

Figure 6–10. Bronchopneumonia. The bronchiole and surrounding alveoli are filled with polymorphonuclear neutrophils. Florid pneumonia such as this was present in all lung sections sampled, with macroscopic nodules evident in two of six sections. 150x.

Case History

This 36 day old black male infant was reportedly born one month prematurely with a birth weight of 3972 grams. Although the mother said he had had slight respiratory problems since birth, he was seen by a nurse 2 weeks prior to death with no problems noted at that time. The mother was a diet controlled diabetic. He was found unresponsive in his crib two hours after he had been put to sleep.

At autopsy he weighed 3800 grams with minimal subcutaneous fat. The lungs were focally consolidated and thick purulent exudate was expressed from bronchioles. Microscopically there was diffuse bronchopneumonia (Fig. 6–11). The Pathology Study Panel agreed with the diagnosis of bronchopneumonia.

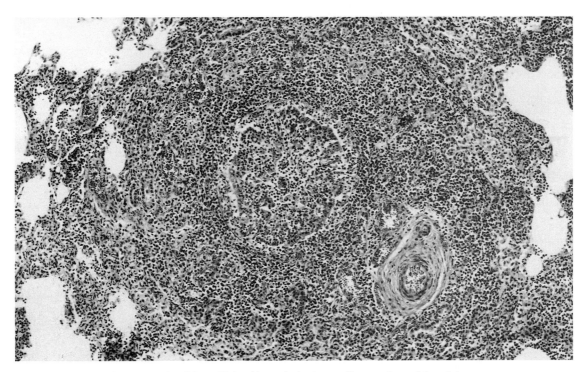

Figure 6–11. Bronchopneumonia. A bronchiole with pus in the lumen. Surrounding acini contain numerous polymorphonuclear neutophils. Florid bronchocentric inflammation was evident in four of five lung sections submitted; the fifth section had minimal numbers of inflammatory cells. 75x

Case History

This 7 month old Hispanic male was born prematurely at 32 weeks gestation and was appropriately low birth weight (1532 grams). He reportedly had lung problems since birth. The circumstances surrounding his terminal event are not clear; it is known only that he apparently convulsed at home and became unresponsive. He was admitted to the hospital without vital signs and was revived enough to be maintained in a state of severe shock for 15 hours prior to being pronounced dead. Admitting chest x-ray was negative.

The autopsy revealed a poorly nourished infant without evidence of injury. The lungs grossly and microscopically had widespread bronchopneumonia (Fig. 6–12). There was no record of cultures being done. The case was submitted as death due to bronchopneumonia. The panel agreed.

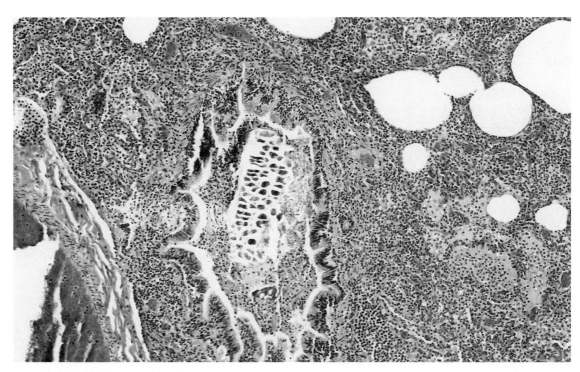

Figure 6–12. Bronchopneumonia. A large vegetable fragment is also present in the bronchiole; whether it was a source of obstruction or secondary to terminal aspiration is unknown. Pus fills the surrounding alveoli. Large confluent patches of bronchopneumonia were evident in three of five lung sections sampled; the remaining two sections had bronchioles filled with pus and focal, patchy pneumonia.   75x

Meningitis

Purulent leptomeningitis is still relatively common in infants and children despite the availability of antibiotic agents capable of killing most of the responsible etiologic agents. Although reported deaths due to infectious diseases in general have decreased 10- to 20-fold since 1935, those due to bacterial meningitis have decreased by only one-half. The incidence of bacterial meningitis in general, and particularly that due to *Hemophilus influenzae* type b and group B beta-hemolytic streptococcus, has increased in recent years.

Bacterial meningitis occurs more frequently in males than in females especially among infants. Conditions that lead to an increased incidence of respiratory infection appear to enhance the incidence of bacterial meningitis.

During the first two months of life the organisms that cause meningitis are most often gram-negative enteric bacilli and group B streptococcus. An increasing number of cases caused by *Listeria monocytogenes* and *Hemophilus influenzae* type b is also being reported among newborns. Among children two months to 12 years of age most bacterial meningitis is due to *Hemophilus influenzae* type b, *Streptococcus pneumoniae,* and *Neisseria meningitidis.*

Signs of bacterial meningitis may be preceded by several days of upper respiratory or gastrointestinal infection. Particularly in young infants, signs of meningeal inflammation may be minimal; only irritability, restlessness, and poor feeding may be noted. Fever is usually but not always present.[28]

At autopsy the pathologist may find a meningeal exudate of varying density distributed widely about the brain. It accumulates around the veins over the convexity of the cerebral hemispheres, in the depths of the sulci, in the sylvian fissures, around the cerebellum, and is often most marked over the circle of Willis. Sometimes, however, the exudate is minimal and initially overlooked by the pathologist during the gross examination, and seen for the first time during examination of microscopic sections.

The spinal cord may be encased in pus, and there may be ventriculitis as well. The leptomeningeal inflammatory process may involve the walls of small arteries and veins with resultant thrombosis. Venous occlusion occasionally produces hemorrhagic necrosis of the cortex and underlying white matter. Another complication is occlusion of major venous sinuses, and there may be necrosis of the cerebral cortex in the apparent absence of thrombi.[48]

On microscopic examination, one finds a typical neutrophilic exudate in the subarachnoid space with varying amounts of fibrin. In more severely affected areas, the entire subarachnoid space is filled with such exudate.[8]

Acute aseptic meningitis, such as is illustrated in Figure 6–15, is attributable to viruses in the vast majority of instances. Enteroviruses account for approximately 80% of all cases of aseptic meningitis; the most common specific types are Coxsackie virus B5 and echoviruses 4,6,9, and 30.

The clinical presentation in viral meningitis is much like that of bacterial meningitis, but the course is generally less fulminant. In most instances the illness is self-limiting; with none of the life-threatening complications of purulent meningitis; however, the disease may be severe and progressive and lead to disability or death.

Histologically, the leptomeningeal infiltrate is predominantly lymphocytic rather than neutrophilic.

Case History

This black female infant was born at term, but with a birth weight of only 1617 grams. She was severely growth retarded in utero. She was three months old when she died. According to her mother she had a "cold" at the time of her death and was being given nose drops. She was in bed with her mother at the time that she was found dead, lying on her back and unresponsive.

The leptomeninges must have been markedly thickened and opaque. The case was submitted as an explained death due to bacterial meningitis. The Pathology Study Panel concurred that this was an explained death due to bacterial meningitis (Fig. 6–13).

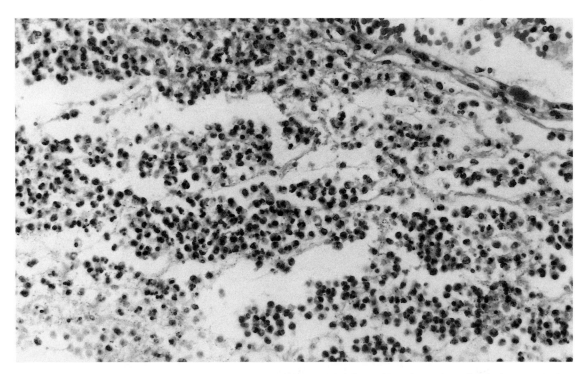

Figure 6–13. Acute bacterial meningitis. The leptomeninges are heavily infiltrated by polymorphonuclear leukocytes. 250x

Case History

This black male infant was born prematurely, at 35 weeks of gestation, with an appropriate birth weight for gestational age, 2230 grams. He was seven months old when he died.

The case was submitted as an autopsy control with the diagnosis of meningitis. The neutrophils in the leptomeninges are not numerous, as in the previous case, and are accompanied by some lymphocytes (Fig. 6–14). However, the panel agreed that this was an explained death due to meningitis and that it was acute and probably not viral.

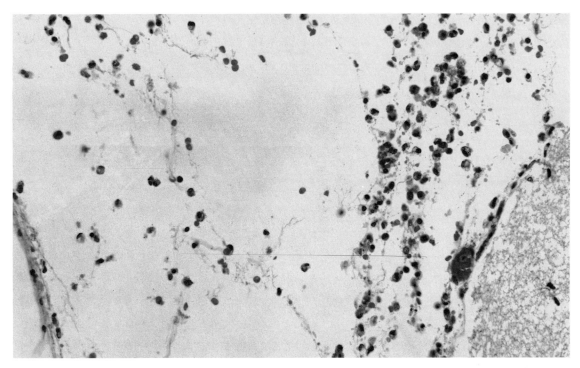

Figure 6–14. Acute bacterial meningitis. Although the leptomeninges contain far fewer neutrophils than appear in Figure 6–13, they are sufficiently numerous to support the diagnosis of meningitis. 250x

Case History

This black female infant was born prematurely, at 35 weeks of gestation, with a birth weight of 2639 grams. Her mother was said to be a heroin addict who had stopped using heroin after the fourth month of her pregnancy. The baby was not reported to have been ill prior to her death at 13 days of age. The baby was found dead in bed with her mother, four and one half hours after her last feeding.

In this case there is a lymphocytic rather than a neutrophilic exudate (Fig. 6–15). Acute viral meningitis like this is a self-limiting disease with none of the life-threatening complications that occur in pyogenic meningitis. It is likely that no gross changes in the leptomeninges were appreciated at autopsy. Although this case was submitted as an explained death, the Pathology Study Panel classified it as SIDS.

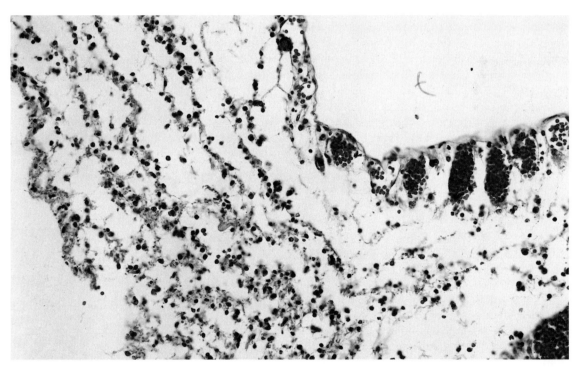

Figure 6–15. Viral meningitis. The leptomeninges, though thin, contain an impressive number of lymphocytes. Neutrophils are not included in this exudate; this is typical of the inflammatory process in viral meningitis. . 160x

Boric Acid Poisoning

Although it has been reported in the literature, boric acid poisoning is an extremely uncommon cause of sudden and unexpected death in infants, especially after the first week of life. In the past, such deaths occurred when boric acid powder was mistakenly used in place of powdered milk formula in preparing the infant formula in a few hospital nurseries. In each such instance, several of the infants in the nursery died simultaneously.

Also, pure boric acid powder has been used commonly by mothers in the treatment of severe diaper rash. When the infant's skin is completely denuded over large areas, it is possible for the boric acid to be absorbed in sufficient quantities to poison an infant. A few such cases have been reported.[23]

There are only two features of boric acid poisoning apparent during the gross autopsy: bright red discoloration of the skin of the palms of the hands and a denuded diaper area heavily coated with white powder.

There is, however, a typical histologic lesion that can be seen in sections of the pancreas in infants with boric acid poisoning. It consists of single, relatively large, round, homogeneous, cytoplasmic inclusion bodies, in pancreatic acinar cells, which appear blue in sections stained with hematoxylin and eosin.[31]

There was no case of boric acid poisoning in the NICHD Cooperative Study of SIDS Risk Factors. The illustrative case and microscopic section (Fig. 6–16) presented here were taken from the files of one of the Pathology Study Panel members.[64] In this case the cytoplasmic inclusion bodies alerted the pathologist to the suspected boric acid poisoning. Subsequently a representative of the medical examiner's office was sent to the home to talk with the infant's mother; he discovered that she had been using pure boric acid powder to treat her baby's advanced diaper rash. At autopsy, the denuded diaper area was caked with white powder.

Case History

This white female infant was born at term, weighing 3430 grams. She was thought to be in good health until the day before death when her mother noticed purple mottling of her face. At 2:00 am on the day she died she did not take her bottle well, was "breathing very hard", and vomited. Later she became unresponsive. She was dead by the time her mother got her to the hospital.

The medical examiner's autopsy revealed reddened palms and soles and a severe diaper rash with denudation of most of the skin in the diaper area; in addition, the entire diaper area was heavily coated with caked, white powder. Microscopic sections of the pancreas revealed extensive cytoplasmic vacuolization of acinar cells, and within those vacuoles, distinct inclusions (Fig. 6–16). Later investigation revealed the fact that the infant's mother had been using pure boric acid powder to "treat" the baby's ulcerated diaper rash.

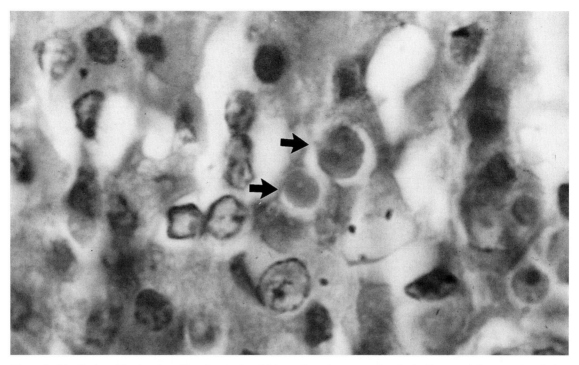

Figure 6–16. Boric acid poisoning. Near the center of this section of pancreas (marked with arrows) there are two dark grey, homogeneous cytoplasmic inclusions; these were blue in hematoxylin and eosin stained sections. 60x

Encephalitis

Encephalitis, inflammation of the brain, is an extremely uncommon cause for sudden and unexpected death in infants who have been apparently well. The diagnosis can be established with absolute certainty only by microscopic examination of the brain.

The etiologic agents capable of causing encephalitis in infants of this age are many and can be divided into four principal categories: (1) viral infections; (2) non-viral infections; (3) parainfectious, postinfectious, or allergic; (4) unknown.[17]

Included in the first category are mumps, measles, the enterovirus group, rubella, and the herpes virus group. The most common type of viral encephalitis in the first year of life is eastern equine. Even this is rare because most infants are protected from the insect vector. But, during epidemics, as many as 20% of the victims may be infants under one year of age.[57] The disease is devastating; it has a high mortality and, if the infant survives, severe sequelae usually ensue.[26]

In the second category of non-viral infections are rickettsia, *Mycoplasma pneumoniae,* and spirochetes.

In the third category the intact, infectious agent is not isolated in vitro from the nervous system. It is postulated that, in this group, the influence of cell-mediated antigen-antibody complexes plus complement produces the tissue damage. This kind of encephalitis is associated with some specific diseases in which the agent itself may also cause some degree of direct damage to the central nervous system; included in this group are measles, rubella, mumps, and pertussis.[17] Some vaccines have also been implicated including rabies, measles, influenza, and vaccinia. The claims that pertussis vaccine can produce encephalitis in infants of this age are not supported by histologically proven cases in the literature.[45-47]

The last category, cause unknown, constitutes more than two-thirds of the cases of encephalitis reported to the Centers for Disease Control in Atlanta.[26]

Clinical manifestations of encephalitis vary greatly in severity. Some children appear to be mildly affected, if at all, and then die suddenly. Others experience high fever and violent convulsions. In most instances, however, they have what appears to be an acute systemic illness with fever, screaming spells, and vomiting. There may be signs of an associated upper respiratory infection. During the acute stage of disease the brain is edematous.

Initially, tissue sections of the brain reveal congestion of, and a neutrophilic infiltrate in, the leptomeninges. In the brain itself, there are perivascular cuffs of neutrophils accompanied by perivascular tissue necrosis with myelin breakdown, neuronal disruption in various stages including, ultimately, neuronophagia and endothelial proliferation or necrosis. Thrombosis of small vessels is common. Infants who survive the first few days have marked destruction of neuronal elements. Mononuclear cells, lymphocytes, and plasma cells replace the polymorphonuclear leukocytes in the lesions of the brain. Viral studies are indicated if there is any suspicion of encephalitis. Immunofluorescent and electron microscopic studies may provide critical diagnostic information.[42]

No cases of encephalitis were encountered in the NICHD study, even among the various groups of control infants or explained deaths.

Ludwig's Angina

Cellulitis in the neck (cervical cellulitis) is also referred to as Ludwig's angina. It is purulent spreading inflammation around the submaxillary gland, beneath the jaw, and about the floor of the mouth. It is usually due to streptococcal infection.[11,55]

The disease is not common but was identified in one of the 15 cases originally submitted as a potential SIDS case, but then classified by the Pathology Study Panel as an explained death. In this case, there was abundant edema and a heavy infiltrate of polymorphonuclear leukocytes in the various sections taken in the region of the pharynx, trachea, and thyroid. A second case of cellulitis in the neck was submitted as one of the 65 explained deaths.

Case History

This black male infant was born very prematurely, at 29 weeks of gestation, with a birth weight of 1419 grams. He was ten weeks old when he died. The baby had a history of jaundice at birth for which he was treated. He was apparently doing well at home until 6:00 p.m. on the day before death; at that time he began to cry and was restless. He was given a bottle and went to sleep an hour later. The following morning he was found dead.

At autopsy gross examination revealed pleural petechiae, but the inflammatory process in the neck was not documented. The case was submitted as SIDS. However, the Pathology Study Panel determined that there was sufficient inflammation in the soft tissue of the neck (Fig. 6–17) to have been responsible for the child's demise. In addition, the baby may also have been septic.

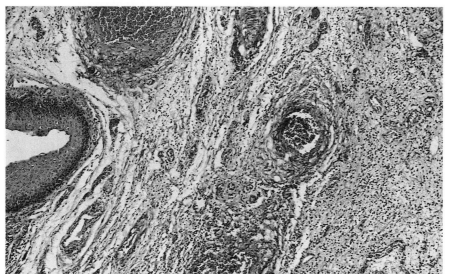

Figure 6–17. Cellulitis in the neck. This is a section through the wall of the pharynx. All of the loose connective tissue beneath the squamous epithelium is edematous and heavily infiltrated with polymorphonuclear leukocytes. 60x

Case History

This white male infant was born at term weighing 3459 grams. He was 20 months old when he died. He had had a mild upper respiratory tract infection for a few days, with a fever of up to 104° the night prior to his death.

This quality control case (Fig. 6–18) was reviewed by the Pathology Study Panel and designated as an explained death. The cause of death was considered to be cellulitis in the neck (Ludwig's angina).

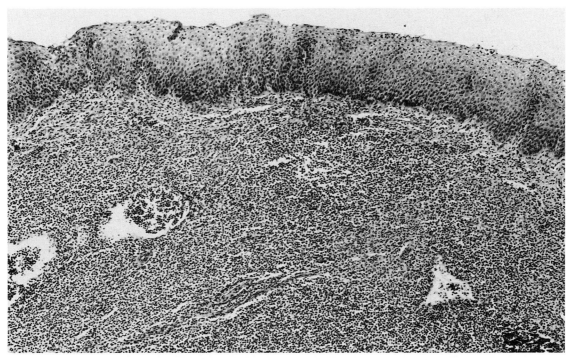

Figure 6–18. Cellulitis in the neck. In this case, the inflammatory infiltrate is much more striking than in Figure 6–17. There is less edema and there are many more neutrophils. 60x

Cystic Fibrosis of The Pancreas (In Hot Weather)

Cystic fibrosis of the pancreas is occasionally responsible for the sudden and unexpected death of an infant via the mechanism of excessive salt loss in hot weather. This phenomenon occurs on account of the abnormally high salt content of the sweat of patients with the disease.

There are few gross anatomical clues to this diagnosis in infants. Principal among them are generalized, advanced fatty change of the liver (which may be perceived and diagnosed correctly by the radiologist) and strikingly diminished size of the gallbladder.

Much more readily appreciated are the microscopic hallmarks of the disease, particularly in infants, in the pancreas and gastrointestinal tract. Sections of the pancreas reveal not only inspissation of secretions in dilated ducts and acini but, also, widespread, early, interstitial fibrosis. In the small bowel and, to a lesser extent, the colon, one observes inspissation of pink-staining secretion in crypts and occasional cystically dilated glands as well. Neither the typical pulmonary nor hepatic changes are apt to be apparent in babies; however, there is often striking fatty change throughout the liver.[3, 13, 16, 18, 19, 25, 54, 56]

Figure 6–19 is from a published case,[66] as no such cases were included in the NICHD SIDS Cooperative Epidemiological Study.

Case History

This white female infant was born at term weighing 3680 grams. She thrived for a time but then began to lose ground developmentally as she became pale and irritable. Later she started to "spit up" her feedings and her legs became puffy. Eventually she refused all feedings and became so irritable that she was unable to sleep. However, she never experienced diarrhea.

When she was admitted to the hospital, at the age of five months with anasarca and fever, her sodium was 125 mmols/L. Despite what seemed to be adequate therapy, she went into renal failure and died (Fig. 6–19).

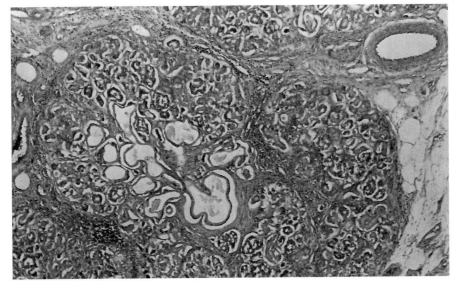

Figure 6–19. Cystic fibrosis of the pancreas. This is a section of the pancreas from an infant who died unexpectedly of cystic fibrosis. The characteristic features are the striking dilatation of acini and ducts and their content of inspissated secretion (pink in hematoxylin and eosin stained sections). 40x

CAUSES FOR SUDDEN EXPLAINED INFANT DEATHS DETERMINED AT GROSS AUTOPSY, BY HISTORICAL DATA AND/OR BY ANCILLARY STUDIES

The Battered Infant

The battered infant is not necessarily readily recognized upon gross external examination, particularly if the infant's skin is deeply pigmented. Bruises, for example, may not be immediately apparent. Occasionally, they can be identified with certainty only when the skin is incised revealing the telltale hemorrhage beneath. At times, the first indication of trauma appears as the scalp is being reflected and hemorrhage is identified. In any instance in which abuse is suspected, the pathologist should document carefully all areas of injury. The inside of the infant's mouth should be inspected, especially the area between the upper anterior gingiva and the interior of the upper lip, as tears of the frenulum are common in abuse.

Whole body X-rays are helpful, occasionally revealing completely unsuspected old or recent fractures which might not otherwise have been identified. It is especially important to inspect the head in search not only of fractures but, also, old and recent subdural hemorrhages and cerebral edema with evidences of increased pressure, e.g., the inferior cerebellar pressure cone.[33, 36, 38, 40, 52, 62, 68]

In the so-called "shaken baby syndrome," one expects to see retinal hemorrhages, although they are not specific for that entity. If they are suspected, it is best to remove the eyes, fix them, and section them appropriately for microscopic examination.[14, 24, 39]

Suffocation

Sometimes infants are suffocated deliberately. It is easy for an adult to press his or her hand against the infant's nose and mouth to accomplish that end. In those cases, findings at autopsy may not be different from those seen in the typical SIDS; the two are not usually distinguishable, either grossly or microscopically.

Accidental suffocation occurs all too frequently. One of the most common causes is the soft, delicate, supple sheet of clear plastic that dry cleaners use to drape over the clothing they deliver to their customers. This product is ubiquitous and is often thoughtlessly left near or in an infant's crib. If it happens to lie against an infant's face, it tends to adhere to the skin, particularly if the skin is moist and if the baby inhales against the plastic. This is one of the accidents that may become evident only in the course of careful investigation at the scene.

Despite the lack of good scientific evidence, infants in the first year of life probably do not suffocate accidentally from contact with ordinary bed clothing (of either the adult or infant type). A normal infant, including a neonate, will lift and move his head as necessary to maintain an adequate airway. It is also probable that neither adult blankets nor pillows will suffocate a normal baby in the first year of life. Waterbeds have been implicated as a potential cause of suffocation, but there is no proof that such accidents do occur. If, indeed, that possibility is entertained in any given case, a number of factors must be taken into consideration in arriving at that conclusion: the age and body weight of the baby, the degree to which the water bed is expanded, the position of the body, i.e., prone or supine, the location of the body on the bed, and the maturity of the infant, i.e., his capacity to lift or turn his head, etc. The matter is not a simple one in any case.

So-called overlaying (usually by the mother) has been suggested as a cause of accidental suffocation of babies (even back to Biblical times as in the Book of Solomon and the story about the woman whose baby died in the night "because she overlaid it"). However, most adult caretakers, especially mothers, have a "sixth sense," even in sleep, which will arouse them should the threatened infant move to defend his airway or even cry. But this protective mechanism might be expected to fail if the adult involved were drugged or intoxicated or if the infant were brain damaged.

It is important for the pathologist to keep in mind, as mentioned above, that autopsy findings in both suffocation with a soft object and SIDS are virtually the same. One cannot distinguish between them.

Congenital Heart Disease

Not many forms of congenital heart disease mimic SIDS. Most of those potentially fatal for infants produce clearly evident signs, such as cyanosis or rapid breathing, during the life of the infant for quite a long time before death. However, there are three congenital heart lesions that do lead to sudden and unexpected death in apparently well babies: congenital aortic valvular stenosis, total anomalous pulmonary venous return, and endocardial fibroelastosis (or sclerosis).[4]

Aortic stenosis, whether congenital (in children) or acquired (in adults), is a classic cause of sudden and unexpected death. Hence, among infants under one year of age, it is necessarily a major element in any list of "rule-outs" or exclusionary diagnoses for SIDS.[15, 22, 53]

Typically, an infant born with this lesion may seem well upon discharge from the newborn nursery. Occasionally, the typical murmur is not detected on physical examination at that time, and there may be no signs or symptoms of illness following discharge. A few weeks thereafter, the baby may be found suddenly lifeless in his crib.

A careful autopsy, in such a case, will reveal characteristic congenital narrowing of the aortic valve, the result of distal fusion of the cusps. The aortic orifice may be only a minute opening in a firm fibrous diaphragm within which remnants of cusps cannot be identified, or the stenosis may result from a thickened, tricuspid, bicuspid, or unicuspid valve. The thickening, which is often produced by nodular, opalescent, semi-cartilaginous excrescences, may practically occlude the functional orifice.

In such cases, the right atrium, ventricle, and pulmonary artery are large. The ductus arteriosus is widely patent. The aorta is small and may bear an associated coarctation. The left ventricle and often the left atrium are small; the wall of the former is often thickened and its endocardium is sometimes thickened and opaque.

Total anomalous pulmonary venous return can be overlooked at gross autopsy unless the pulmonary venous drainage is inspected. The abnormal pulmonary venous return can be supradiaphragmatic or infradiaphragmatic. The former can present in the postneonatal period as sudden death. [4, 67]

Endocardial sclerosis may be overlooked by the autopsy pathologist when the characteristic white opacification of the endocardium is minimal. In equivocal cases, the pathologist need only contrast the endocardial lining of the left ventricle with that of the right; normally both should be of the same hue. If the left is appreciably more white and opaque than the right, it is abnormal. By the time a child dies of the disease, the heart has usually become globular in its dilatation, which is quite apparent in its overall external configuration, and the interior of the apical portion of the left ventricle is typically rounded rather than normally pointed.

An interventricular septal defect alone, or even in combination with a patent ductus arteriosus, is not expected to cause an infant of this age to die suddenly, unless the defect is exceptionally large.

Intracranial Arteriovenous Malformation

An arteriovenous malformation consists of a tangle of abnormal vessels of various sizes that have the characteristics of both arteries and veins; 90% of arteriovenous malformations are intracranial. Of these, half are located on the surface of the brain and the other half are deep inside the cerebral hemispheres.

The vascular channels of those located within the brain are separated from one another by glial tissue in which one can find evidence of either recent or old bleeding. There are arteries supplying the tangled mass of vessels and there are identifiable veins draining it.

Most instances of hemorrhage from these vascular malformations occur in persons between the ages of 10 and 30; however, in rare instances a hemorrhage of that type can cause the death of an infant.[41,49,61]

Gastroenteritis with Dehydration and Fluid and Electrolyte Imbalance

Infants in the first year of life are extremely susceptible to fluid loss and electrolyte imbalance. Babies less than one year of age can become seriously dehydrated very quickly and die as a result of either protracted vomiting and/or diarrhea. Babies are very different from adults in this regard.[20,29,30,58]

Often parents themselves do not grasp the seriousness of the problem and, as a consequence, fail to seek medical help until their infant is moribund.

At autopsy, the body of an infant who has succumbed to dehydration exhibits few telling morphologic features of that state. The eyes are deeply sunken, and in picking up a fold of relatively thin skin between thumb and forefinger one can ascertain (if the infant's body is not yet cold) that the skin "tents"; it will remain in the pinched position demonstrating loss of normal skin turgor. A history of either vomiting or diarrhea or both will substantiate the gross autopsy observation. Also, the stomach may be empty and the large bowel contain only liquid material.

The best means of supporting this gross diagnosis, however, is chemical analysis of the vitreous humor. In cases of acute gastroenteritis, it is difficult to make a firm microscopic diagnosis. In instances of protracted diarrhea with malabsorption and in some cases of starvation, however, there may be characteristic microscopic changes in the small bowel with loss of villi (Figs. 6–20).

Case History

This Hispanic female infant was born at term with a birth weight of 4000 grams. She was born in Mexico and arrived in the United States eight days before her death at the age of two months. The mother reported that she had been well and very responsive until three days before her death when she became ill, droopy and listless. She was taken for a sick baby visit three days before her death with the chief complaints of cough and diarrhea. Her weight at that outpatient visit was 3685 grams. She was diagnosed as having both an upper respiratory illness and gastroenteritis. Antibiotics were prescribed, and she was discharged to her home. The mother was asked to bring her baby back to be hospitalized if her condition did not improve in the next 24 hours. She was not taken back for care.

This case was initially submitted as SIDS but later turned-around in the field and changed to bronchopneumonia. The pathology study panel noted evidence of bronchitis, bronchopneumonia, and enteritis (Fig. 6–20). Also, it was evident that the infant had been stressed for some time since there was advanced lymphocytic depletion of the thymus. This death was probably due to gastroenteritis but was not labelled as an explained death by the panel because of the lack of a death investigative report in the records and missing information in the autopsy report.

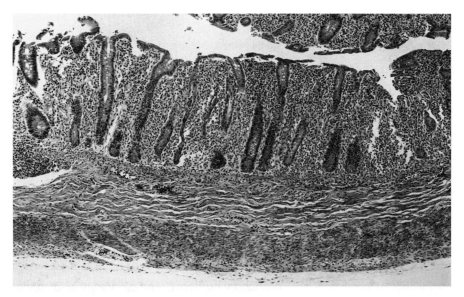

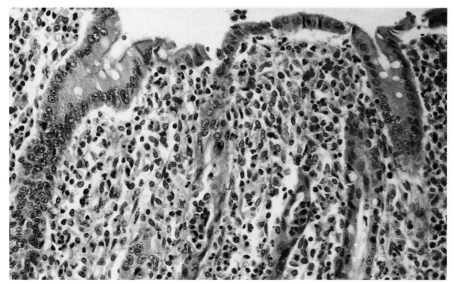

Figure 6–20
Malabsorption.
A(upper): This is a full-thickness, cross section of the wall of the small bowel from an infant two months of age. Note the absolute disappearance of all villi to the extent that the mucosal surface appears flat. Flattening of the surface can be seen in a number of different malabsorption states, including nontropical sprue and even in starvation; although quite abnormal, it is nonspecific. 60x
B (lower): In this higher magnification of A it becomes apparent that many of the abundant cells in the lamina propria are polymorphonuclear leukocytes. This infant probably had enteritis at the time of death. 250x

Starvation, Neglect, and Failure to Thrive

It is sometimes difficult for the pathologist to distinguish among starvation, neglect, and failure to thrive. When an infant who has died is found to be cachectic, especially if the body is dirty, it is often assumed that the baby was either neglected or maltreated. The adequacy of medical care of the infant becomes an issue. In some cases, however, investigation reveals that the caretaker did not realize the life-threatening condition of the infant.

In such instances, the pathologist's final diagnosis must be made with all of the facts at hand, including a complete medical history for the child from birth to death, full information involving the circumstances leading up to the death, and a thorough necropsy including examination of all pertinent microscopic slides.[1,9,10,21,35,63]

MASSIVE ASPIRATION OF GASTRIC CONTENTS

There is no unanimity of opinion, even among pediatric pathologists, with regard to the significance of massive aspiration, usually of gastric contents, and its role in the cause of infant death.

There may be several explanations for the presence of gastric content in the upper airway other than the infant's own regurgitation and aspiration during life.

It is possible to force the gastric contents of an infant, who has already died, up into the esophagus and pharynx and, subsequently, down into the airway by means of attempts at resuscitation, e.g., compression of the lower part of the chest and upper abdomen during artificial respiration.

Another hypothetical mechanism concerns the transport of the body after death. It has been demonstrated radiologically that gastric contents can be displaced from the stomach into the esophagus and pharynx by tilting the body, head down. It may also be possible to cause this same liquid material to then flow down into the larynx and trachea by tilting the body in the other direction.

Lastly, and probably most importantly, some pathologists are convinced that an infant who is physiologically intact will not inhale liquid material in his pharynx but rather will spit it out. This results in the familiar phenomenon of "spitting up" which occurs so frequently in normal infants. Even if the baby should aspirate a little, it is likely that he will then cough to clear his airway, provided he has the physical capability to do so.

Pediatric pathologists commonly find gastric contents in the upper airway in autopsies of infants who have clearly succumbed to a variety of recognized mortal lesions (Figs. 6–21 and 6–22). The mere presence of gastric contents in the airway probably does not, of itself, explain the death of an infant. None of the deaths in the NICHD SIDS Cooperative Epidemiological Study was attributed to massive aspiration.

Case History

This black female infant was born at 42 weeks gestation and was growth retarded, weighing only 2156 grams. Her death at eight months of age was caused by intentional suffocation while in the care of someone other than her mother.

Ultimately, cardiopulmonary resuscitation was attempted. In all microscopic sections of the lung (Figs. 6–21 and 6–22) many bronchioles were plugged with foreign material, much of which was clearly recognizable as partly digested food including muscle fibers and adipose tissue. Exactly how that material got into the airways is not clear; it may have been, as discussed previously, forced there by attempts at artificial respiration, under the circumstances, accidental spontaneous aspiration seems unlikely.

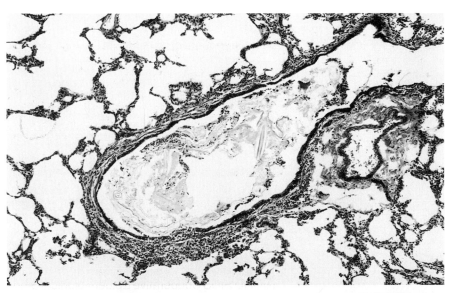

Figure 6–21.
Aspiration of gastric
contents. A bronchiole,
the lumen of which is
filled with amorphous
material, which may be
milk, and two strands of
what appear to be fibers
of some sort. 60x

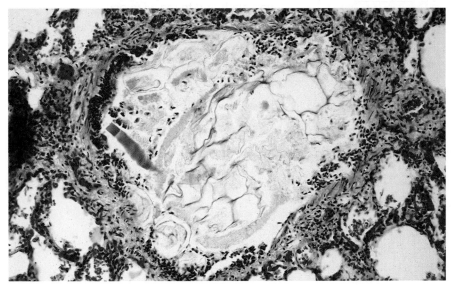

Figure 6–22.
Aspiration of gastric
contents. This is a
cross section of a
bronchiole completely
filled with aspirated
gastric content. On the
left there is a single
muscle fiber, devoid of
nuclei, and on the right
is a sizeable piece of
adipose tissue, also
devoid of nuclei. 160x

REFERENCES

1. Adelson L. Homicide by starvation, the nutritional variant of the "battered child." JAMA 186:458-60, 1963.

2. Aherne W, Bird T, Court SD, Gardner PS, McQuillin J. Pathological changes in virus infections of the lower respiratory tract in children. J Clin Pathol 23:7-18, 1970.

3. Andersen DH. Cystic fibrosis of the pancreas and its relation to celiac disease. Am J Dis Child 56:344-99, 1938.

4. Arey JB. Chapter 7: Malformations of the valvular, supravalvular, and intravalvular regions. In: Cardiovascular Pathology in Infants and Children. Philadelphia: W.B. Saunders Co., 1984, pp 173-90.

5. Arey JB. Endocardial sclerosis, in Chapter 8: Malformations of the endocardium, myocardium, and pericardium. In: Cardiovascular Pathology in Infants and Children. Philadelphia: W.B. Saunders Co., 1984, pp 191-4.

6. Arey JB. Myocarditis, in Chapter 8: Malformations of the endocardium, myocardium, and pericardium. In: Cardiovascular Pathology in Infants and Children. Philadelphia: W.B. Saunders Co., 1984, pp 324-34.

7. Arey JB. Rhabdomyomas, in Chapter 16: Tumors of the heart and pericardium. In: Cardiovascular Pathology in Infants and Children. Philadelphia: W.B. Saunders Co., 1984, pp 372-6.

8. Arey JB, Sotos J. Unexpected death in early life. J Pediatr 49:523-39, 1956.

9. Barbero GJ. Failure to thrive, in Chapter 5: General considerations in the care of sick children. In: Behrman RE, Vaughan VC, eds. Nelson Textbook of Pediatrics, 13th ed. Philadelphia: W.B. Saunders Co., 1987, pp 210-1.

10. Barbero GJ, Shaheen E. Environmental failure to thrive: A clinical view. J Pediatr 71:639-41, 1967.

11. Barkin RM, Bonis SL, Eighammer RM, Todd JK. Ludwig's angina in children. J Pediatr 87:563-5, 1975.

12. Becker AE, Anderson RH. Pathology of congenital heart disease. London: Butterworths, 1981.

13. Bodian M. Fibrocystic disease of the pancreas. New York: Grune and Stratton, 1953.

14. Caffey J. The whiplash shaken infant syndrome. Pediatrics 54:396-403, 1974.

15. Campbell M, Kauntze R. Congenital aortic valvular stenosis. Br Heart J 15:179-94, 1953.

16. Claireaux AE. Fibrocystic disease of the pancreas in the newborn. Arch Dis Child 31:22-7, 1956.

17. Cherry JD. Encephalitis, in Chapter 11: Infectious diseases. In: Behrman RH, Vaughan VC, eds. Nelson Textbook of Pediatrics, 13th ed. Philadelphia: W.B. Saunders Co., 1987, pp 556-60.

18. Cotran RS, Kumar V, Robbins SL. Cystic fibrosis (CF, mucoviscidosis), in Chapter 10: Diseases of infancy and childhood. In: Cotran RS, Kumar V, Robbins SL, eds. Robbins Pathologic Basis of Disease, 4th ed. Philadelphia: W.B. Saunders Co., 1989, pp 533-96.

19. Craig JM, Haddad H, Schwachman H. The pathological changes in the liver in cystic fibrosis of the pancreas. Am J Dis Child 93:357-69, 1957.

20. Darrow DC, Pratt EL, Flett J, Gamble AH, Wiese HF. Disturbances of water and electrolytes in infantile diarrhea. Pediatrics 3:129-56, 1949.

21. Davis JH, Rao VJ, Valdes-Dapena M. A forensic approach to a starved child. J Forens Sci 29:663-9, 1984.

22. Doyle EF, Arumugham P, Lara E, Rutkowski MR, Kiely B. Sudden death in young patients with congenital aortic stenosis. Pediatrics 53:481-9, 1974.

23. Ducey J, Williams DB. Transcutaneous absorption of boric acid. J Pediatr 43:644-51, 1953.

24. Dykes LJ. The whiplash shaken infant syndrome. What has been learned? Child Abuse Negl 10:211-21, 1986.

25. Farber S. Pancreatic function and disease in early life. V. Pathologic changes associated with pancreatic insufficiency in early life. Arch Pathol 37:238-50, 1944.

26. Farber S, Hill A, Connerly ML, Dingle JH. Encephalitis in infants and children caused by the virus of the eastern variety of equine encephalitis. JAMA 114:1725-31, 1940.

27. Fechner RE, Smith MG, Middlekamp JN. Coxsackie B virus infection of the newborn. Am J Pathol 42:493-505, 1963.

28. Feigin RD. Acute bacterial meningitis beyond the neonatal period, in Chapter 11: Infectious diseases: Bacterial infections. In: Behrman RH, Vaughan VC, eds. Nelson Textbook of Pediatrics, 13th ed. Philadelphia: W.B. Saunders Co., 1987, pp 569-73.

29. Finberg L. Dehydration in infants and children. N Engl J Med 276:458-60, 1967.

30. Finberg L. Hypernatremic (hypertonic) dehydration in infants. N Engl J Med 289:196-8, 1973.

31. Fisher RS. Intracytoplasmic inclusions in the pancreas due to boric acid poisoning. Am J Pathol (Abstract) 27:745, 1951.

32. Gold AP, Freeman JM. Depigmented nevi. The earliest sign of tuberous sclerosis. Pediatrics 35:1003-5, 1965.

33. Gonzales AG, Vance M, Helpern M, Umberger C. Legal medicine, pathology, and toxicology. New York: Appleton-Century Crofts, Inc., 1954, p 473.

34. Hosier DM, Newton WA. Serious Coxsackie infection in infants and children. Myocarditis, meningoencephalitis, and hepatitis. Am J Dis Child 97:251-67, 1958.

35. Hufton IW, Oates RK. Nonorganic failure to thrive: A long-term follow-up. Pediatrics 59:73-7, 1977.

36. Jones JG. Sexual abuse of children. Current concepts. Am J Dis Child 136:142-6, 1982.

37. Kelly J, Anderson DH. Congenital endocardial fibroelastosis. II. A clinical and pathological investigation of those cases without associated cardiac malformations including a report of two familial instances. Pediatrics 18:539-55, 1956.

38. Kempe CH, Helfer RE, eds. The battered child, 3rd ed. Chicago: University of Chicago Press, 1980.

39. Lambert SR, Johnson TE, Hoyt CS. Optic nerve sheath and retinal hemorrhages associated with the shaken baby syndrome. Arch Ophthalmol 104:1509-12, 1986.

40. Lenoski EF, Hunter KA. Specific patterns of inflicted burn injuries. J Trauma 17:842-6, 1977.

41. Levine OR, Jameson AG, Nellhaus G, Gold AP. Cardiac complication of cerebral arteriovenous fistula in infancy. Pediatrics 30:563-75, 1962.

42. Manz HJ. Pathology and pathogenesis of viral infections of the central nervous system. Hum Pathol 8:3-26, 1977.

43. McAllister HA, Fenoglio JJ. Tumors of the cardiovascular system. In: Atlas of Tumor Pathology, 2nd series. Fascicle 15. Washington, D.C.: Armed Forces Institute of Pathology, 1978.

44. McKinney B. Endocardial fibroelastosis. In: Pathology of the Cardiomyopathies. London: Butterworths, 1974, pp 11-28.

45. Miller DL, Alderslade R, Ross EM. Whooping cough and whooping cough vaccine: The risks and benefits debate. Epidemiol Rev 4:1-24, 1982.

46. Mortimer EA Jr. Assessing benefit-risk ratios: Pertussis vaccine as a case in point. Cleve Clinic Q 49:235-8, 1982.

47. Mortimer EA Jr, Jones PK. Pertussis vaccine in the United States: The benefit-risk ratio. In: Manclark CR, Hill JC, eds. Proceedings of the International Symposium on Pertussis. Rockville, Md.: U.S. Department of Health, Education, and Welfare, DHEW Publ. No. (NIH) 79-1830, 1979, pp 250-5.

48. Morris JH. Acute pyogenic meningitis, in Chapter 29: The nervous system. In: Cotran RS, Kumar V, Robbins SL, eds. Robbins Pathologic Basis of Disease, 4th ed. Philadelphia: W.B. Saunders Co., 1989, p 1392.

49. Morris JH. Arteriovenous malformations of the brain, in Chapter 29: The nervous system. In: Cotran RS, Kumar V, Robbins SL, eds. Robbins Pathologic Basis of Disease, 4th ed. Philadelphia: W.B. Saunders Co., 1989, p 1408.

50. Nora JJ, Nora AH. Genetics and counseling in cardiovascular diseases. Springfield, Ill.: Charles C. Thomas Publishers, 1978, pp 76-7.

51. Noren GR, Kaplan EL, Staley NA. Nonrheumatic inflammatory cardiovascular disease. In: Moss AJ, Adams FH, Emmanouilides GC, eds. Heart Disease in Infants, Children, and Adolescents, 2nd ed. Baltimore: Williams and Wilkins Co., 1977, pp 559-76.

52. Norman MG, Smialek JE, Newman DE, Horenbala EJ. The postmortem examination of the abused child: Pathological, radiographic, and legal aspects. Perspect Pediatr Pathol 8:313-43, 1984.

53. Ongley PA, Nadas AS, Paul MH, Rudolph AM, Starkey GWB. Aortic stenosis in infants and children. Pediatrics 21:207-21, 1958.

54. Oppenheimer EH, Esterly JR. Pathology of cystic fibrosis: Review of the literature and comparison with 146 autopsied cases. Perspect Pediatr Pathol 2:241-78, 1975.

55. Patamasucon P, Siegel JD, McCracken GH. Streptococcal submandibular cellulitis in young infants. Pediatrics 67:378-80, 1981.

56. Potter EL, Craig JM. Pathology of the fetus and the infant, 3rd ed. Chicago: Year Book Medical Publishers, Inc., 1975, pp 350-3, 365, and 401.

57. Potter EL, Craig JM. Pathology of the fetus and the infant, 3rd ed. Chicago: Year Book Medical Publishers, Inc., 1975, p 506.

58. Robson AM. The pathophysiology of body fluids, in Chapter 5: General considerations in the care of sick children. In: Behrman RE, Vaughan VC, eds. Nelson Textbook of Pediatrics, 13th ed. Philadelphia: W.B. Saunders Co., 1987, pp 172-90.

59. Stern RC. Acute bronchiolitis, in Chapter 13: The respiratory system. In: Behrman RE, Vaughan VC, eds. Nelson Textbook of Pediatrics, 13th ed. Philadelphia: W.B. Saunders Co., 1987, pp 897-8.

60. Stern RC. Bacterial and viral pneumonias, in Chapter 13: The respiratory system. In: Behrman RE, Vaughan VC, eds. Nelson Textbook of Pediatrics, 13th ed. Philadelphia: W.B. Saunders Co., 1987, pp 899-905.

61. Stern L, Ramos AD, Wigglesworth FW. Congestive heart failure secondary to cerebral arteriovenous aneurysm in the newborn infant. Am J Dis Child 115:581-7, 1968.

62. Sturner WG. Chapter 11: Pediatric deaths. In: Curran WJ, McGarry AL, Petty CS, eds. Modern Legal Medicine, Psychiatry, and Forensic Science. Philadelphia: F.A. Davis Co., 1980, pp 226-8.

63. Trube-Becker E. The death of children following negligence. Social aspects. J Forens Sci 9:111-5, 1977.

64. Valdés-Dapena M, Arey JB. Boric acid poisoning: Three fatal cases with pancreatic inclusions and a review of the literature. J Pediatr 61:531-46, 1962.

65. Valdés-Dapena MA, Hummeler K. Sudden and unexpected death in infants. II. Viral infections as causative factors. J Pediatr 63:398-401, 1963.

66. Valdés-Dapena M, Poole C, Worley L. A clinical-radiologic-pathologic conference: Failure to thrive, anemia, and anasarca. J Pediatr 94:1005-9, 1979.

67. Wigglesworth JS. Abnormalities of venous return, in Chapter 11: The Cardiovascular system. In: Perinatal Pathology, Vol. 15, in Major Problems in Pathology. Philadelphia: W.B. Saunders Co., 1984, pp 216-7.

68. Wilson EF. Estimation of the age of cutaneous contusions in child abuse. Pediatrics 60:750-2, 1977.

69. Winstanley DP. Sudden death from multiple rhabdomyomata of the heart. J Pathol Bacteriol 81:249-51, 1961.

70. Wright HT, Okuyama K, McAllister RM. An infant fatality associated with Coxsackie B virus. J Pediatr 63:428-31, 1963.

CHAPTER **7**

INCIDENTAL OR INCONSEQUENTIAL LESIONS

INTRODUCTION

There are a number of lesions commonly encountered in cases of sudden infant death syndrome (SIDS) that, of themselves, could not possibly account for the infant's death. Some of these lesions are clearly congenital and others are obviously acquired. They are nevertheless irrelevant to the death of the baby and are presented in order that they will be recognized as such and not be mistaken for potential morbid or mortal lesions.

For the sake of simplicity these lesions are presented by organ system, including in each category both those which are congenital and those which are acquired.

The order of the organ system presentation corresponds to that in Chapter 3, Normal Histology of the Infant in the Postneonatal Period. Within each system, the lesions are dealt with as follows: (1) cellular injury and adaptation; (2) inflammation and repair; (3) fluid and hemodynamic derangements; (4) neoplastic lesions; (5) environmental lesions.

HEART

Patchy Interstitial Fibrosis

Occasionally the pathologist finds a patch of interstitial fibrosis in the myocardium that does not seem to be related to any historical or morphologic feature of the case. It must be assumed, then, that some incident occurred during the life of the infant that resulted in a focus of local death of muscle and subsequent scarring. Of itself, a tiny lesion of this sort, if not associated with the conduction system, could scarcely represent the cause of the death of an infant and would therefore be designated an incidental finding.

Case History

This white male infant was born at term, weighed 3090 grams at birth, and had no history of illness. He died at three months of age. His mother described only a little difficulty with his spitting up formula. He was found dead about four hours after his last feeding. He had been seen by his pediatrician for a regular well-baby visit on the day of his death and was found to be growing and developing normally. This case was originally felt to be a SIDS but was later turned around in the field with a diagnosis of interstitial pneumonia. However, after review by the Pathology Study Panel the case was reclassified as SIDS (Fig. 7–1).

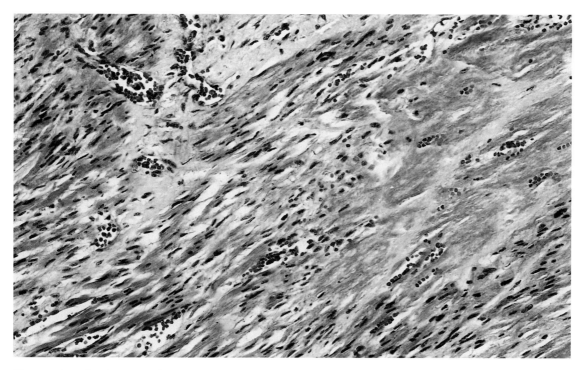

Figure 7–1.   Focal scarring of the myocardium. In the center and left lower corner is an almost solid sheet of avascular, acellular, dense fibrous connective tissue; the remainder is normal heart muscle.   160x

Calcium Deposit in a Papillary Muscle

When a tiny deposit of calcium is found in the very center of a papillary muscle the assumption is that at some time that infant experienced an episode of hypoxemia. That insult results in local death of myocardium, characteristically centrally in the distal portion of a papillary muscle because that portion receives blood flow last. A lesion of this size should be considered an incidental finding since it is much too small and insignificant to have altered the function of the heart.

Case History

This white female infant was born post-term, at 43 weeks of gestation, weighing 3515 grams. She died at four months of age. She had been in good health. The case was classified as SIDS (Fig. 7–2).

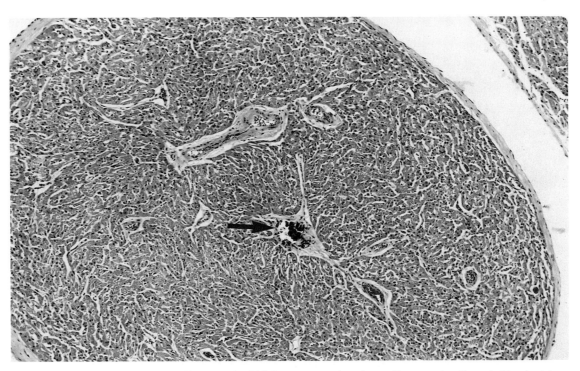

Figure 7–2. Calcium deposit in a papillary muscle. This is a cross section of a papillary muscle with central focal calcium deposition. At the tip of the arrow is a tiny aggregate of calcium at what is presumed to have been a minute focus of necrosis at some earlier time. 160x

Iatrogenic Lesions/Needle Track Marks

Infants who have experienced life-threatening episodes are often taken quickly to the nearest emergency room, where the physician may administer substances, such as epinephrine, into the heart. Cardiac injections sometimes induce intramyocardial bleeding, visible in microscopic sections of the heart muscle as localized accumulations of blood, forcing adjacent tissues apart. When the myocardium reveals these characteristic signs of epinephrine injection, there are, in some instances, corresponding large ecchymoses in adjacent epicardium. These accumulations exceed the size of the petechiae often encountered in the epicardium in SIDS deaths. This type of lesion does not occur in a baby of this age as a natural phenomenon.

Case History

This white female infant was born at term, 40 weeks of gestation, weighing 2863 grams. She died at 36 days of age. When it was realized that she was near death, cardiopulmonary resuscitation was attempted. A single needle mark in the skin of the chest was noted at autopsy. This case was classified as probable SIDS (Fig. 7–3).

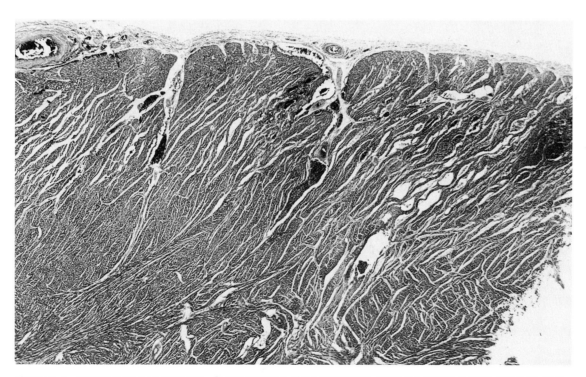

Figure 7–3. Needle track in myocardium. On the right side of the photograph, there is a cluster of clear, colorless, clefts in the myocardium paralleling muscle fibers and marking the site of injection. 15x

Case History

This black female infant was born at term with a birth weight of 3459 grams. She had been in good health before her death at 24 days of age. She was found unresponsive about five hours after last having been seen alive. She was rushed to the emergency room, where she was pronounced dead. Her death was designated a SIDS (Fig. 7–4).

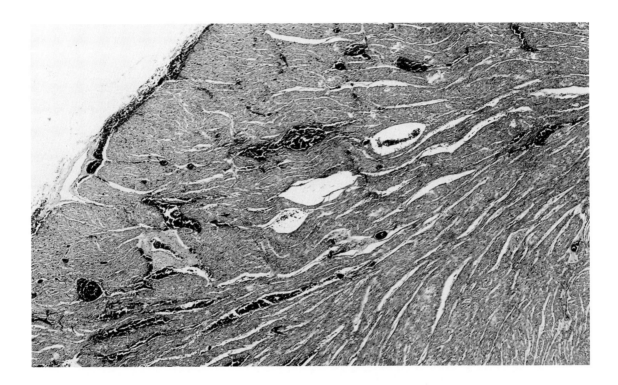

Figure 7–4. Needle track in myocardium. It is apparent here that both blood and some other fluid have dissected between muscle bundles and out into the epicardium. The several cleft-like and rounded spaces in the middle of the photograph appear to have contained some fluid other than blood. 25x

Epicardial Hemorrhage

Just as pleural and thymic petechiae are common features of a "typical" SIDS autopsy, so also are these same tiny hemorrhages in the epicardium. They probably reflect the same pathogenetic mechanism. However, intracardiac injections, during the agonal period, are apt to give rise to focal, single, somewhat larger collections of blood within the visceral pericardium.

Case History

This black male infant was born at term, small-for-gestational age with a birth weight of only 2041 grams. He died at nine weeks of age. He was found dead five hours after his last feeding. His death was classified as SIDS (Fig. 7–5).

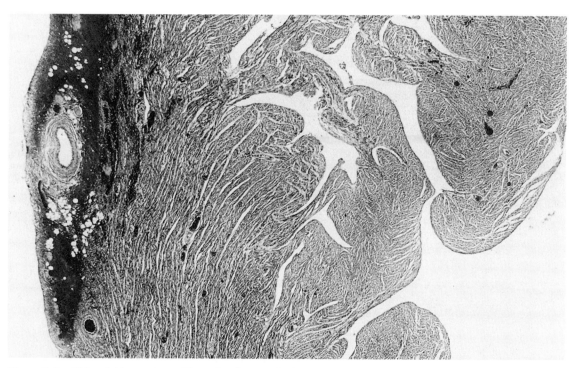

Figure 7–5. Epicardial hemorrhage. The epicardium, on the left, is markedly hemorrhagic and some blood has also infiltrated underlying muscle. This lesion is likely iatrogenic. 15x

Ischemic Necrosis

Infants who are hypoxemic for any reason are likely to have infarcts of the myocardium at autopsy. Infants with pneumonia or on artificial life-support systems are often hypoxemic; the effect of this is evident at autopsy in softening of the brain and in foci of ischemic necrosis of the myocardium. Both the brain and the heart muscle are extremely susceptible to oxygen deficiency. Acute necrosis, with the architecture intact, and with no reactive inflammation, affirms that this incidental lesion is of very recent origin.

The site of ischemic necrosis in the heart in infants is usually the tip of the papillary muscle because that is the last part of the myocardium to receive blood. This anatomic and physiologic circumstance is also responsible for focal calcium deposits in the same place.

Case History

This Hispanic female infant was born at term and weighed 3289 grams. Clinically, it was thought that she had died of pneumonia and, in fact, postmortem examination confirmed the clinical determination of pneumonia as the cause of death (Fig. 7–6).

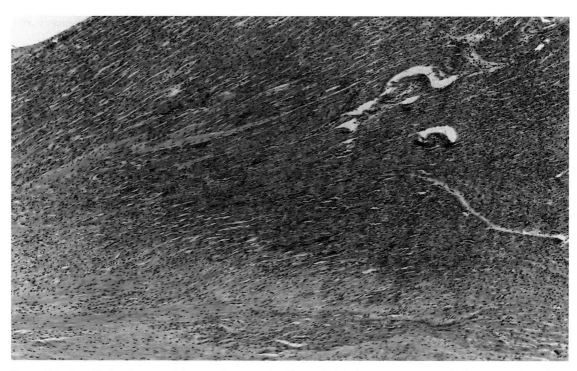

Figure 7–6. Focal ischemic necrosis in a papillary muscle. The central dark grey area, surrounded by engorged small vessels, is a very recent and focal infarct of the myocardium. It is the result of local ischemia, similar to, but more recent than, that which caused the calcium deposits seen in Figure 7–2. 100x

SYSTEMIC INFECTIONS

Cytomegalovirus Infection

It is not at all uncommon to encounter, as an incidental finding, at autopsy, the typical large cells of cytomegalovirus infection in both newborns and older infants. This infection may be acquired before, during, or after birth. The incidence is higher among lower socioeconomic groups.

When the infection is introduced into a family, it is likely that every susceptible member will develop the infection eventually, usually in the absence of recognizable disease. The virus is present in saliva, the secretions of the upper respiratory tract, spermatozoa, white blood cells, milk, urine, and feces. Contact with any of those sources may result in transmission of the infection.

The great majority of babies who have the infection, either congenital or acquired, remain asymptomatic. Very few become ill with the disease and even fewer die of it. The presence of a small number of characteristic cytomegalic cells at necropsy is not significant. They appear most often in the lungs and kidneys. Characteristically, in the kidney the presence of these cells is heralded by a focal, heavy infiltrate of lymphocytes (Fig. 7–9).

Immunodeficient children and some newborns succumb to the disease. Neonates with the generalized disease have widespread petechiae and hepatosplenomegaly. Other manifestations of cytomegalovirus infection include jaundice, purpura, microcephaly, cerebral calcifications, and chorioretinitis.

Case History

This black female infant was born at term weighing 3147 grams. She had been in good health, except for a minor eye infection two weeks before her death at three months of age. Her death was both sudden and unexpected. Autopsy revealed an early pneumonia and this incidental pulmonary cytomegalovirus infection. This case was classified a SIDS (Fig. 7–9).

Figure 7–7. Cytomegalovirus infection. This is a bronchiole at three different powers demonstrating cytomegalovirus infection. A (upper, facing page): Projecting from the otherwise smooth, thin, epithelial lining of the central bronchiole there are four prominent cells, each of which is large enough to be distinguished, even at this low power. 60x B (middle, facing page): In addition to the four large cells attached to the epithelial lining, there is one other cytomegalic cell floating in the lumen. 160x C (lower, facing page): In addition to the large nuclear mass, there is a crescent-shaped cluster of minute cytoplasmic inclusions aggregated along the bottom of the most prominent cell. 400x

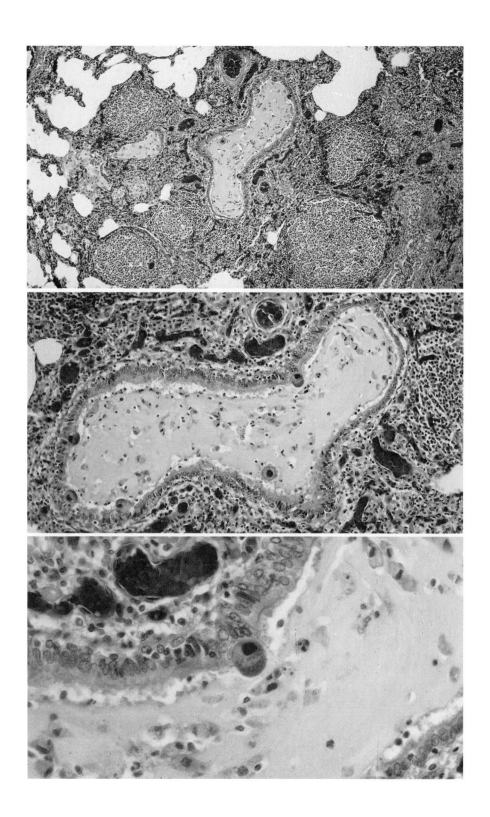

Case History

This white male infant was born at term weighing 2840 grams. He was almost two months old when he died. He had a history of noisy breathing and "breathing problems" since birth. He had also had one episode of pneumonitis. On the day of his death, his mother was wheeling him in his stroller outdoors; when she arrived home she found that he was dead. His death was designated a SIDS.

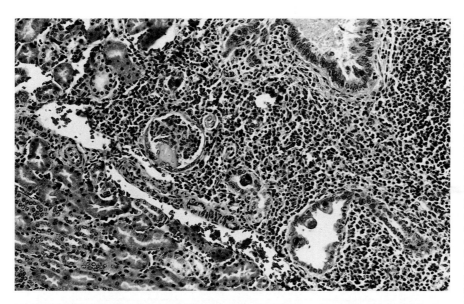

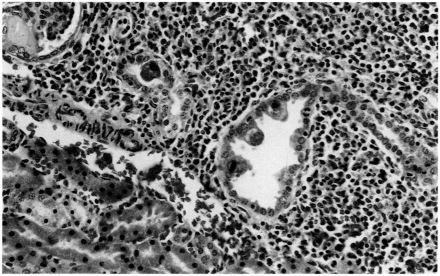

Figure 7–8.
Cytomegalovirus infection in the kidney. A (upper): This photomicrograph shows typical aggregates scattered in the cortex. They are characterized by the presence of innumerable, crowded lymphocytes where epithelial elements would be expected to be. The affected cells are most often apparent in the lining epithelium of tubules. One such dilated tubule appears in the right lower corner of this picture; at least three of its lining cells have been transformed by the cytomegalovirus. 160x
B (lower): An enlargement of the right lower quadrant of Figure 7–8A showing to better advantage the individual cytomegalic cells. 250x

Case History

This Hispanic male infant was born post-term, at 42 weeks of gestation, weighing 3270 grams. He was one and a half months old when he died. He was in good health prior to his sudden and unexpected death. The case was classified as SIDS (Fig. 7–9).

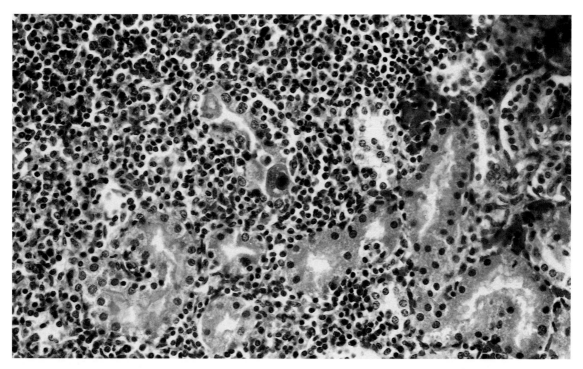

Figure 7–9. Cytomegalovirus infection in a kidney. This photograph shows clearly the morphology of a typical cytomegalic cell. For a single cell to be designated as affected by or bearing the cytomegalovirus, it should be many times larger than nearby epithelial cells of the same type. It also must display a central, intranuclear, dense, darkly stained body (viral forms by electron microscopy), surrounded by a clear halo, which is in turn rimmed by a delicate single dark line representing the nuclear membrane. Smaller cytoplasmic inclusions are usually apparent as well but can be seen only at higher magnification. A focal, heavy infiltrate of lymphocytes is also present, and is often seen in a kidney infected with cytomegalovirus. 250x

UPPER AIRWAY

Minimal to moderate inflammation of various parts of the upper airway (i.e., epiglottis, larynx, trachea, and bronchi) is found in approximately one-third of SIDS autopsies. It is generally agreed that lesions such as this would not be expected to take the life of an otherwise healthy infant in the first six months of life. Because babies of this age frequently experience upper airway inflammation and usually recover, such inflammatory processes, of minimal to moderate degree, when encountered at autopsy are considered inconsequential.

Epiglottitis

Life-threatening epiglottitis caused by *Hemophilus influenzae* does not occur in infants in the age range typical for SIDS (less than one year old), but has been seen occasionally in older infants (between one and two years of age).[6] On the other hand, mild viral inflammation is common at this age and relatively unimportant from the clinical standpoint.

Case History

This black female infant was born at term weighing 3175 grams. She had been well prior to her death at the age of three months. She was found dead in a supine position six hours after last having been seen alive. Her death was designated a SIDS (Fig. 7–10).

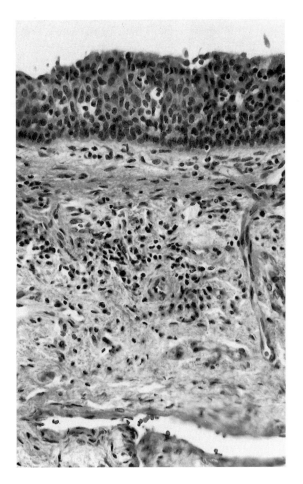

Figure 7–10. Epiglottitis. Just beneath the epithelium covering the epiglottis, which is partly respiratory and partly squamous, is a mild inflammatory exudate consisting almost exclusively of lymphocytes. This degree and type of inflammation is common in SIDS deaths in different parts of the upper airway, including the epiglottis. 250x

Tracheitis

Mild inflammation of tracheal mucosa is a common finding in SIDS autopsies. It may be viewed as part of the spectrum of viral infection of the upper airway. Of itself, it is of little clinical significance.

Case History

This black male infant was born at term weighing 3430 grams. He was almost five months old when he died. His mother reported that he had been well except for a cold in the two weeks prior to his death. This case was classified as probable SIDS (Fig. 7–11).

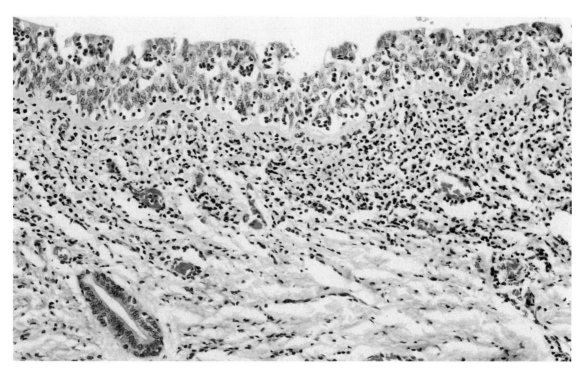

Figure 7– 11. Tracheitis. Just beneath the basement membrane there is a broad band of lymphocytic infiltration. 160x

LUNG

Bacterial Colonization

Sudden infant death syndrome occurs most frequently in the middle of the night. Because the body often lies at room temperature for hours afterward, it is common to find colonies of bacteria in the lung, where probably a few pedestrian agents had been at the moment of the child's death. In the dark, warm, moist, and richly proteinaceous medium, bacteria multiply rapidly so that histologic sections of lung may reveal round or oval masses of bacteria scattered about, often confined to an anatomical space such as the lumen of a blood vessel or an alveolus. In either case the logical assumption is that they were not there in masses at the moment of the baby's death and that they cannot be implicated in the etiology of the death.

In some instances, the bacteria cluster about an aspirated droplet of gastric contents; at other times, one can recognize an aspirated squamous cell, perhaps from the mouth, in the middle of the colony. Presumably, in those instances, the bacteria arrived in the lung together with the aspirated material or cell.

Case History

This Hispanic male infant was born at 38 weeks of gestation weighing 3010 grams. He was eight and a half months old at death. He had gastroenteritis for a few days before he died. His death was designated a SIDS (Fig. 7–12).

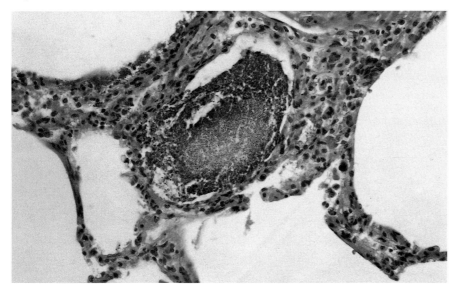

Figure 7–12. Postmortem bacterial colonization of lung. An oval mass of what appear to be cocci in an alveolar space appears in the center of the photograph. A colony of this size, in the absence of any inflammatory cells, is clearly incidental. 250x

Case History

This Hispanic female infant was born at 42 weeks of gestation with a weight of 3912 grams. She was three and a half months old when she died. Prior to her death she had a runny nose.

She was found dead, lying prone, her face in a pillow, just a few minutes after last having been seen alive. This case was classified as SIDS (Fig. 7–13).

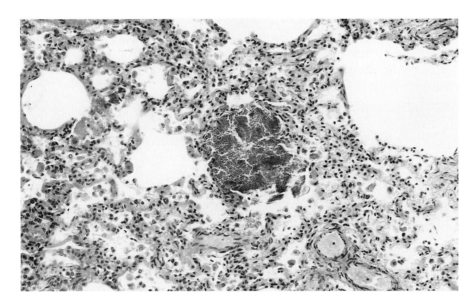

Figure 7–13.
Postmortem bacterial colonization of lung.
A (upper). There is a rounded colony of bacteria in an alveolus in the center of the photograph. 160x
B (lower): Higher magnification makes it clear that these are cocci. 250x

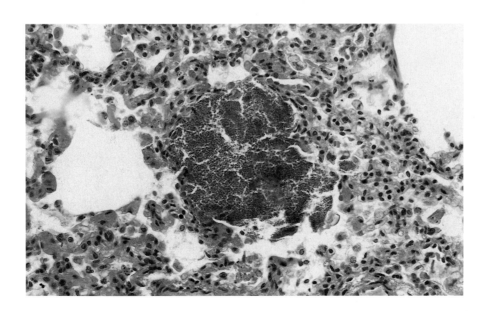

Patchy Overaeration

When attempts are made to resuscitate an infant, after the child has ceased respiration and has apparently died, air is forced into the lungs and trapped there. The infant lung has unique elasticity, which causes it to collapse after death. Presumably, in some cases, portions of lung proximal to the artificially induced air bubbles collapse and do not permit air in distal sites to flow out spontaneously. The histologic pattern created by postmortem "assisted pulmonary ventilation" is distinctive. It is characterized by the presence of widely separated, unnaturally round, smooth bubbles of air that far exceed the size of a normal alveolus or alveolar duct in that same section. There is also striking collapse of the lung between the "bubbles." This iatrogenic pattern is best perceived at very low magnification.

Case History

This Hispanic male infant was born at term with a birth weight of 3203 grams. He died at seven months of age. He had had a "cold" for one month prior to death. The case was classified as probable SIDS (Fig. 7–14).

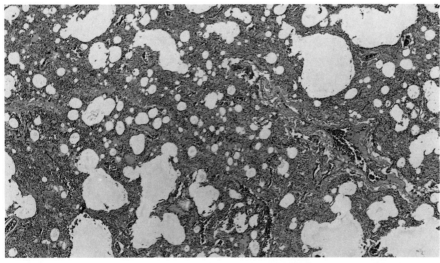

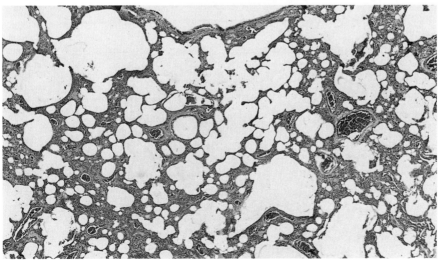

Figure 7–14. Patchy overaeration. This unique pattern of alternating overaeration and atelectasis is the result of agonal or postmortem assisted pulmonary ventilation. A (upper): The key feature of this incidental "lesion" is the distinctive, perfectly round profiles of the air spaces. 25x B (lower): In this tissue sample overaeration is a more prominent feature than atelectasis, whereas the opposite is true in Figure 7–15A. 25x

Case History

This black male infant was born at term and weighed 3440 grams. He died at six months of age. He had a cold at the time he died and was being treated for that. The case was classified as SIDS (Fig. 7–15).

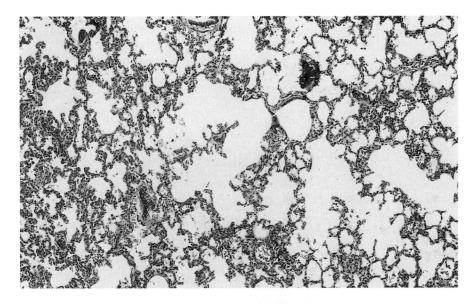

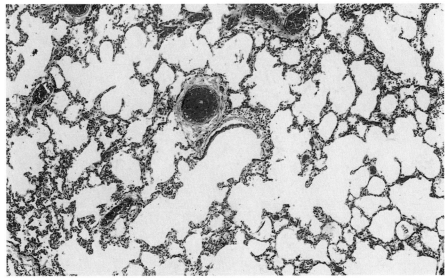

Figure 7–15.
Overexpansion of air spaces. Sometimes the forceful intro-duction of air into the lungs expands an entire acinus including the terminal bronchiole, alveolar duct, and alveoli. The morphologic result is a pattern of wide-open, branching air passages. A (upper): Over-expansion of air spaces demon-strating the typical branching of what are probably alveolar ducts. Compare the width of one of these branching airways in the center of the field, with the width of an apparently normal air space in the left lower corner. The smooth contours are a clue to the fact that they have been produced artificially, as normal infant alveoli in death are the shape of crumpled paper bags. 60x B (lower): This photograph demon-strates a markedly expanded terminal respiratory bronchiole communicating with an alveolar duct; both of them are patho-logically distended. Note the small size and irregular shapes of the normal air spaces in the left lower corner. 60x

Subpleural Emphysema

This is a special form of coalescence of air space that has been seen, especially in newborn babies who have spent some time in neonatal intensive care nurseries. It is associated with the use of assisted pulmonary ventilation in the neonatal intensive care nursery. However, it may be produced in other ways as well. It may be associated with prematurity.

The pattern is distinctive and consists of a single band of excessively expanded air spaces directly beneath the pleura. The individual enlarged spaces are elongate, and most of them are arranged side-by-side with their long axes at right angles to the pleura.

This lesion[20] was first observed in the early 1980's and later found in at least two of the infants in the NICHD study. Both had been born prematurely; both survived for about three and a half months. Apparently, the lesion itself has no deleterious clinical implications.

Case History

This black male infant was born prematurely, at 30 weeks of gestation, weighing 1106 grams. He was found dead in bed with his mother five hours after his last feeding at 16 weeks of age. This case was classified as SIDS (Fig. 7–16).

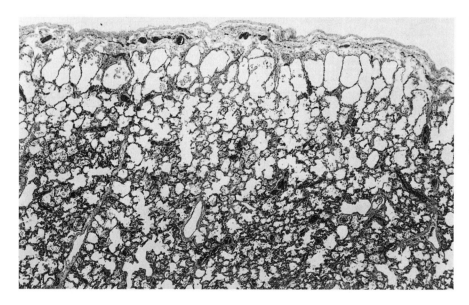

Figure 7–16. Subpleural emphysema. Illustrated here is this distinctive lesion in an infant lung. It is a subpleural band of excessive alveolar expansion. The palisade these spaces create is unique. 25x

Case History

This black male infant was born prematurely, at 35 weeks of gestation, weighing 1920 grams. He died at the age of three and a half months. His death was designated a SIDS.

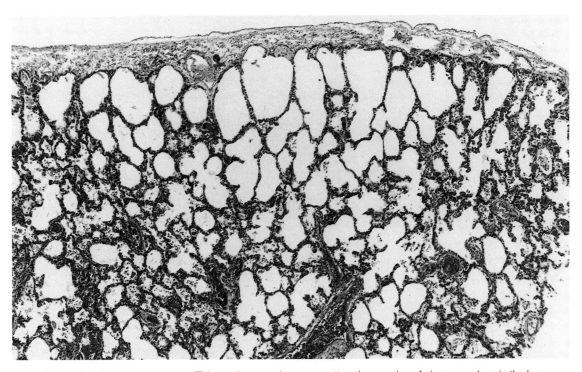

Figure 7–17. Subpleural emphysema. This section reveals some scattered expansion of air spaces deep in the lung. However, the remarkable subpleural band of elongate spaces all parallel to one another, and arranged at right angles to the pleura, is readily distinguished from the rest. 40x

Interstitial Pulmonary Emphysema

Whenever attempts are made to assist breathing, particularly in infants, and particularly if mechanical respirators are used, air can be forced into interstitial tissues in septa, around vessels. Large numbers of air bubbles in interlobular septa impair respiration by two mechanisms: (1) the air bubbles "splint" the septa, making them rigid, less flexible than normal, and (2) the "locked-in" air bubbles take up space in the thorax; if large enough and numerous enough, they can even compress surrounding alveoli.

In babies who die suddenly and unexpectedly at home, interstitial emphysema may be produced either by those persons present at the site who attempt mouth-to-mouth resuscitation, by medical personnel (with or without mechanical respirators), or by both.

In some cases, air bubbles in the septa are quite round, but in most instances, they are oval and arranged in the long axis of the septum. Sometimes they are clearly in connective tissue; in other instances they are within lymphatic channels; endothelial cells can be identified at their margins. Occasionally, it is difficult to decide whether a given set of enlarged lymphatics represents lymphangiectasia or air in lymph vessels. In most such instances, review of septa in a number of sections will clarify the issue. These lesions are easily overlooked. Hence, the autopsy pathologist should scan all lung sections at low power at the beginning of every microscopic study, looking for them systematically.

Case History

This black female infant was born prematurely, weighing only 1404 grams. She died at two and a half months of age. She remained in the hospital for one month after birth but was reported to have been well during that time. She was found dead in her bassinet at home two hours after last having been seen alive. The case was classified as SIDS (Fig. 7–18).

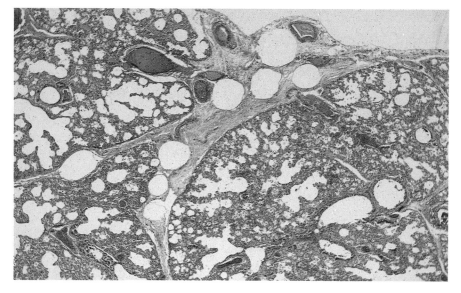

Figure 7–18. Interstitial pulmonary emphysema. In the middle of the photograph are at least eight perfectly round air bubbles trapped within connective tissue septa. It is said that this phenomenon can be produced in infants by their own powerful attempts to breathe, in pulmonary hyaline membrane disease, for example. However, nowadays it is probably more often induced by artificial ventilation, either mouth-to-mouth resuscitation or mechanical ventilatory assistance. 25x

Case History

This white male infant was born at term, at 38 weeks of gestation, weighing 2750 grams. He was 41 days of age when he died. He was reported to be in good health prior to his sudden death. He was simply found unresponsive while in bed with both of his parents. Cardiopulmonary resuscitation was attempted. His death was designated a SIDS (Fig. 7–19).

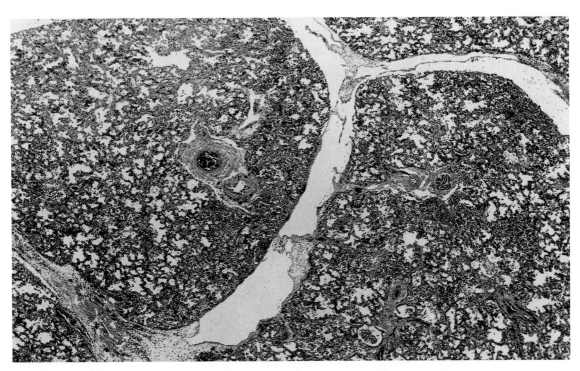

Figure 7–19. Interstitial pulmonary emphysema. In the left lower corner of the figure is a small hemorrhage within a septum and in the vicinity of interstitial emphysema; this association occurs frequently, presumably because small vessels in the septum are torn by the force of the entrance of air into the tissues. In the vertically oriented septum, in the middle of the picture, air appears in a long lymphatic vessel; the endothelial lining of the vessel is apparent at the lower end and on the right side. Superiorly, air seems to be located both within and out of such vascular channels. 25x

Macrophages in Alveoli

In almost any infant autopsy, a few scattered macrophages can usually be found in otherwise normal pulmonary alveoli. Small clusters of them are usually considered to be "within the range of normal" or not having any special significance. They are presumably the result of incidental, small episodes of aspiration, probably of fluid material.

Case History

This white male infant was born at term weighing 3842 grams. He was placed in a foster home and subsequently adopted. He died at five and a half months of age. He was in an infant seat, in a car, at the time of death. The case was classified as SIDS (Fig. 7-20).

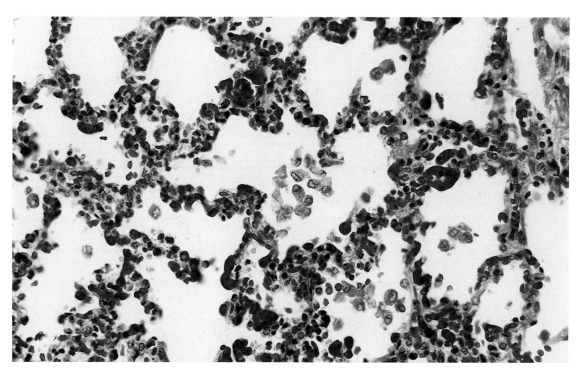

Figure 7–20. Macrophages in alveoli. In this picture there are approximately 12 open alveoli. In three of them, there are small clusters of up to 11 macrophages. No other liquid or solid material appeared here or elsewhere in these lungs. It is impossible to determine what etiologic factor induced the presence of the macrophages and, by themselves, they are of no consequence. 250x

Acute Aspiration of Gastric Content, Milk

It is not unusual to find rather homogeneous or amorphous, bluish-staining material in a few alveoli, alveolar ducts, bronchioles, and even bronchi in the lungs of infants who die suddenly and unexpectedly. It is assumed that this substance represents milk consumed by the child during the hours preceding death, which later found its way up the esophagus, and down into the airways.

The same material is found in the same places in autopsies on children of a similar age who die in hospitals. Some pediatric pathologists believe that it reflects an in vivo process and they will sign out such cases as "death due to massive aspiration of gastric content." Others are disinclined to accept the notion that an infant who is otherwise relatively well would permit that sort of insult to the airway. It is their belief that, if an infant's physiologic responses in the head and neck are intact, the baby will automatically spit out the vomitus rather than inhale it. They contend that only obtunded reflexes would allow massive aspiration to occur. They look upon such aspiration in an otherwise normal infant as an agonal event, the result of dysrhythmias in the complex interaction between breathing and swallowing that occur *while* the child is dying. They do not accept massive aspiration of vomitus as a cause of death.

Another possibility is that the milky fluid gets into the airway after death. Postmortem experiments with human bodies have shown that fluid in the stomach can be caused to move by gravity from the stomach into the pharynx and then down into the airways simply by repositioning the body. The body of an infant is more likely than that of an adult to be tilted into a head-down position between the time of death and the time of autopsy.

It also seems likely that vigorous attempts at resuscitation during the agonal or early postmortem period may displace gastric contents into the pharynx and airway.

Alternatively, if an infant actually does inhale vomitus, especially repeatedly, it is presumed that he or she must be suffering from a pathologic condition that would permit aspiration of foreign matter. It follows then that such a child is, to some extent, neurologically handicapped. In fact, children with brain damage do aspirate regurgitated matter regularly; to prevent that, they are, in many instances, hospitalized and subjected to fundoplication.

Case History

This white male infant was born at term, at 38 weeks of gestation, weighing 2770 grams. Although he was reported to be gaining weight slowly, there was no history of recent illness. He was 35 days old when he died. The case was classified as probable SIDS (Fig. 7–21).

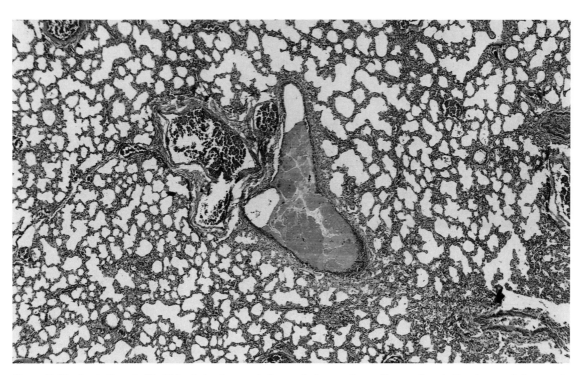

Figure 7–21. Aspiration of milk. This photomicrograph demonstrates a rather uniform pattern in the sizes and shapes of alveolar ducts and alveoli. It would appear that neither agonal nor postmortem attempts at resuscitation were made in this case because we see here none of the perfectly round, excessively large "bubbles" of air found in such instances. However, the one large bronchiole in the center of the picture is almost entirely filled with homogeneous material, which was light blue in hematoxylin and eosin stains. This is how milk, recently aspirated, looks in routine microscopic sections.* 25x

* NOTE: In this case, it would appear that the infant had a recurring problem with aspiration because, in other sections of lung, there were "milk granulomas" as well, attesting to at least one earlier episode (See Figure 7–27, p. 182).

Case History

This black male infant was born at 37 weeks of gestation weighing 2730 grams. He was eight weeks old at death. His death was designated a SIDS (Fig. 7–22).

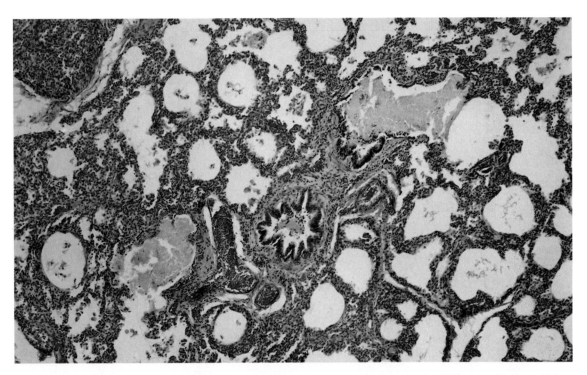

Figure 7–22.   Aspiration of milk. On each side of the central bronchiole, milky fluid completely fills a terminal bronchiole and an alveolar duct. The milk may have been aspirated as an agonal event or accidentally during resuscitation. 60x

Case History

This Hispanic female infant was born at 42 weeks of gestation with a weight of 3912 grams. She was three and a half months old when she died. Prior to her death she had had a runny nose. She was found dead, lying prone, her face in a pillow, just a few minutes after last having been seen alive. This case was classified as SIDS (Fig. 7–23).

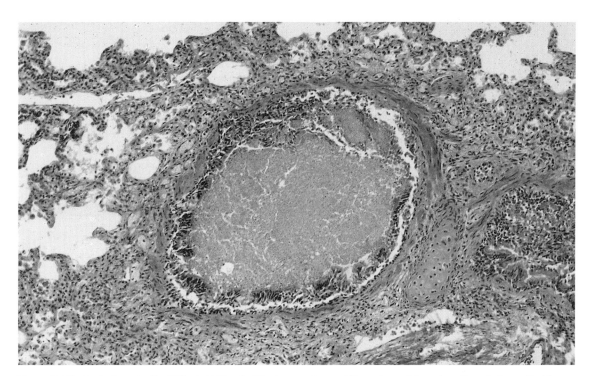

Figure 7–23. Aspiration of milk. Milky fluid fills all of the lumen of a small bronchus. A bar of cartilage in the wall of the bronchus is evident in the photograph, on the right. 100x

Case History

This black female infant was born at 37 weeks of gestation with a birth weight of 2750 grams. She was two months old when she died. She had diarrhea for two days before death but no other illnesses. She was in bed with her mother when found unresponsive, lying prone, with her head turned to one side. This case was classified as SIDS (Fig. 7–24).

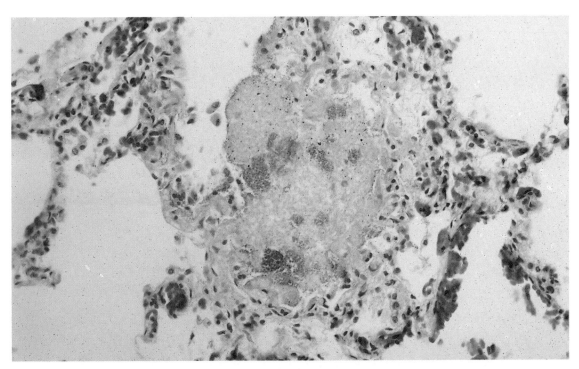

Figure 7–24. Aspiration of milk. This figure illustrates a single air space which is about half filled with milk. The several discrete aggregates of tiny gray to black dots in it are colonies of bacteria, which probably multiplied after the death of the baby, having been present singly or in small groups within the fluid at the time of aspiration. 250x

Acute Aspiration of Solid Material

In older infants who have begun to eat solid food, the same sort of mechanism or mechanisms responsible for the "aspiration" of milky gastric content may be responsible for the appearance of particles of solid food in small airways.

Case History

This Asian male infant was born at 42 weeks of gestation with a birth weight of 3912 grams. He was 16 weeks old at death. He was said to have had "fluid on his lungs" after birth. He was fed before being put down on the sofa on the day of his death and was found there, unresponsive, three hours later. Despite attempts at resuscitation he died at that time. His death was designated a SIDS (Fig. 7–25).

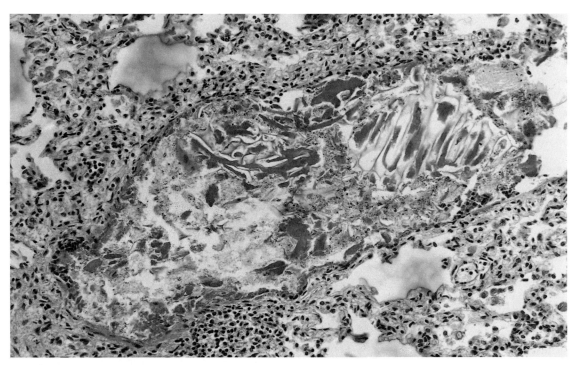

Figure 7–25. Aspirated solid matter. The anatomical structure in the center of the photograph is probably a bronchiole, denuded of its lining epithelium. Its lumen is entirely filled with "aspirated" material; although much of it is amorphous, there are also arcs and bands of some solid material in it. A small amount, around the middle of the photograph, appears to be vegetable in nature. 160x

Case History

This black male infant was born prematurely with a weight of 2296 grams. He died at ten weeks of age. He was hospitalized once for bronchiolitis, and at that time, an electrocardiogram showed sinus tachycardia. On the day of death he had been vomiting. He died on the way to the hospital. His death was designated a SIDS (Fig. 7–26).

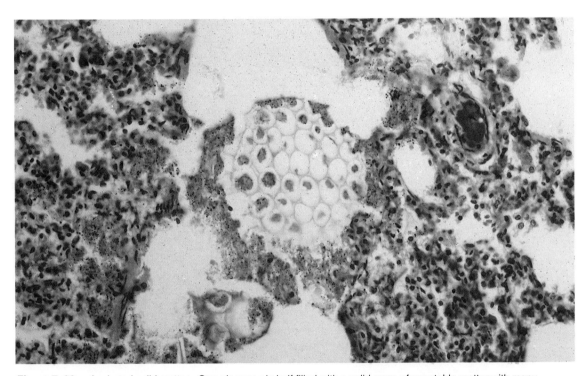

Figure 7–26. Aspirated solid matter. One air space is half filled with a solid mass of vegetable matter with many uniform, sharply demarcated cells. This is interpreted as being "aspirated" gastric content. 250x

Solitary "Aspiration Granulomas"

On occasion, sections from an infant autopsy reveal a single "milk granuloma" in an otherwise unremarkable lung. This lesion probably reflects an isolated incident rather than a continuing or chronic problem (see Figs. 8–15 through 8–18, Chronic Aspiration, Chapter 8, "The Gray Zone"). When a granuloma is isolated and solitary it is assumed that the infant's integration of swallowing and breathing was normal and that the lesion is not of any clinical or pathological consequence.

Case History

This white male infant was born at term, at 38 weeks of gestation, weighing 2770 grams. He died at 35 days of age. Although he was reported to be gaining weight slowly, there was no history of recent illness. This case was classified as probable SIDS (Fig. 7–27).

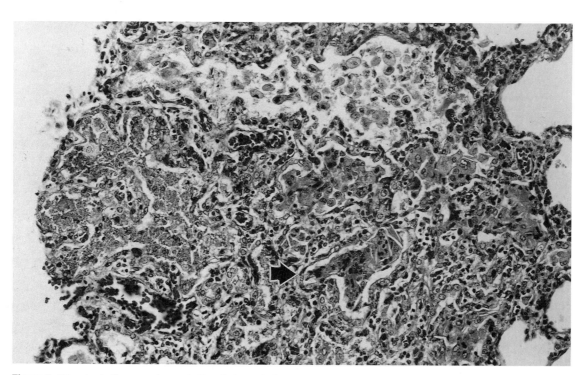

Figure 7–27. Aspiration granuloma. In the photograph there are several aggregates of macrophages. One of them, marked with an arrow, contains a small mass of amorphous dark colored material with cholesterol clefts in it. 160x

Case History

This white male infant was born at term with a birth weight of 3204 grams. He died at the age of two months. He was found dead six and a half hours after last having been seen alive. His death was designated a SIDS (Fig. 7–28).

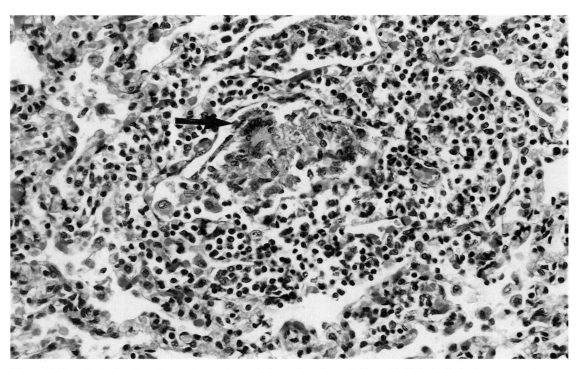

Figure 7–28. Aspiration granuloma. A granuloma similar to that shown in Figure 7–27, but with far fewer macrophages and one possible multinucleated giant cell (arrow). 250x

Case History

This Asian male infant was born at term with a birth weight of 3480 grams. He was almost two months old when he died. This case was classified as SIDS (Fig. 7–29).

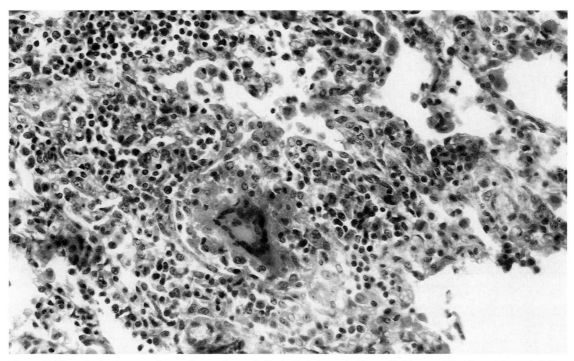

Figure 7–29. Aspiration granuloma. A granuloma similar to that shown in Figure 7–28 except that it contains a definite giant cell, apparently of the Langhans type. 250x

Case History

This white male infant was born at term weighing 3501 grams. He was one year and three months of age at death. He died of miliary tuberculosis (Fig. 7–30).

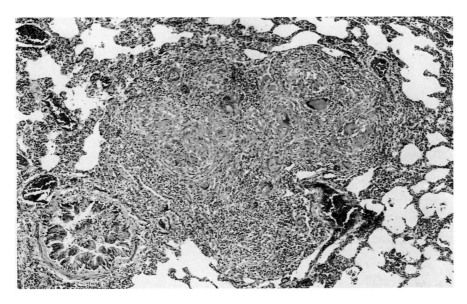

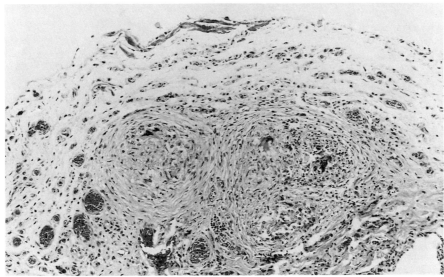

Figure 7–30.
Tuberculous granuloma of the lung. Both of these photographs are of tuberculous granulomas of the lung and are presented here for purposes of contrast with the preceding figures. The tubercles depicted in these two figures are more solid, compact, and epithelioid in nature than are those produced by the aspiration of milk. They do not contain the typical amorphous gray material centrally which represents aspirated milk, nor do they bear cholesterol clefts. Also, the aggregate of granulomas in Figure 7–30A is not subpleural, as milk granulomas usually are. Instead, this cluster of granulomas is immediately adjacent to a bronchiole of fair size, obviously at some distance from the pleura. A (upper): 60x B (lower): 100x

Bronchiolitis, Minimal

Frequently, a baby who dies of SIDS will be reported as having had an upper respiratory infection at the time of death or for a few days before death.

In such cases, bronchiolitis may be observed in microscopic sections of the lung at necropsy, i.e., one or two affected bronchioles in one or two of the five sections. Sometimes the infiltrate consists of lymphocytes, and cuffs the bronchiole like a dark cylinder. Less commonly, the infiltrate consists of, or includes, neutrophils. These cellular infiltrates are usually heaviest around the epithelial lining and only a few cells seem to be migrating through it. On occasion there are crowds of these cells in the lumen, sometimes mixed with mucus.

When affected bronchioles are few in number, as described above, and not dramatically inflamed, it is unlikely that this lesion alone can have accounted for the baby's death. Very few of the many babies diagnosed by their physi-cians as having bronchiolitis die. The mortality among hospitalized patients with bronchiolitis due to respiratory syncytial virus infection is about two percent.[8] However, the case fatality rate for all acute bronchiolitis in infants is below one percent.[9] When death does occur in such a mild case, it must be assumed that unknown, unrecognized factors were fundamentally responsible for the death, and the infant's demise remains basically unexplained because no one knows what those unknown elements are.

Case History

This black male infant was born at term weighing 3130 grams. He was ten months old when he died. He had a history of frequent colds and had had a severe one accompanied by difficulty in breathing the day before death. This case was classified as SIDS with bronchiolitis (Fig. 7–31).

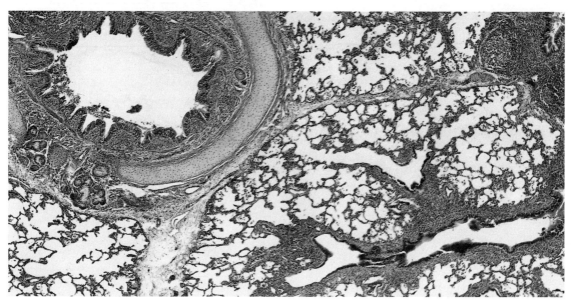

Figure 7–31. Bronchiolitis. There is a bronchus, cut in cross section, in the left upper corner of this photograph and another, sectioned longitudinally, in the right lower corner. The wall of each is thickened by the presence of a peripheral cuff of inflammatory cells, most of which are lymphocytes. The lumina are empty. Essentially all bronchioles, including terminal respiratory bronchioles, had a similar degree of lymphocyte cuffing. The amount of lymphoid tissue is slightly more than expected for this baby's age. The presence of bronchioles such as these indicates that the baby had bronchiolitis when death occurred, but it is difficult to attribute the death of an apparently healthy baby to a lesion as minor as this. 25x

Case History

This baby was Filipino, a female, two and a half months of age at death. She had been born at term weighing 2835 grams. She had a "tight cough" for a week before death. Her condition was improving when she was found unresponsive in her bassinet, three and a half hours after having last been seen alive. Her death was designated a SIDS with bronchiolitis (Fig. 7–32).

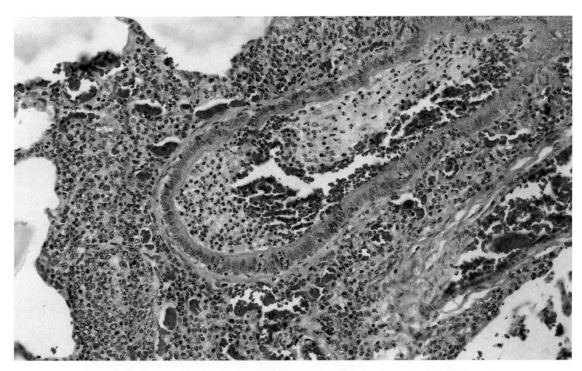

Figure 7–32. Bronchiolitis. This photograph shows inflammatory cells not only around the wall of the bronchiole and in it, but also in the epithelium and in the lumen, where they are mixed with mucus. The majority of these inflammatory cells seem to be neutrophils rather than lymphocytes. Essentially all large bronchioles of all five lung sections showed these changes; however, the smaller bronchioles were not involved, and there was no evidence of bronchpneumonia. 160x

Bronchopneumonia, Minimal

Occasionally, infants who succumb to SIDS have early or minimal bronchopneumonia at the time. The essential question in these cases is whether or not the disease was sufficiently grave to have caused death. More often than not, it appears to be a lesion an otherwise healthy infant ought to have survived. In such instances, it is our custom to designate the death as being unexplained and, therefore, in accordance with the definition of SIDS.

Case History

This black female infant was born at term and weighed 3147 grams. She died at three months of age. She was apparently in good health except for an eye infection two weeks before death. She was found dead, quite unexpectedly, in a supine position. This case was classified as SIDS (Fig. 7–33).

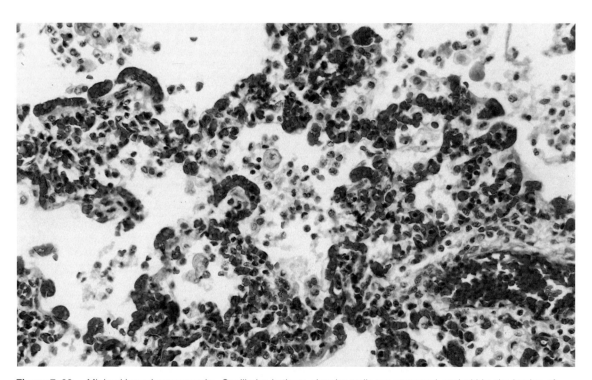

Figure 7–33. Minimal bronchopneumonia. Capillaries in these alveolar walls are engorged, and within the lumina of alveoli there are moderate numbers of neutrophils and macrophages. This was an isolated finding in only one section of lung. 250x

SPLEEN

Extramedullary Hematopoiesis

Extramedullary hematopoiesis (EMH) occurs in several organs in infants of this age, apparently in response to anemia or hypoxemia. Other common sites of extramedullary hematopoiesis are liver and thymus (see Figs. 7–44, 7–45, and 7– 54).

Case History

This black male infant was born at 26 weeks of gestation with a weight of 710 grams. He died at three months of age. He had a slight cold for three days prior to death but there was no other history of recent illness. He was found dead in bed with his mother six and a half hours after his last feeding. His death was designated a probable SIDS (Fig. 7–34).

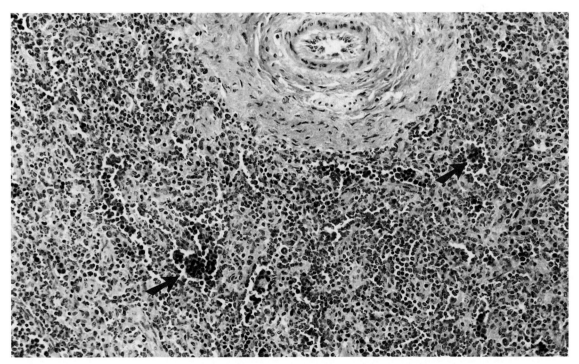

Figure 7–34. Extramedullary hematopoiesis in the spleen. This photomicrograph shows the splenic red pulp with a single medium-sized artery near the middle of the top. Scattered below it, to the right of the middle and downward, are approximately eight clusters (two marked with arrows) of small dark nuclei, very sharply demarcated and seeming to have scarcely any cytoplasm. These are clumps of developing erythrocytes. 160x

KIDNEY

Focal Subcapsular Scars

Focal subcapsular scars are common lesions, even in infants. Each represents a past local injury. They usually have no serious clinical implications and they do not contribute to death.

Case History

This white male infant was born prematurely at 36 weeks of gestation and weighed 2041 grams. He died when he was almost four months old. This case was classified as probable SIDS (Fig. 7–35).

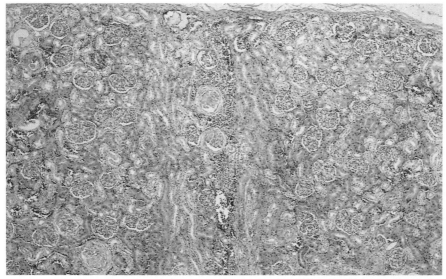

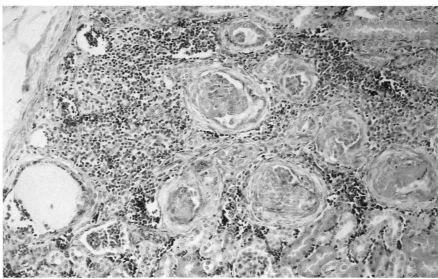

Figure 7–35. Focal subcapsular scar in the kidney.
A (upper): These lesions are usually pyramidal with their bases against the capsular surface of the organ. The one in this photograph is quite slender and elongate. The tiny cyst next to it, just below the capsule, is no doubt causally related to it. One of the larger glomeruli to the left of the scar also has suffered in the common insult with pericapsular scarring and scarring of the glomerular tufts as well. 60x
B (lower): Taken from the same case, this photomicrograph illustrates a similar subcapsular scar at considerably higher magnification. The background of lymphocytes in connective tissue is a constant feature of such lesions. The six or so still recognizable glomeruli within the lesion display various stages of scarring and obliteration. 160x

Subcapsular Microcysts

Occasional subcapsular microcysts in the kidney are not of particular significance, any more than are occasional sclerotic glomeruli. The presence of many, however, should arouse suspicion concerning their association with other congenital abnormalities, diseases, or syndromes.

Case History

This white female infant was born at 37 weeks of gestation and weighed 2820 grams. She was two months old when she died. She had a cold for a week before death and was found dead five hours after last having been seen alive. Her death was designated a SIDS (Fig. 7–36).

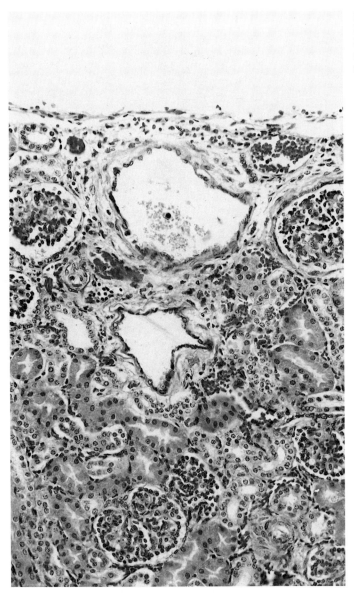

Figure 7–36. Subcapsular microcysts of the kidney. Just beneath the capsule of the kidney are two tiny, epithelial-lined cysts. It is not unusual to find a few such cysts in a section of otherwise normal kidney. 160x

Focal Calcium Deposits

Focal deposits of calcium are common, inconsequential lesions observed with fair frequency in the cortex of both adult and infant kidneys. They probably represent sites of old injury and focal cell death to which calcium has been bound.

Case History

This black female infant was born at term weighing 3232 grams. She was almost three months old at death. Her death was designated a SIDS (Fig. 7–37).

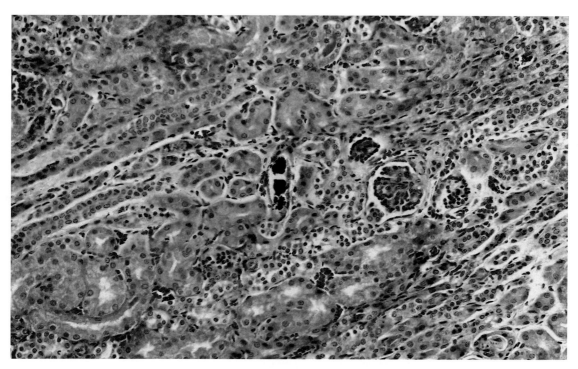

Figure 7–37. Focal calcium deposits. Both this figure and the next one illustrate focal calcium deposits. They were taken from different autopsies. 250x

Case History

This Hispanic female infant was born at term weighing 4000 grams. She was two months old when she died. She had become listless and droopy three days before her death and was diagnosed clinically as having an upper respiratory illness and gastroenteritis. Her death was probably due to gastroenteritis (Fig. 7–38).

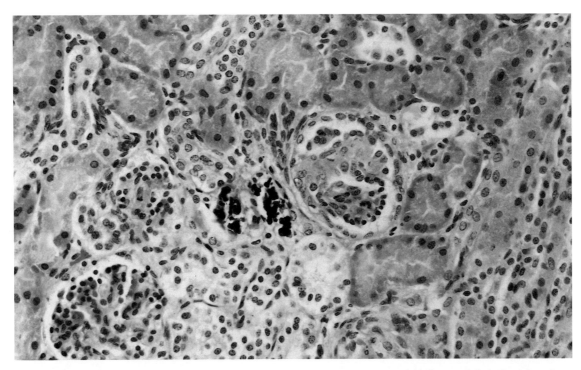

Figure 7–38. Focal calcium deposits. This common, inconsequential lesion occurs fairly frequently in both adult and infant kidneys. 160x

Nodular Renal Blastema

Nodular renal blastema is a relatively common finding in autopsies on infants in the first year of life. These lesions are frequently multiple and usually located just beneath the capsule. Each consists of microscopic clusters of immature metanephric blastema. They were first described in infants with trisomy 18 and in children with Wilms tumor.[3,4] They are also seen in infants with trisomy 13 as well as normal infants.[8]

Case History

This black male infant was born at term with a weight of 3544 grams. He was almost two months old when he died. He had no history of prior illness. His death was designated a probable SIDS (Figs. 7–39 and 7–40).

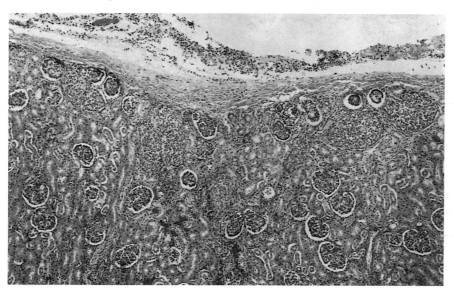

Figure 7–39. Nodular renal blastema. This photomicrograph shows, just beneath the capsule of the kidney, several (at least four) discrete, solid masses of nodular renal blastema. 60x

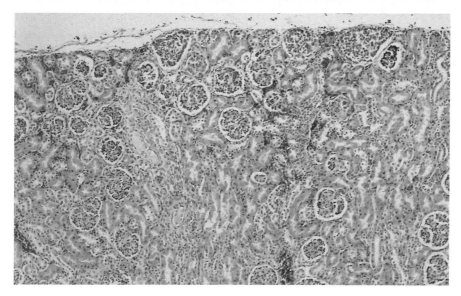

Figure 7– 40. Higher magnification of nodular renal blastema. The lesion is composed of undifferentiated small round to oval cells. 250x

Case History

This white male infant was born prematurely at 34 weeks of gestation and weighed 2084 grams. He was kept in the hospital for two months because of a "breathing problem." He died at four months of age. The case was classified as SIDS (Fig. 7–41).

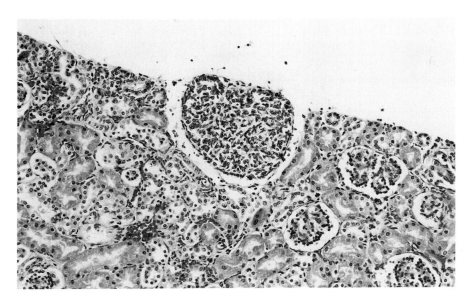
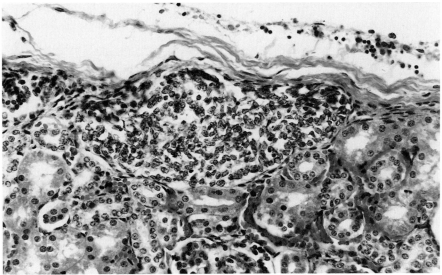

Figure 7–41. Nodular renal blastema. Both of these photographs illustrate nodular renal blastema in the usual place, just beneath the capsule of the kidney.
A (upper): 160x
B (lower): 250x

GASTROINTESTINAL TRACT

Ectopic Rests of Gastric Mucosa in the Esophagus

Ectopic rests of gastric mucosa in the esophagus have no clinical significance. They are frequently recognized grossly in infant autopsies appearing as tiny, discrete, sharply demarcated, slightly elevated, slightly granular, ovoid, light pink patches, against the white of surrounding esophageal mucosa, at the level of the larynx. They are usually located anteriorly and average 2-3 mm in greatest dimension in the newborn. They do not seem to be in any way related to Barrett's esophagus because they are never located in the lowest third of that organ.[16]

Case History

This white female infant was born at term with a birth weight of 3856 grams. She was six weeks old when she died. Her death was designated a probable SIDS (Fig. 7–42).

Figure 7–42. Ectopic rests of gastric mucosa in the esophagus. These two photographs illustrate a typical example of this common choristoma. It is apparent here that the patch of gastric mucosa is characteristically neither wide nor deep.
A (upper, facing page): 15x
B (lower, facing page): 40x

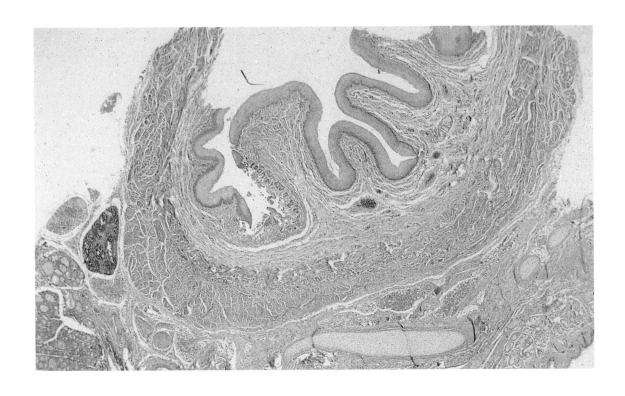

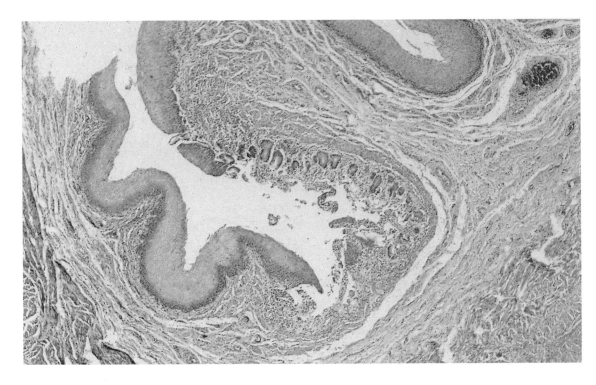

Inflammation of the Cardioesophageal Junction

Inflammation of the cardioesophageal junction is rare in infants who die of SIDS. One of the routine sections provided to the panel in every case was a longitudinal section of this junction. For many years, it has been assumed that some infants who die of sudden infant death syndrome do so because of repetitive gastroesophageal reflux, resulting in spasmodic airway obstruction. This hypothesis still has not been proved or disproved. The studies that would be required to support it are extremely difficult to mount. Of the 757 singleton SIDS cases in the NICHD study, it was possible to obtain only two convincing cases of cardioesophageal inflammation. However, a more thorough scrutiny of the entire series of sections by an authority on the subject of reflux effects on the lower end of the esophagus might reveal histologic details that were missed by the Pathology Study Panel.

In the two cases in this group, it is interesting to note that the inflammatory process is predominantly lymphocytic.

Case History

This black female infant was born at 38 weeks of gestational age with a birth weight of 2551 grams. She was said to have been in good health before her death. She was found dead in her crib at three and a half months of age. This case was classified as definite SIDS (Fig. 7–43).

Figure 7–43. Cardioesophageal junction with heavy lymphocytic infiltration. A (upper, facing page): This picture provides a low-power view of the distal end of the esophagus immediately above the stomach. Note that there is a heavy infiltrate of lymphocytes in the lower part of the mucosa between the basement membrane of the epithelium and the muscularis mucosae. The cause and clinical significance of this esophagitis remain unknown to us. It may have been caused by chronic reflux of gastric content. 60x   B (lower, facing page): This is an enlargement of the central portion of Figure 43A. At this magnification, inflammatory cells can be discerned *within* the epithelium as well as below it. 250x

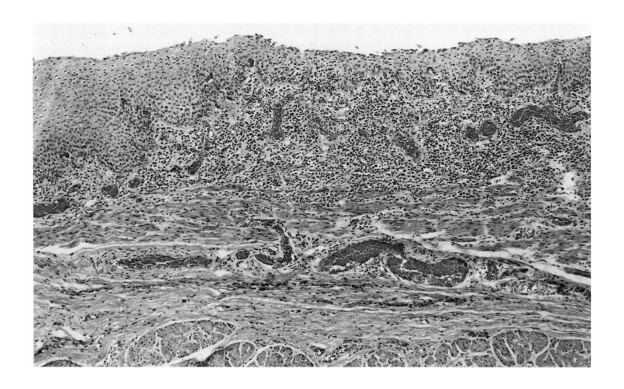

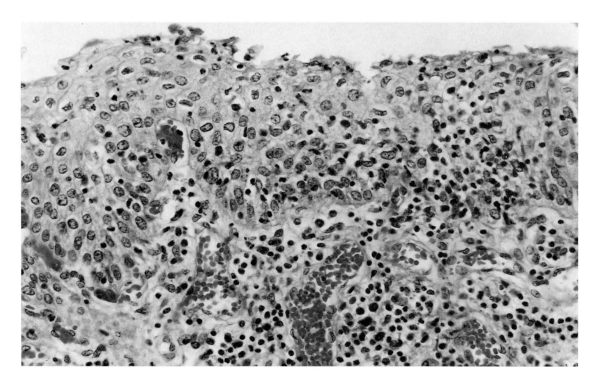

LIVER

Extramedullary Hematopoiesis

Many infants who succumb to SIDS have aberrant foci of hematopoiesis within the hepatic parenchyma. This abnormal production of red cells occurs more frequently among infants who die of SIDS than it does among normal babies.[1,2] This has been shown not only for infants of the same postnatal age, but also for those of the same postconceptual age.

How these foci are to be interpreted remains a question. One might speculate that some SIDS infants are anemic or chronically hypoxemic for other reasons.[13,14,17,18,21]

Case History

This black male infant was born at 26 weeks of gestation with a weight of 710 grams. He died at three months of age. He had a slight cold for three days prior to his death but there was no other history of recent illness. He was found dead in bed with his mother six and a half hours after his last feeding. His death was designated a probable SIDS (Fig. 7–44 and 7–45B).

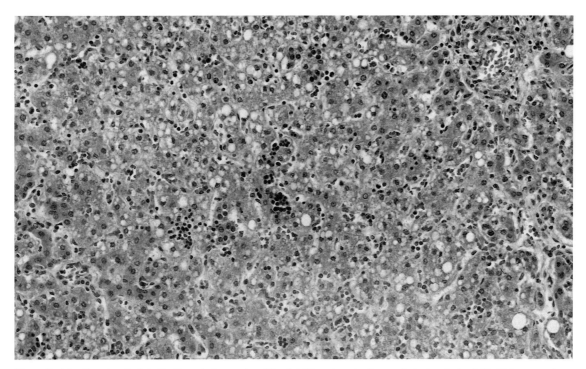

Figure 7–44. Hematopoiesis in the liver. In the center of the field there is a single, small cluster of about 10-15 tiny, round, dense, black nuclei. These are developing erythrocytes. See Figure 7–45B for higher power view of this case. 160x

Case History

This black male infant was born with a low birth weight, 2126 grams, at 37 weeks of gestation. The baby's mother had been treated for hypertension during pregnancy. Nevertheless, the infant was purported to have been in good health prior to his death at 41 days of age. He was found unresponsive, face down in his crib, ten hours after having last been seen alive. This case was classified as SIDS (Fig. 7–45A).

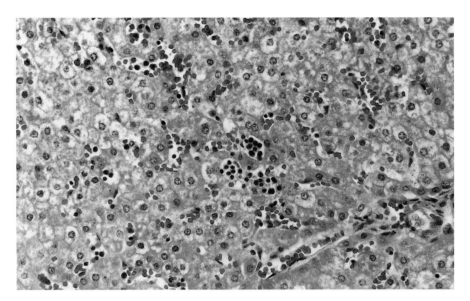

Figure 7–45.
Hematopoiesis in the liver. The previous figure, and these two, show, at progressivley increasing degrees of magnification, typical islands of hemato-poiesis (here, mostly erythropoiesis) in the infant liver.
A (upper): 250x
B (lower): This is an enlargement of the central portion of Figure 7–44. 400x

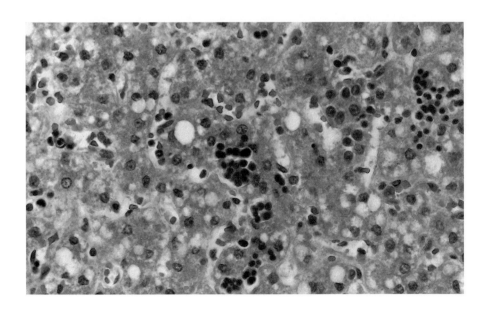

Fatty Change

Mild to moderate fatty change in the liver, seen microscopically is not an uncommon accompaniment of SIDS and has no special clinical significance that we are aware of. However, it is said that nutritional deprivation produces fatty change in the liver. In an infant of this age, a relatively short period of fasting, such as might occur during an episode of gastroenteritis, could have produced the effect illustrated here (Fig. 7–46).

Case History

This black male infant was born at term, at 41 weeks of gestation, weighing 3033 grams. He had diarrhea just before death. A doctor had seen the baby for that problem but had sent him home with his mother. The baby was not considered to be seriously ill. He was found unresponsive in his crib seven hours after his last feeding. He was 52 days old when he died. The case was classified as SIDS (Fig. 7–46).

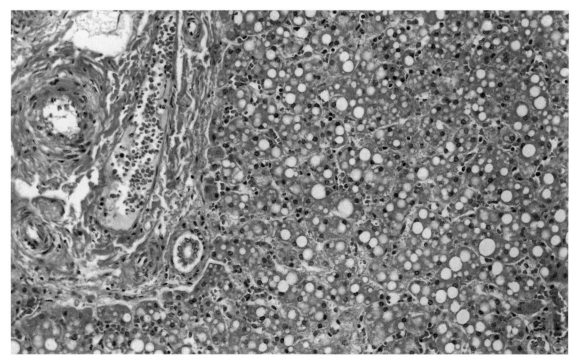

Figure 7–46. Fatty change in the liver. Individual, intracytoplasmic lipid vacuoles are large and push nuclei to the edges of cells. 160x

Hemangioma

Hemangioma of the liver is a recognized finding in infant autopsies. These lesions are hamartomas and, in babies, are usually small, less than 1 cm in greatest diameter. To the naked eye they appear to be dark purple and discrete, with slightly sunken and spongy cut surfaces. Each is made up of a congerie of capillary-like or sinusoidal channels, lined by flattened endothelial cells. Although they are not encapsulated, they do have sharp margins.

Case History

This white male infant, the second-born of twins, was delivered at 34 weeks of gestation with a weight of 2098 grams. He was almost six months old when he died. His death was designated a SIDS (Fig. 7–47).

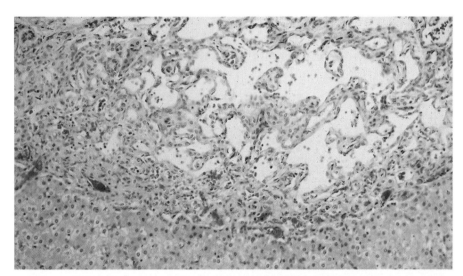

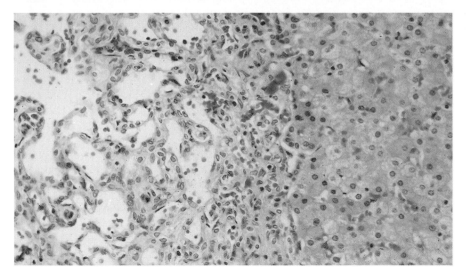

Figure 7–47. Liver, hemangioma. These two photographs demonstrate a hemangioma of the liver, at medium and high magnification.
A (upper): 160x
B (lower): 250x

PANCREAS

Ectopic Splenic Tissue in the Tail of the Pancreas

Tiny spherical accessory spleens are commonly encountered in autopsies on newborn infants, usually in the vicinity of the hilus of the spleen. Less common is the sort of arrangement in which one of those extra little spleens is nestled within the distal end of the tail of the pancreas. In some instances, such islands are separated from pancreatic tissue; however, sometimes, as is illustrated here, there is no clear separation.

Case History

This white male infant was born post-term at 43 weeks of gestation with a weight of 3190 grams. He died at 14 months of age. His clinical history was apparently normal; however, he had measles two weeks before his death. The case was designated a SIDS (Fig. 7–48).

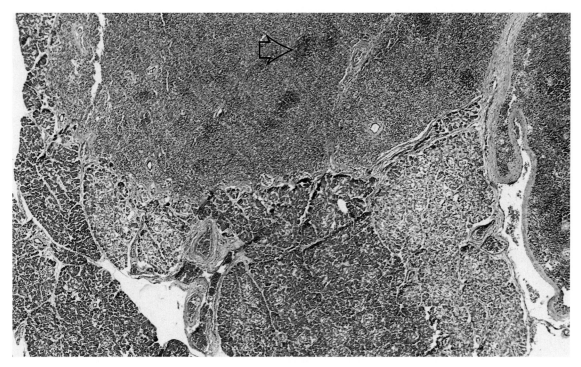

Figure 7– 48. Nodule of aberrant splenic tissue within the pancreas. The lobulate structure in the lower half of the photograph represents the tail of the pancreas. The more or less homogeneous gray mass in the upper half, with its inferior convexity almost blending with the pancreas, is an aberrant nodule of splenic tissue embedded in the tip of the tail of the pancreas. The darker gray patches in the splenic tissue (open arrow) represent white pulp or malpighian corpuscles. 25x

ADRENAL

Hemorrhage into and Calcification of the Medulla of the Adrenal

Adrenal hemorrhage occurs with some frequency in newborns, especially in relation to breech and other forms of traumatic delivery.[5, 7, 19] The exact cause of these hemorrhages has never been established; they may be due to trauma (in some cases, this may be concluded from accompanying clinical and pathological features), anoxia, or severe stress, as in overwhelming infection.

Calcification of central hematomas of the adrenal has been identified roentgenographically and, also, at autopsy in older infants and children, which indicates that not all adrenal hemorrhages are fatal.

Both recent adrenal hemorrhage and calcification of an old adrenal hematoma were encountered in infants in the NICHD study who were ultimately classified as SIDS.

Case History

This black female infant was born at term weighing 3742 grams. She was found dead in her crib when she was two months old. This case was classified as SIDS (Fig. 7–49).

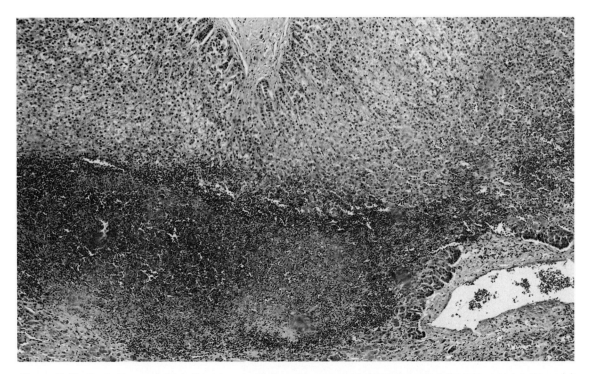

Figure 7–49. Central hemorrhage in the adrenal. All along the upper half of this photograph there is normal cortex and, in a midline dip, some of the capsule of the gland. Just below the middle of the picture there is a band of hemorrhage, which seems to have originated in the medulla; along its right-hand margin a little of the medullary tissue is still recognizable, adjacent to a sizeable blood vessel. 60x

Case History

This black male infant was born very prematurely at 30 weeks of gestation with a birth weight of 1177 grams. His mother had high blood pressure throughout her pregnancy. He remained in the hospital for two months until his weight reached five pounds. He did not have a normal weight gain after discharge from the hospital. He was found dead two hours after a feeding when he was three months old. There had been a previous sibling who died of SIDS three years before his death. The case was designated a SIDS (Fig. 7–50).

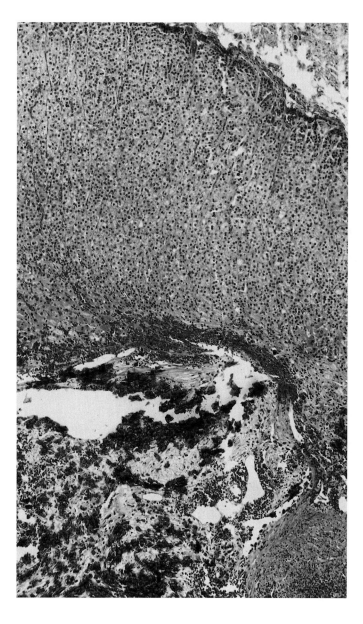

Figure 7–50. Calcification of an old central hematoma in the adrenal of an infant. Normal cortex of the adrenal occupies the upper half of the photograph. In the lower left corner in the medulla of this adrenal are numerous clusters of very darkly stained crystalline material, which is calcium, deposited in an old hematoma. 60x

Cytomegaly

The fetal portion of the neonatal and infant adrenal cortex may contain giant cells, especially centrally.[15] They may be few or many and are associated with erythroblastosis fetalis and the Beckwith-Wiedemann syndrome.[12] Adrenal cytomegalic cells also are encountered commonly in infants of diabetic or prediabetic mothers (together with pancreatic islet cell hyperplasia and hypertrophy and clinical hypoglycemia). The same change may be seen in the fetal zone of adrenal rests in other parts of the body. It has been encountered in an ectopic adrenal rest at the hilus of the testis.[1] There are no specific gross changes that signal the presence of the lesion.

In most of the cases in this series, when both adrenals were examined, only one was affected, although in some cases both were. The affected cells are so striking and the nuclei so large and darkly stained that they can be discerned at very low magnification. The cells are polyhedral and measure up to 50 microns in diameter.

Adrenal cytomegaly has been observed in white and black newborn infants weighing from 400 grams up to 4,500 grams. In the NICHD study population, they were found in infants between two and three months of age.

Case History

This Hispanic female infant was born at term with a birth weight of 3062 grams. The baby was found dead in her crib when she was two months old. The case was classified as SIDS (Fig. 7–51).

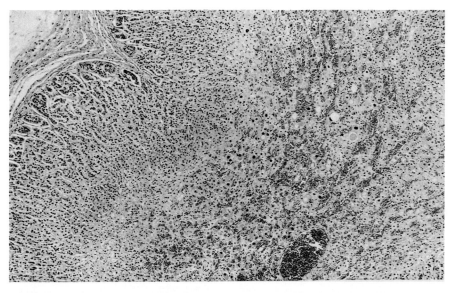
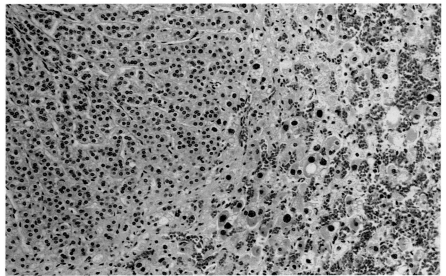

Figure 7–51. Adrenal cytomegaly.
A (upper): The adrenal cortex is on the left, and a bit of the medulla with a central vessel in the lower right corner of this photograph. Above and to the left of the engorged vessel, there are countless large black dots representing the nuclei of cytomegalic adrenal cortical cells. These nuclei are many times larger than their normal counterparts on the left. 60x B (lower): This photograph is an enlargement of the central portion of Figure 7–51A. 160x

Case History

This black female infant was born two months prematurely with a birth weight of 1814 grams. She died at two and a half months of age. She was apparently well, and was in bed with her mother when she was found dead almost four hours after having been fed. The case was designated a SIDS (Fig. 7–52).

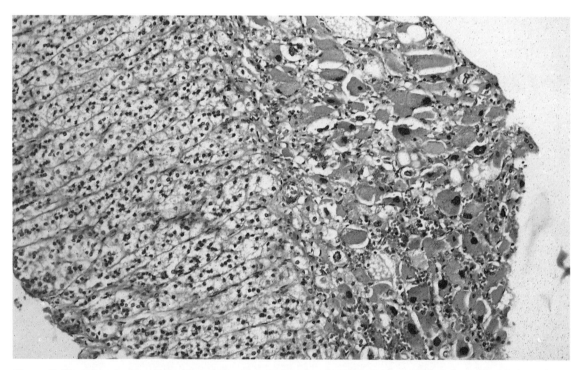

Figure 7–52. Adrenal cytomegaly. Normal, vacuolated adrenal cortical cells are seen on the left; on the right is the fetal zone, virtually transformed into a sheet of cytomegalic cells. At this magnification, one can appreciate the marked variability in shape as well as the large size, dark color, and variable intracellular position of the nucleus. In most instances the nucleus is pressed against one side of the cell. 160x

Neuroblastoma-in-Situ

Occasionally, in a neonatal autopsy, a small clump of neuroblasts or a miniature neuroblastoma is found, nestled in the medulla of an otherwise normal adrenal. These masses may be large enough to be perceived with the naked eye. On histologic examination they appear to be made up of crowded, tiny, dark staining cells, reminiscent of lymphocytes, with almost no visible cytoplasm.[11]

Case History

This black female infant was born at term, 40 weeks of gestation, and was small-for-gestational age, weighing only 2325 grams. She had a cold for a week before her death at 24 days of age. She was sleeping with her mother the night of her death and is said to have cried out during her sleep. Later she was found dead, lying on her side. This case was classified as SIDS (Fig. 7–53).

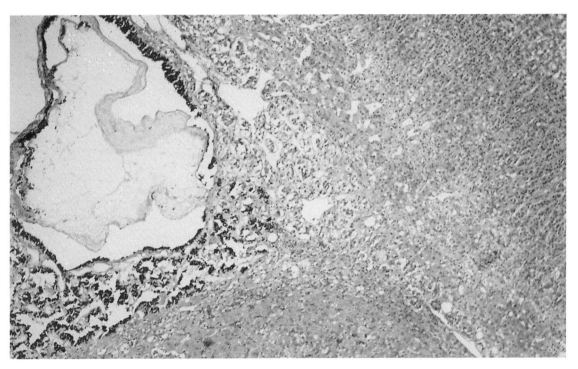

Figure 7–53. Neuroblastoma in situ, in the adrenal. The lighter staining portion of this photographic image represents the almost plexiform medulla, oriented obliquely across the photograph from the upper left to the lower right corner . The open ring surrounded by small, darkly stained cells just to the left of the medulla represents a tiny neuroblastoma. The reason for the central space in it, in this instance, is unclear; the space may represent the site of prior central necrosis within the mass. 60x

THYMUS

Extramedullary Hematopoiesis

Foci of extramedullary hematopoiesis are often found within the thymus in autopsies of premature infants. They are most prominent in septa. When they occur, hematopoiesis is likely to be found in other organs as well, especially the liver, spleen, and the adrenal.

Case History

This Hispanic male infant was born at term with a weight of 4026 grams. He died at three months of age. He was found dead during his nap, only one hour after having been seen alive. The case was classified as SIDS (Fig. 7–54).

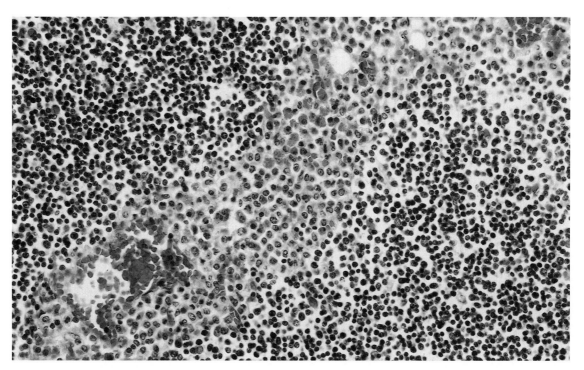

Figure 7–54. Extramedullary hematopoiesis in the thymus. The hematopoietic cells here appear to be mostly myeloid; they form a band, oriented across the picture, from the lower left to upper right corner. Above and below the band there are crowds of small lymphocytes. 250x

CENTRAL NERVOUS SYSTEM

Recent Subarachnoid Hemorrhage

Sometimes an infant autopsy reveals tiny patches of fresh hemorrhage into the leptomeninges, in the absence of any other intracranial bleeding. Such small hemorrhages are produced, in all probability, by anoxia and not by trauma.

Case History

This Hispanic female infant was born prematurely at 32 weeks of gestation and weighed 1304 grams. She was almost three months old when she died. She was fundamentally well from birth until her death. Her death was designated a SIDS (Fig. 7–55).

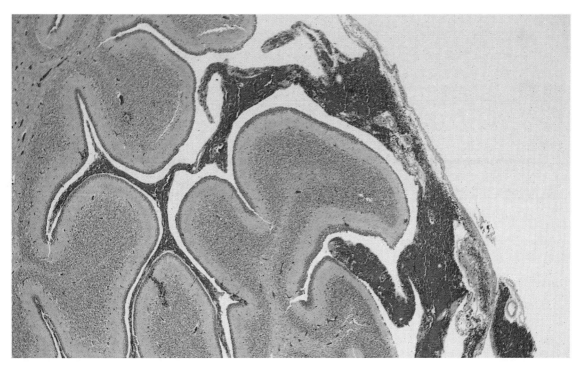

Figure 7–55. Subarachnoid hemorrhage. This is a section through cerebellar folia showing recent subarachnoid hemorrhage. 25x

Case History

This Hispanic female infant was born at 39 weeks of gestation and weighed 2693 grams. She was well from birth and was found dead face down in her crib, one hour after feeding, at two and a half months of age. The case was classified as SIDS (Fig. 7–56).

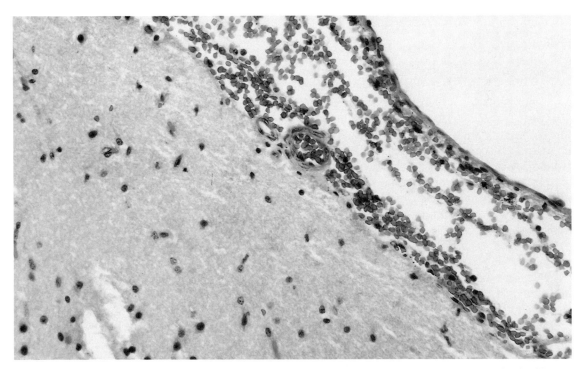

Figure 7–56. Subarachnoid hemorrhage. Intact erythrocytes are seen between the pia mater and the arachnoid. There is no evidence of chronicity here. 250x

Pigment-laden Macrophages in the Leptomeninges

Pigment-laden macrophages in the leptomeninges of infants in the first months of postnatal life may reflect either primary or secondary hemorrhage at that site. Neither the primary nor the secondary form is usually associated with trauma.

Primary hemorrhage into the subarachnoid space in newborns is usually mild and consists principally of slight extravasation of red cells into the areas around major blood vessels. This is almost invariably the result of anoxia and is not caused by mechanical injury.

Intraventricular hemorrhage is a common cause of morbidity and mortality among infants born prematurely. When blood in this lesion leaves the ventricular system via the foramina of Luschka and Magendie in a child who survives, it enters, secondarily, into the subarachnoid space where it may be picked up by wandering macrophages. This type of hemorrhage is probably the most common origin of the hemosiderin in pigment-laden macrophages within the leptomeninges.

The large, dark cells high in the leptomeninges in Figure 7–57 are macrophages heavily laden with hemosiderin. When located in the vicinity of the foramina of Luschka and Magendie, they probably reflect extension of old intraventricular hemorrhages. If they appear over the cerebral hemispheres, they are more than likely anoxic in origin.

Case History

This white male infant was born prematurely at 32 weeks of gestation and weighed 2060 grams. Normal weight for that gestational age would have been about 1500 grams. The infant's excessive weight was attributable to anasarca; the baby was hydropic on account of erythroblastosis fetalis. The infant was hospitalized for two and a half months following birth. He was both deaf and blind and was being seen regularly by physicians. He died when he was almost four months old. His death was attributed to multiple congenital anomalies (Fig. 7–57).

Figure 7–57. Leptomeninges bearing pigment-laden macrophages. A (upper, facing page): 160x B (lower, facing page): 250x

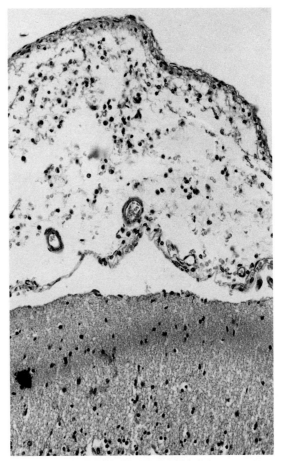

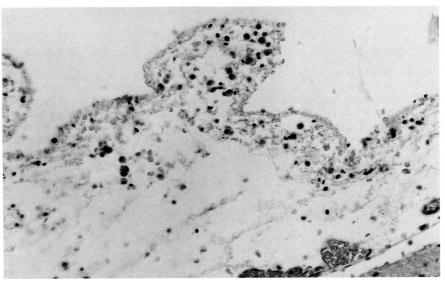

Residua of Old Germinal Matrix Hemorrhages

There are two types of lesions that linger in the area of the germinal matrix to mark the sites of perinatal hemorrhage there. The first is a focal cluster of small glial cells admixed with *pigment-laden macrophages*. The second is a sort of *pseudocyst* surrounded by a slender band of glial cells. Sometimes these cystic lesions are rounded, but many times they are collapsed and elongate. They may have pigment-laden cells in their walls. They are usually located below and very close to the angle of the lateral ventricle. Of themselves, neither of these lesions has any clinical significance or correlates.

Case History

This black female infant was born very prematurely at 29 weeks of gestation and weighed 1219 grams. She remained in the hospital for one month after birth. She died at two months of age. Her death was designated a SIDS (Fig. 7–58).

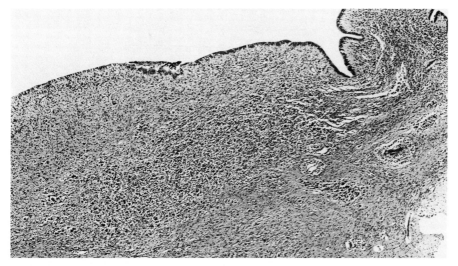

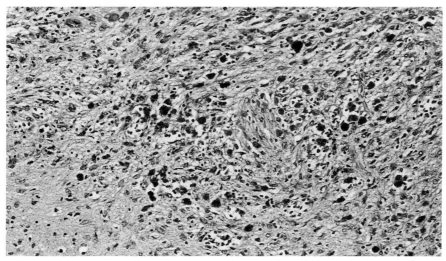

Figure 7–58. Clusters of pigment-laden macrophages in the brain. A (upper): Deep to the ependyma, there are several aggregates of large, dark cells; these are hemosiderin-laden macrophages, remnants of an old perinatal paraventricular hemorrhage. 40x
B (lower): This photograph is from the same case as Figure 7–58A. It illustrates, at higher magnification, the cell types at the site of a typical cluster. 160x

Case History

This black male infant was born at term with a birth weight of 3487 grams. He was found dead in bed at two months of age. His death was designated a SIDS (Fig. 7–59).

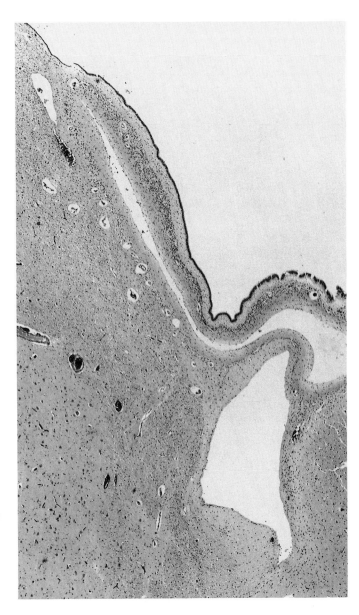

Figure 7–59. Paraventricular pseudocyst. In the brain, immediately below the ependymal lining of the lateral ventricle are two pseudocysts. The upper one is slender and elongate and parallels the ependymal lining above it. Even at this magnification, a halo of glial cells can be seen surrounding that lesion. To its right is a second, more expanded, triangular pseudocyst. Each is the end result of a focal, perinatal, germinal matrix hemorrhage at that site. 25x

---

BLOOD

Sickling of Red Cells

Some sickle cells may be found in microscopic sections from any series of autopsies involving black infants and children. These are erythrocytes that have a somewhat elongate shape and very sharply pointed ends. It is the latter feature that best distinguishes this type of cell. No normal red cell ever has needle-sharp, pointed ends no matter how deformed it becomes, but red cells from patients with the sickle cell trait do have this feature, particularly in severe oxygen deprivation. It can be assumed that any patient in the agonal state experiences terminal hypoxemia. However, the mere finding of sickled cells, even in a number of organs, does not indicate that the patient had sickle cell disease, or that he or she died of the disease.

Pediatric hematologists believe it highly improbable that an infant under six months of age would or could die of sickle cell disease because their relative levels of residual fetal hemoglobin are so high. Even the very first clinical manifestations of the disease do not usually appear until the latter part of the first year.[10] Consequently, the autopsy observation of moderate numbers of sickled cells in an infant who has succumbed to SIDS, especially in the first half of the first year of life, probably indicates only that the baby had sickle cell trait.

Case History

This black male infant was born at term with a weight of 3580 grams. He died when he was five and a half months old. His death was classified as SIDS, although because he was five and a half months old and because there are so many red cells sickled in this spleen, it seems possible that he might have died in the midst of a sequestration crisis (Fig. 7–60).[10]

Figure 7–60. Sickling of red cells in the spleen. A (upper, facing page): This figure illustrates widespread sickling of erythrocytes in the red pulp of the spleen. 400x B (lower, facing page): Sickling of red cells in the lung. This figure was taken from the same case and shows two isolated red cells within a pulmonary alveolus; they seem to have escaped through the wall of a capillary. Both cells are elongate and the one in the center has a typical needle-sharp, pointed end. 1,000x

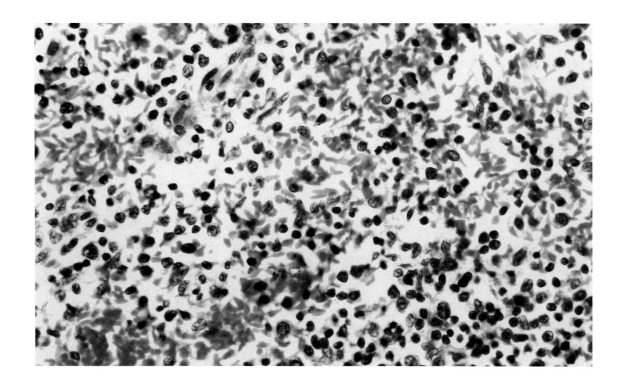

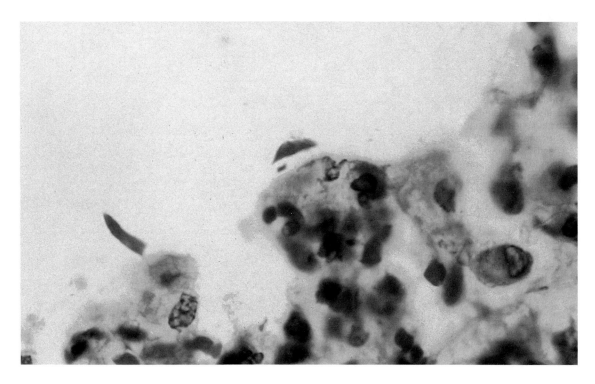

Case History

This black female infant was born at term with a birth weight of 3400 grams. She died when she was 15 days old. She had been sleeping in bed with her mother when she was found dead. Her death was designated a SIDS (Fig. 7–61).

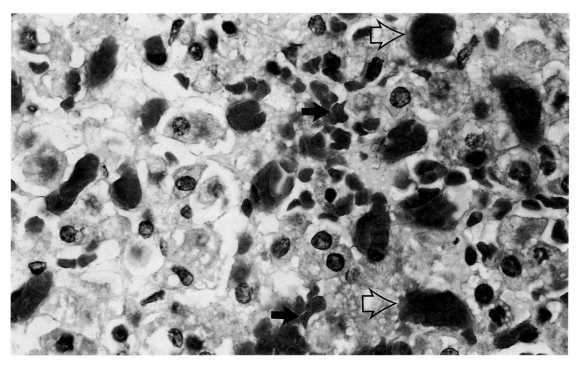

Figure 7–61. Sickling of red cells in the liver. This picture shows a little fatty change in individual liver cells and two of the histologic features of sickling. The first is the presence of elongate erythrocytes and erythrocytes with needle-sharp, pointed ends (solid arrows). (In this instance, the altered cells are not as numerous, absolutely or relatively, as in the preceding case. This is probably no more than sickle trait, although it is not possible to be certain of that at autopsy, following fixation of the tissues, since the baby was only 15 days of age at death). A second feature and one that is often helpful in first alerting the pathologist to the sickling condition, is the unusual packing of red cells in small vessels to the extent that the contours of the individual cell are lost (open arrows). This extraordinary "stacking" of flattened, elongate cells is eye-catching. 630x

REFERENCES

1. Arey JB. Adrenal cytomegalic cells in adrenal rest at hilus of testis. Personal communication, 1989.

2. Behrman RE, Vaughan VC. Acute bronchiolitis, in Chapter 13: The respiratory system. In: Behrman RE, Vaughan VC, eds. Nelson Textbook of Pediatrics, 13th ed. Philadelphia: W.B. Saunders Co., 1987, pp. 897-8.

3. Bove KE, Koffler H, McAdams AJ: Nodular renal blastema. Definition and possible significance. Cancer 24:323-32, 1969.

4. Dehner LP. Pediatric Surgical Pathology, 2nd ed. Baltimore: Williams and Wilkins, 1987, pp. 649-52.

5. DeSa JD, Nicholls S. Haemorrhagic necrosis of the adrenal gland in perinatal infants: A clinico-pathological study. J Pathol 106:133-49, 1972.

6. Franciosi RA. Hemophilus influenzae epiglottitis. Personal Communication, 1989

7. Hill EE, Williams JA. Massive adrenal hemorrhage in the newborn. Arch Dis Child 34:178-82, 1959.

8. Keshgegian AA, Chatten J. Nodular renal blastema in trisomy 13. Arch Pathol Lab Med 103:73-5, 1979.

9. McIntosh K. Infections due to respiratory syncytial virus, in Chapter 11: Infectious Diseases. In: Behrman RE, Vaughan VC, eds. Nelson Textbook of Pediatrics, 13th ed. Philadelphia: W.B. Saunders Co., 1987, pp. 680-2.

10. Pearson HA. Sickle cell hemoglobinopathies, in Chapter 15: Diseases of the blood: Hemolytic anemias due to hemoglobinopathies. In: Behrman RE, Vaughan VC, eds. Nelson Textbook of Pediatrics, 13th ed. Philadelphia: W.B. Saunders Co., 1987, pp. 1049-51.

11. Potter EL, Craig JM. Pathology of the Fetus and the Infant, 3rd ed. Chicago: Year Book Medical Publishers, Inc., 1975, p.202.

12. Potter EL, Craig JM. Pathology of the Fetus and the Infant, 3rd ed. Chicago: Year Book Medical Publishers, Inc., 1975, p.333-5.

13. Naeye RL. Hypoxemia and the sudden infant death syndrome. Science 1974;186:837-8.

14. Naeye RL. Sudden infant death. Sci Am 1980;242:56-62.

15. Valdés-Dapena M. Histology of the Fetus and the Newborn. Philadelphia: W.B. Saunders Co., 1987, pp. 133 and 144-5.

16. Valdés-Dapena M. Histology of the Fetus and the Newborn. Philadelphia: W.B. Saunders Co., 1987, pp. 195 and 206.

17. Valdés-Dapena M. The morphology of the sudden infant death syndrome: an overview. In: Tildon JT, Roeder LM, Steinschneider A, eds. Sudden Infant Death Syndrome. New York: Academic Press, 1983, pp. 169-79.

18. Valdés-Dapena M. A pathologist's perspective on possible mechanisms in SIDS. Ann NY Acad Sci 533:31-6, 1988.

19. Valdés-Dapena M. Iatrogenic disease in the perinatal period. Pediatr Clin North Am 36: 67-93, 1989.

20. Valdés-Dapena M, Huff D. Subpleural emphysema. Personal communication, 1989.

21. Valdés-Dapena M, Gillane MN, Ross D, Catherman R. Extramedullary hematopoiesis in the liver in sudden infant death syndrome. Arch Pathol Lab Med 103:513-5, 1979.

Sudden Infant Death Syndrome

CHAPTER *8*

"THE GRAY ZONE"

INTRODUCTION

The statement that pathology is not an exact science is applicable in many instances of sudden and unexpected infant deaths. For example, two able pathologists examining the same set of microscopic sections from a case of bacterial pneumonia may come to totally different conclusions. One may decide that the cause of death is pneumonia and the other, that the lesion is not severe enough or is insufficient to have caused death. The term "gray zone" is used as a category for those situations (cases) in which it is difficult to state whether or not a specific microscopic lesion is sufficiently severe to have caused death.[1,22,25,33]

Cognizant of the difficulty in achieving concordance for a diagnosis of death, an a priori system was established for the microscopic review by the Pathology Study Panel. This system allowed each pathologist to record his or her observations on a form, which listed specific lesions (e.g., congestion, inflammation, petechiae, etc.) for each organ and allowed quantitation of those (and other) findings. Significant lesions were then dichotomized by organ system into those likely to be morbid and those likely to be mortal. Within this framework, the three pathologists independently developed remarkably similar microscopic criteria for the diagnosis of SIDS. Thus, at the end of the first review (of only microscopic findings) a consensus for the cause of death was reached for the vast majority of cases. After the microscopic reviews had been completed, additional criteria based on scene investigation, background information, and autopsy findings were established.[15,29,34]

The entire review process reflected the rationale used in making decisions such as how much bronchiolitis is required to declare a lesion mortal. The ability to reach consensus as to the cause of death for these "gray zone" cases reflects the strength of this review system. Undoubtedly, these difficult and somewhat subjective decisions will continue to plague pathologists reviewing "gray zone" cases in the future. However, application of the classification system used by the Pathology Study Panel for the NICHD study and reference to the illustrative cases presented here may be helpful in this difficult process.

Classification of Significant Lesions

Significant lesions can be classified as morbid or mortal lesions. Morbid lesions are those which, by themselves, are probably not fatal. Mortal lesions are those which, by themselves, would cause death (Table 8–1). These categories do not represent rigid criteria and should be applied within the context of the circumstances of the case.

Table 8–1. **Significant Morbid* and Mortal Lesions**

Organ	Morbid	Mortal or Possibly Mortal
Heart	Ischemic necrosis, especially at tips of papillary muscles	Myocarditis (viral)
		Endocardial fibroelastosis
	Foci of hemorrhage in epicardium and/or myocardium	
Lung	Mild to moderate bronchopneumonia	Pneumonia, advanced, with many neutrophils in many clusters of alveoli and seen in in many tissue sections
	Mild to moderate interstitial pneumonia	
	Congestion	
	acute: engorgement of capillaries, etc.	
	chronic: hemosiderin-laden macrophages	
	Edema	Bronchopulmonary dysplasia
	Tracheitis	
	Bronchitis	
	Bronchiolitis, patchy	Bronchiolitis—extensive
	Patchy atelectasis	
	Clusters of squames in alveoli (leftover from an episode of fetal anoxia)	
	Emphysema and interstitial emphysema	
	Abundant macrophages in alveoli	
	Granulomas, few	
	Abundant mucus in airways	
Liver	Extramedullary hematopoeisis	
	Fatty change	
	Triaditis, lymphocytic	
	Cholestasis in liver cells, or canaliculi	
	Hamartomas	
	hemangioma	
	bile duct hamartoma	

Table 8-1. *Continued*

Kidney	Cytomegalic inclusions, within cells, in some tubules Glomerular sclerosis, scattered So-called "immaturity" of glomeruli Foci of nephroblastomatosis	
Pancreas	Simple dilatation of acini	Changes of cystic fibrosis (i.e., dilatation of acini and ductules) with inspissation of secretions, when accompanied by appropriate morphologic changes in gut, lung, etc.
	Apparent hyperplasia of islets of Langerhans and/or scattered isolated islet cells	Unquestionable hypertrophy (or atypia) of islet cells accompanying unquestionable hyperplasia
Brain	Residue of old focal germinal matrix hemorrhage	Encephalitis Meningitis
	Perivascular hemorrhage	Arteriovenous malformation, intracranial
	Congestion	Cerebral edema
Spleen	Extramedullary hematopoiesis	Universal sickling in all organs in a child more than 11 months of age (sequestration crisis)
Blood	Moderate sickling in vessels in a variety of organs in infants less than 6 months of age	Universal sickling in all organs in a child more than 11 months of age (sequestration crisis)

*Morbid lesions imply any pathologic lesion, some of which may be incidental/inconsequential lesions.

ACUTE BRONCHIOLITIS

Acute bronchiolitis is a viral illness. It is common among infants in the first two years of life with a peak incidence at about six months.[13] Like SIDS it occurs most often during winter and early spring and is reported both sporadically and epidemically.[31] The respiratory syncytial virus is the most common cause of acute bronchiolitis, accounting for more than 50% of cases.[5, 6, 7, 9] Other etiologic agents include the parainfluenza 3 virus, mycoplasma, some adenoviruses, and occasionally other viruses.[18] The source of the infection is usually another family member with a minor respiratory illness.[8, 11]

The disease is characterized by bronchiolar obstruction as the result of thickening of the bronchiolar wall on account of edema and inflammatory cell infiltration there. The obstruction is compounded when there is mucus and cellular debris in the lumen. Because resistance to airflow in a tube is inversely related to the cube of the radius (r^3) of the lumen, even slight thickening of the wall in an infant may have a profound effect on air flow. The result is impaired exchange of gases in the lung.

Affected infants are first noted to have a mild upper respiratory tract infection with serous nasal discharge and sneezing. Usually these symptoms last several days and may be accompanied by a fever of 101°–102° F. Loss of appetite, gradual development of respiratory distress, and a wheezy cough may follow later. In mild cases, symptoms disappear in one to three days. In severe cases the symptoms develop within hours and the course may be protracted.[37]

The most critical phase of the illness occurs two to three days after the onset of symptoms. At that time the very small infant may have apneic spells. Because of tachypnea, affected babies are apt to become dehydrated; this is attributed to loss of water vapor and the infant's inability to drink fluids. Nevertheless, recovery is usually complete within a few days and mortality is less than 1%.

In any series of sudden infant deaths, the pathologist will encounter only a few cases of bronchiolitis.[18] In most of these cases, only one or two affected bronchioles will be apparent in one or two lobes and, if other factors are consistent, the death may be considered a SIDS. At other times, however, many bronchioles are inflamed and there seems little doubt that the disease caused the baby's death. In between those two extremes are the gray zone cases in which the pathologist cannot decide whether the bronchiolitis is or is not responsible for the baby's death.

Case History

This black male infant was born prematurely at 36 weeks gestation and weighed 2098 grams. He remained in the hospital for ten days after birth and, according to his mother, vomited frequently. He weighed 3632 grams at the time of his death. He had a cold and runny nose for several days before his death at the age of 28 days. Autopsy revealed very few affected bronchioles and minimal pneumonitis. The death was designated a probable SIDS (Fig. 8–1).

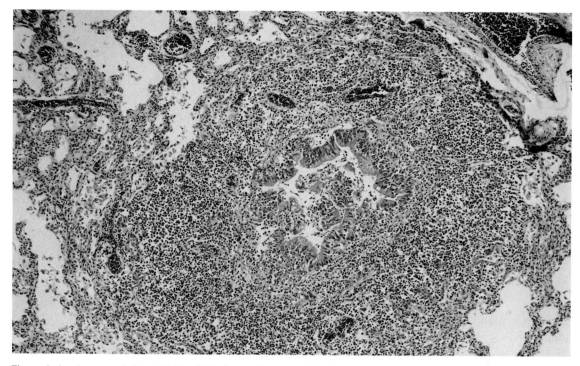

Figure 8–1. Lung, acute bronchiolitis. This picture shows marked thickening of the wall of a bronchiole in a case of bronchiolitis; the inflammatory cells involved are all lymphocytes and they almost completely obscure the smooth muscle there. Bronchiolitis was evident in approximately 25-50% of all bronchioles on two of three lung sections; the third section was essentially normal. Notice that there is no exudate in adjacent alveoli. 60x

Case History

This white male infant was born at only 32 weeks of gestation with a birth weight of 1410 grams. He was the first-born of twins and died at two months of age. He had respiratory distress syndrome at birth. At a well-baby checkup two weeks before death (six weeks of age) he weighed 2155 grams. He had a cold prior to death. His twin, who was in the crib with him at the time of his death, survived. This case was designated as a SIDS (Fig. 8–2).

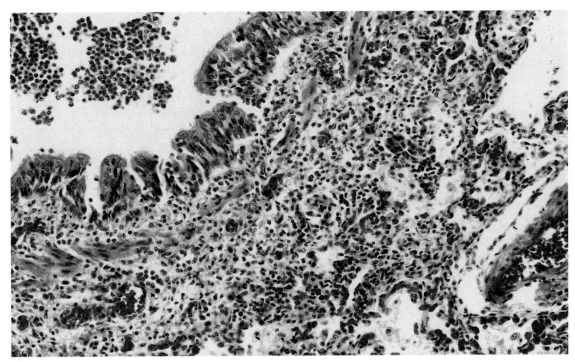

Figure 8–2. Lung, acute bronchiolitis. This figure, at higher magnification than the case in Figure 8–1, shows one segment of the wall of an affected bronchiole. Notice that the inflammatory cells are lymphocytes and that some of these cells are in the lumen of the airway and among lining epithelial cells. There are also a few macrophages in surrounding alveoli. Approximately 50% of all bronchioles in all lung fields showed similar changes. A very early patchy pneumonia was evident in one lung section.160x

Case History

This black male infant was born at term with a birth weight of 3580 grams. He died at five and one half months of age. His mother reported that he had been exposed to measles within the last two weeks of life and, also, that he had recently been immunized. He had a cold for more than two weeks prior to his death and became listless and droopy in the last 24 hours prior to his death. He had been taken for a sick baby visit one day before dying with the chief complaint of a cold. He weighed 8165 grams at this sick visit. The next day his mother called the doctor twice because the baby had a cough, was "congested," and had a temperature (39.8 ° C).

This case was originally submitted as a SIDS, but the cause of death was turned around in the field to acute tracheobronchitis. Acute and subacute tracheobronchitis were noted on the microscopic review; however, the panel determined that these lesions were insufficient to constitute a cause of death for a healthy baby of this age. This death was re-classified as SIDS (Figs. 8–3 and 8–4).

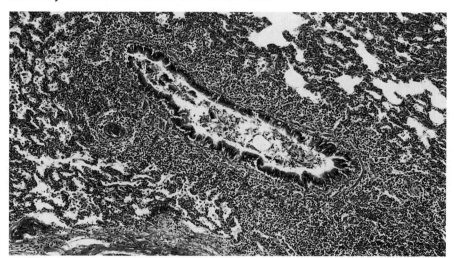

Figure 8–3. Lung, acute bronchiolitis. This is a single bronchiole with a wide cuff of lymphocytes, typical of bronchiolitis. 60x

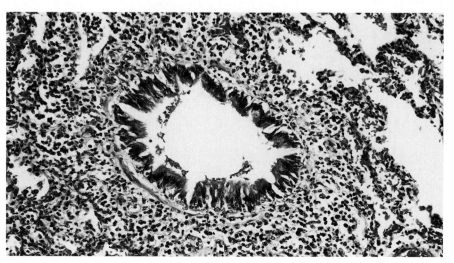

Figure 8–4. This high power photograph of the same patient's lung shows a very tiny bronchiole with a thin band of smooth muscle in its wall. There are, however, fairly large numbers of lymphocytes in the wall, which thicken the wall perceptibly. Only a minority of small bronchioles in two of four lung sections showed the inflammation seen in these two photomicrographs (Figs. 8–3 and 8–4). 160x

Case History

This white male infant was born at term with an appropriate birth weight, 3969 grams. He died when he was almost 13 months old. He was seen during a sick baby visit ten days before his death for measles and a cough. He received medication after his sick visit, and his mother reported that he had neither cough or fever on the day that he died. He was at his baby-sitter's home and was discovered in the crib, unresponsive, less than 45 minutes after last having been seen alive.

Lesions of the type seen in Fig. 8–5 were scattered about the several microscopic sections of lung; there was no question but that the child had broncholitis, probably viral, at the time of death. Nevertheless, because the lesions seemed insufficient, of themselves, to have caused the death of an otherwise healthy and asymptomatic child, this case was classified as SIDS (Figs. 8–5 and 8–6).

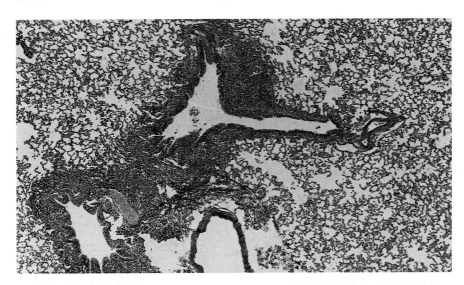

Figure 8–5. Lung, acute bronchiolitis. These two bronchioles demonstrate heavy inflammatory cell infiltration of their walls and the surrounding connective tissue. Most of the infiltrate consists of lymphocytes. 25x

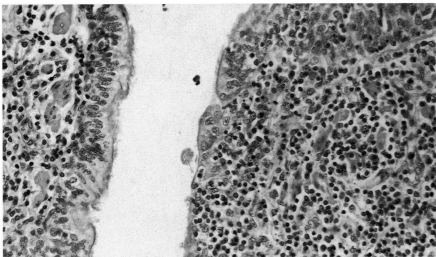

Figure 8–6. In this figure, at higher magnification, it is clear that the involved inflammatory cells are lymphocytes. Only two large bronchioles in five total lung sections showed these changes. The lungs were otherwise histologically unremarkable. 250x

Case History

This black female infant was born at term, weighing 2977 grams. She had a cold for a week before her death at almost five months of age.

This case was originally submitted as SIDS but, subsequently, was turned around in the field, and the cause of death changed to pneumonia. The Pathology Study Panel did not be-lieve that the degree of pneumonia present was sufficiently serious as to have caused the infant to die, nor did they feel the bronchiolitis seen in Fig. 8–7, even in combination with a mild pneumonia, was extensive enough to cause death. This death was re-classified as SIDS (Fig. 8–7).

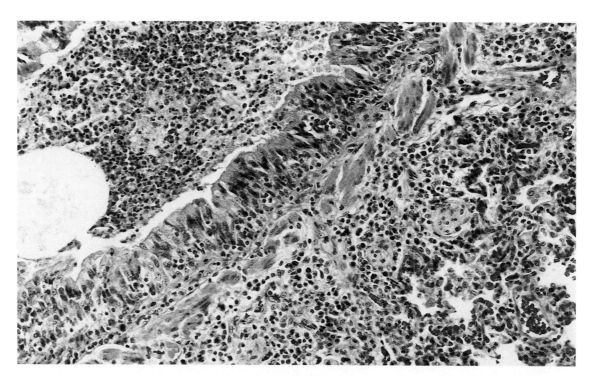

Figure 8–7.   Bronchiolitis. There is pus in the lumen of this single small bronchiole and a mixed infiltrate in the wall and in the lining epithelium. The infiltrate in the wall is predominantly lymphocytic. This change was evident in a minority of bronchioles in all five lung sections sampled. 160x

PNEUMONIA

Pneumonia presents the best example of lesions that fall into the gray zone. Whenever a pathologist discovers this disease during an infant autopsy, the immediate question is whether the amount and severity of pneumonia present was sufficient to have taken the life of an otherwise healthy infant. This decision is always a "judgment call" as what may seem a mortal lesion to one physician is not to another.

There is little point in classifying pneumonias in infants according to anatomical distribution because, for practical purposes, the vast majority, in infants, are bronchopneumonias. [32] Although some pneumonias are confluent, involving almost all of a lobe or two, they are almost never truly lobar. In addition, extremely few are interstitial. It is more useful to classify infant pneumonias according to the etiological agent. Most of those seen at autopsy are bacterial; very few are of viral etiology. Other types of infection are rare in infants.

Primary bacterial pneumonia is much less common than secondary, i.e., complicating minor upper respiratory infection. The bacterial agents one expects to encounter among post-neonatal infants are Pneumococci, Staphylococci, and *H. influenzae* for which the associated case fatality rates are low. [14, 19, 26]

Viral pneumonia, on the other hand, is most often produced by respiratory syncytial virus, parainfluenza virus, adenovirus, or enterovirus. The majority of infants with viral pneumonia recover uneventfully. [32]

Case History

This black female infant was born at term with an appropriate birth weight of 3147 grams. She died at three months of age. She had apparently been in good health, except for an eye infection when she was one month old which was treated at a local hospital. The baby was unexpectedly found dead.

The case was originally submitted as a typical SIDS. The Pathology Study Panel found early pneumonia in one focus of the lung, together with evidence of cytomegalovirus infection. They designated the case as a SIDS with early pneumonia (Fig. 8–8).

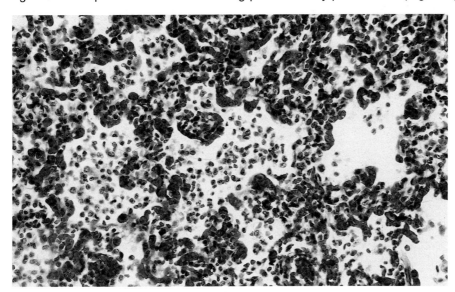

Figure 8–8. Bronchopneumonia. Most of the air spaces in this field contain pus. The capillaries in alveolar walls are markedly engorged. This was the only focus of pneumonia seen with five sampled lung fields. 250x

Case History

This black male infant was born at term with a birth weight of 3130 grams. He was ten months old when he died. He had a history of frequent colds and one recent severe upper respiratory infection for which he was being given medications at the time of his death. He had experienced some difficulty with breathing the day before death. He was taken to the local hospital where he was diagnosed as having pneumonia. The next day he was dead on arrival at the hospital.

This case was submitted originally as a SIDS, but later turned around in the field as a death due to bronchopneumonia. The Pathology Study Panel agreed that there was sufficient evidence of pneumonia combined with the more extensive bronchiolitis in the various sections of the lung to have accounted for the death of the child (Fig. 8–9).

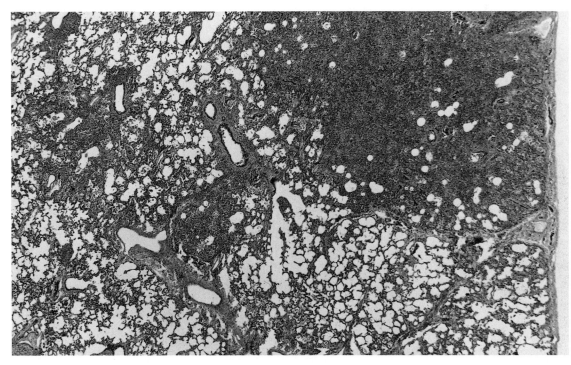

Figure 8–9. Bronchopneumonia. There is an area of consolidation in the right upper corner, directly below the pleura. This is not due to atelectasis because the pleura is not depressed; it is, instead, due to filling of alveoli with pus. The area of pneumonia involved one low power field (4x objective, 10x ocular) of one lobe only; however, broncholitis was also evident in large bronchioles in all five lung sections sampled. 15x.

Case History

This Hispanic male infant was born at 40 week gestation, weighing 3232 grams. He had a head cold for two days prior to his death at the age of 38 days. He was found dead in his crib two hours after a feeding.

This case was submitted as SIDS. The Pathology Study Panel felt this was a clear example of sudden infant death syndrome since, clinically, the child had not been seriously ill and, pathologically, the lesions in the lung were insufficient to have accounted for the baby's death (Fig. 8–10).

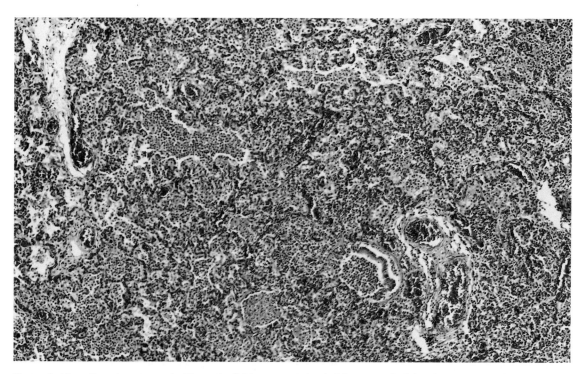

Figure 8–10. Bronchopneumonia. The entire field appears to be dark because all of the air spaces and airways are filled with pus. The dark nuclei of individual neutrophils are visible, especially in the lumen of the bronchiole above and to the left of center. Two lobes sampled showed evidence of bronchopneumonia - one showed consolidated pneumonia; the other, a microscopic focus only. The remaining three lobes showed bronchioles with pus within their lumens, but no pneumonia. 60x

Case History

This black male infant was born prematurely, at 36 weeks of gestation, and weighed only 2098 grams. He remained in the hospital for ten days. The baby's mother reported that he "vomited all of his food" from birth on and always had a cold and runny nose. He was found unresponsive in his bed on the day of his death at 28 days of age.

The case was submitted as SIDS. The extent of pathological change in the lungs was considered by the Pathology Study Panel to be insufficient to have caused the death of an otherwise uncompromised infant. The death was classified as probable SIDS (Fig. 8–11).

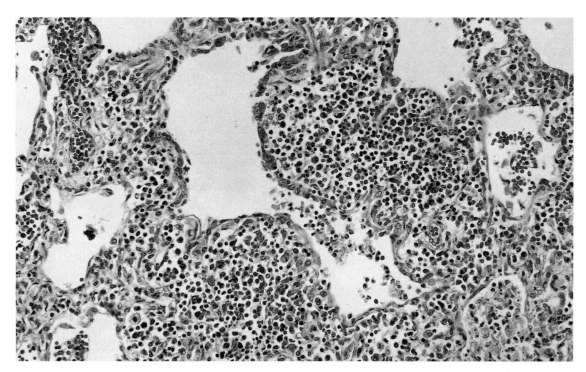

Figure 8–11. Viral pneumonia. Alveolar walls are unquestionably thicker than normal; some of them are as much as ten times normal breadth. They are also markedly hypercellular and the added cells are inflammatory, predominantly lymphocytes and plasma cells. Some alveolar lining cells are swollen. This histopathologic finding was seen consistently in all three lung sections sampled. 160x

MACROPHAGES IN ALVEOLI IN ABNORMALLY LARGE NUMBERS AND EXTENSIVE DISTRIBUTION

In contrast to the circumstances described in Chapter 5, the presence of large aggregates of many macrophages, in many segments of the lung, and in multiple sections suggests a chronic or continuing problem. In the case illustrated previously (Chapter 5, Fig. 5–10) there were only small clusters of a few macrophages in scattered alveoli. However, an infant with an extensive type of lesion has probably been aspirating small amounts of fluid frequently over time. Infants who have suffered brain damage commonly experience difficulty in swallowing effectively and often aspirate small amounts of either their own secretions or regurgitated material. This histologic finding at autopsy raises a serious question about the normality or physiologic capability of the infant. It could be interpreted to mean that the baby had less than optimal control of the critical functions involved in alternately breathing and swallowing.

Case History

This black male infant was born at term, 38 weeks of gestation, but with a birth weight of only 2071 grams, an obvious case of intrauterine growth retardation. He survived for almost nine months with congenital heart disease, a truncus arteriosus with absent left pulmonary artery. On the day of death he cried for ten minutes and then stopped breathing. Ten minutes of resuscitation were undertaken with intubation, Ambu bag, and cardiac massage, to no avail. The panel did not designate this as a SIDS death because of the congenital heart defect. However, some pathologists upon reviewing histologic lesions resembling this have signed such cases out as SIDS (Fig. 8–12).

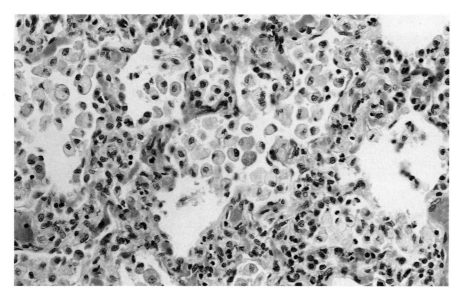

Figure 8–12. Lung, excessive numbers of macrophages in many alveoli. The majority of alveoli shown in this figure contain large numbers of macrophages, certainly more than expected in the typical SIDS case. 250x

EXCESSIVE ASPIRATION OF AMNIOTIC DEBRIS

The fetus who experiences hypoxemia in the latter part of pregnancy – for whatever cause – is apt to "attempt to breathe" (i.e., to make greater inspiratory efforts than are normally involved in the usual, minimal, ongoing, respiratory tidal ebb and flow of fetal life). Because there is so much "dandruff," or exfoliated epithelium from the surface of the skin, suspended in the amniotic fluid at this time, deep inhalation will draw down into the air spaces squames as well as an occasional lanugo hair. Because the fluid inhaled is readily absorbed through the capillaries of the alveolar wall, solid elements, e.g., the squames, tend to become trapped in air spaces and concentrated, particularly if hypoxemia persists for a long period of time.[36] An abrupt, rapidly fatal episode of hypoxemia does not produce this histologic picture. The ordinary, everyday flux of amniotic fluid into and out of the lungs often results in the deposition of a few scattered squamous cells in alveoli but large numbers of them in clusters of air spaces is unquestionably pathologic and reflects the sort of clinical history described above.[17]

If a baby who has experienced protracted intrauterine asphyxia survives for less than 30 days, characteristic clumps of squames may be observed still within alveoli in sections of lung, the water there having been resorbed.

Such episodes of severe, protracted intrauterine hypoxemia frequently damage the central nervous system. Infants who are born following these episodes often have respiratory depression and have very low Apgar scores, at one and five minutes of age. It is conceivable that the central nervous system residua of such damage plays a part in the supposed prebirth disposition of some (or many) infants to SIDS.

When a newborn infant who has suffered severe intrauterine anoxia dies shortly after birth, his death is not essentially respiratory; the volume of lung parenchyma compromised by aspirated debris is insufficient to cause death. Rather, death is the result of the hypoxemic insult experienced by the central nervous system itself during the anoxic episode. Respiration is compromised only secondarily, if at all. Usually, in severe cases, it is simply depressed *centrally*, i.e., the newborn infant does not even try to breathe.[2, 24]

This phenomenon is included in this chapter because the lesion cannot be categorized as not serious. Of itself, it is probably not serious; however, it surely reflects a lesion of the central nervous system that likely predisposes to sudden death in infancy.

Case History

This white male infant was born three weeks postmature with a gestational age stated to be 43 weeks, weighing 3560 grams. He died at 19 days of age. The baby was purportedly never ill. He was simply found dead in his crib, prone, and face to the side. He had been fed seven hours previously. No resuscitation was attempted. This case was designated a SIDS (Fig. 8–13).

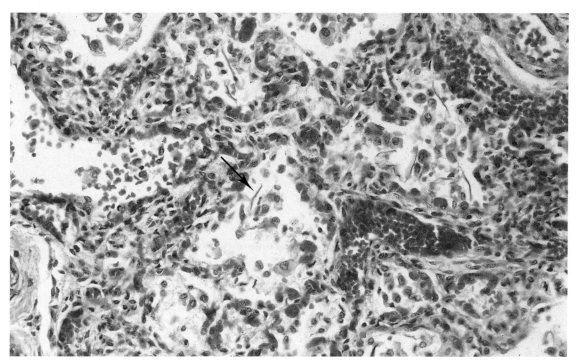

Figure 8–13. Lung, squames in alveoli. All three of these photographs were taken from sections of one infant necropsy. It can be assumed that this baby experienced at least one episode of severe intrauterine fetal anoxia. A (above): In the center of this figure there is a single alveolus containing two squamous cells cut on edge. The upper one is marked with an arrow. Each appears as a discrete, sharply demarcated, delicately wavy, dark line. In hematoxylin and eosin stains squames may be either bright pink or blue. Squames are also seen in the alveoli in the upper middle and upper right regions. 250x

B (upper, facing page): In this photograph there are two large alveoli that contain numerous squames. 250x
C (lower, facing page): The single large air space in the center of this photograph contains an abnormal number of squamous cells, most of them cut on edge. The two alveoli below and to the right of that contain many macrophages and red cells. 250x

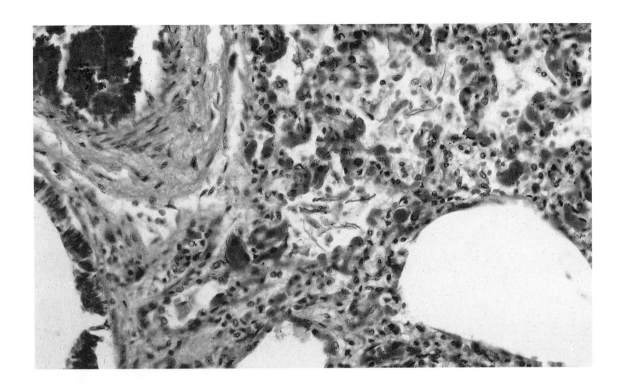

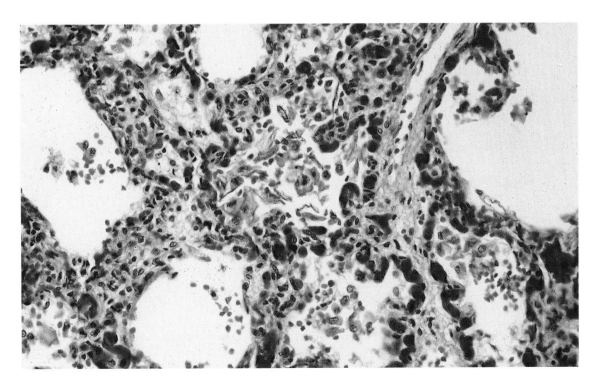

Case History

This black male infant was born at term, 39 weeks of gestation, and experienced intrauterine growth retardation as reflected by a birth weight of only 2128 grams. He died 14 days after birth. He was reported to have been well before death which occurred, unobserved, six and a half hours after his last feeding. In this instance, the case was designated as a SIDS. In retrospect, it would appear that he was a "predisposed" infant (Fig. 8–14).

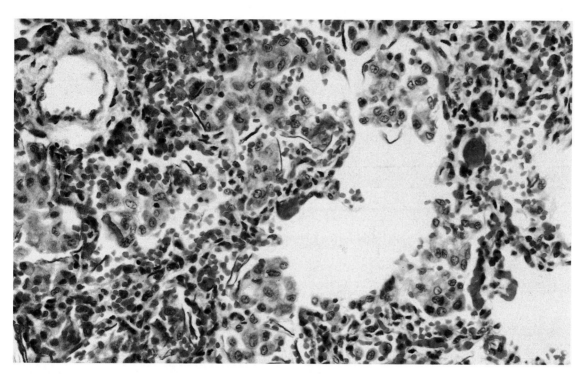

Figure 8–14. Lung, excessive aspiration of amniotic debris. All three illustrations in this figure are sections of lung from an infant who appears to have experienced serious, protracted intrauterine anoxia.
A (above): In this photograph a large air space contains a combination of macrophages and many linear profiles of squamous cells. Some red cells are also present. 250x   B (upper, facing page): In this photograph, the same mix is apparent. Two alveoli, one in the center and one in the upper left corner, are completely filled with this solid material and contain no air. 250x   C (lower, facing page): This is an enlargement of the central portion of Figure 8–14B. In it can be seen the crowded contents of a single alveolus, including squamous cells cut on edge, a cluster of packed macrophages at the bottom, and red cells in the middle left portion of the illustration. 400x

NOTE: Because excessive aspiration of amniotic debris is patchy, what is not shown here are the extensive areas between affected patches like these, in which air spaces are open, clear, and air bearing. Notice that there are no foreign body giant cells, nor any polymorphonuclear leukocytes in these alveoli in response to the squamous cells. The aspiration of solid amniotic debris such as this does not elicit any inflammatory response. Consequently, it is a mistake to speak of "aspiration pneumonia" in newborns because, unless the fluid is contaminated with bacteria, there is no inflammation in the air spaces as a reaction to this solid material alone.

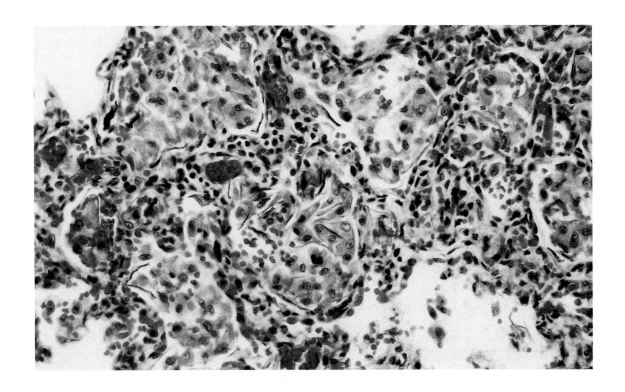

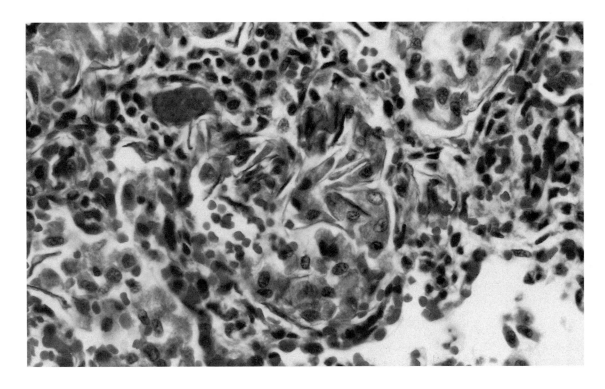

CHRONIC ASPIRATION

Some children, probably those who are either markedly or subtly brain damaged, lack the capability to swallow, especially fluids, without inspiring small amounts of the liquid bolus. These infants have chronic and recurring problems with feeding and respiration; often they are hospitalized for surgical procedures, such as fundoplication, to alleviate or obviate their difficulty.[10,16,23,28]

It appears that some babies with marginal degrees of this same difficulty are never recognized within their short lives as having a disorder that requires medical or surgical attention. Among this group, some die suddenly and unexpectedly and, in their lungs, there is microscopic evidence of their having had repeated episodes of minor aspiration. In some cases, there are focal subpleural accumulations of what looks like milk together with macrophages in pathologically large, peripheral air spaces. For unknown reasons, these intra-alveolar accumulations rarely attract polymorphonuclear leukocytes.[20]

The other type of apparently related morphologic lesion encountered in these cases is the clear-cut, rather discrete granuloma. These also tend to be at the periphery of the lung.

Case History

This black male infant was born prematurely at 34 weeks of gestation and weighed 1986 grams. He experienced respiratory distress syndrome at birth and was later hospitalized for a month with respiratory problems. He died when he was three months old. Autopsy findings were otherwise negative but this case raises serious questions about how such deaths should be signed out by the pathologist. The clinical history and the nature of these lesions suggest strongly that this baby was physiologically, at the very least, subtly handicapped. It is conceivable that such a baby might have been unable to cope with a moderate challenge to his capacity to breathe. By itself, this lesion is probably innocuous, but it does suggest that the infant may have been "predisposed." This case was classified as SIDS (Fig. 8–15).

Figure 8–15. Lung, chronic aspiration. These photographs illustrate a section of the subpleural portion of an infant lung. A (upper, facing page): Vessels in the pleura are dilated and engorged. Immediately beneath the pleura there are unusually dilated air spaces, all filled with rather homogeneous, amorphous, gray material. Toward the right end of the lesion only, that material is admixed with neutrophils. 60x B (lower, facing page): This photograph shows a section of lung from the same infant. At this higher magnification, many macrophages can be seen in the lesion but very few neutrophils are seen. 250x

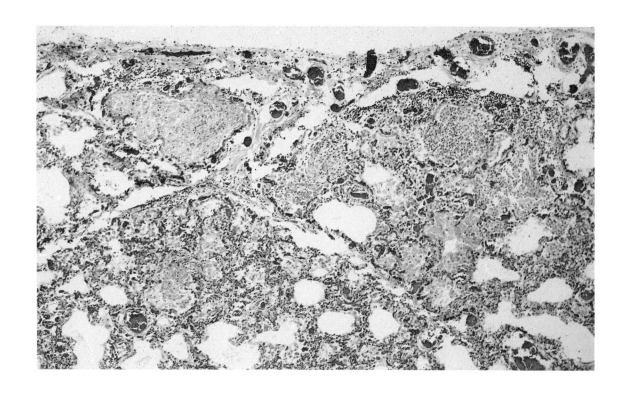

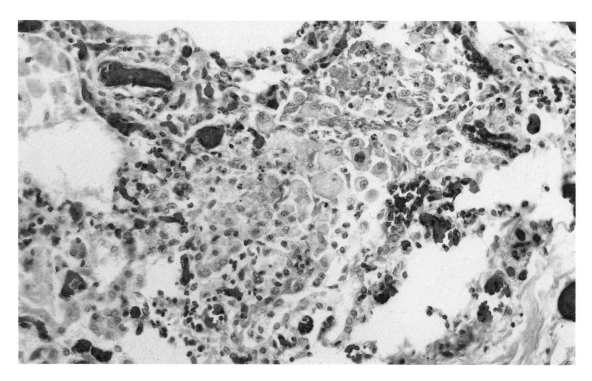

Case History

This Hispanic female infant was born prematurely at 32 weeks of gestation with a birth weight of 1049 grams. She had been diagnosed in the newborn period as having respiratory distress syndrome and remained hospitalized for 47 days. She had apparently recovered from the respiratory condition and did well until her sudden and unexpected death at home at the age of three months. However, this lesion suggests that she had not been entirely well between birth and death. This case was classified as SIDS (Figs. 8–16 and 8–17).

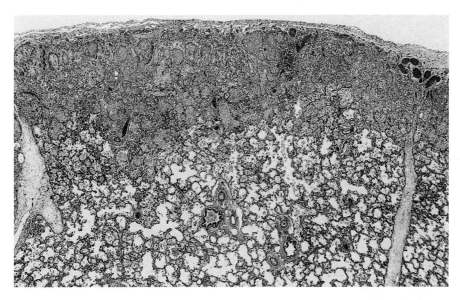

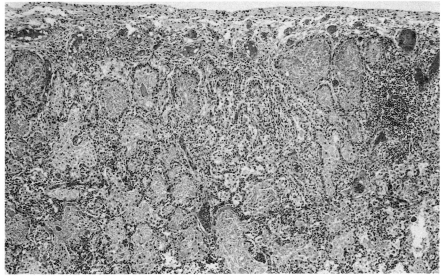

Figure 8–16. Lung, chronic aspiration. All of these illustrations were taken from a lesion in the lung of the same infant.
A (upper): This photograph shows the typical subpleural distribution of the lesion and some engorgement of pleural vessels over it. 25x
B (lower): It is apparent that the affected air spaces are abnormally large; many tend to have their long axes at right angles to the surface. 60x

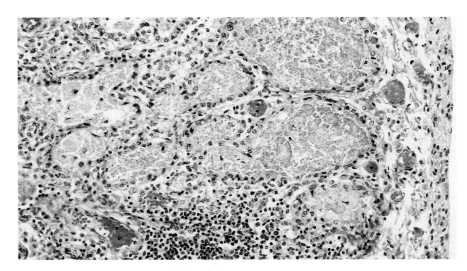

Figure 8–16C. It becomes apparent that the intraalveolar material is rather homogeneous, slightly granular, and accompanied by some macrophages. There is a cluster of lymphocytes along the lower margin. 160x

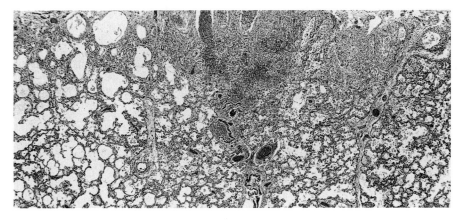

Figure 8–17. Lung, chronic aspiration. These photographs show two sections resembling those illustrated in Figure 8–16. They are from the same infant but are from different portions of the lung. In these, the right-angle orientation of the dilated air spaces to the pleura is even more striking than in the preceding photographs and, for some reason, these accumulations seem to have attracted many more neutrophils.
A (upper): 25x
B (lower): 60x

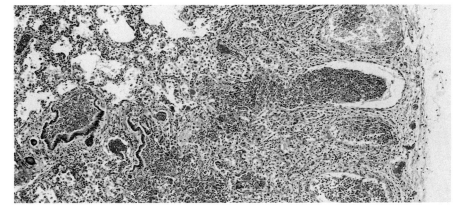

Case History

This white female infant was born prematurely at 35 weeks of gestation with a birth weight of 2240 grams. She had Down syndrome. There was no other history of illness prior to her death at four and a half months of age. She was found dead almost nine hours after having last been seen alive. Her death was classified as a SIDS (Fig. 8–18).

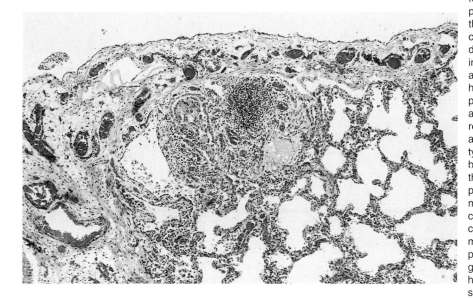

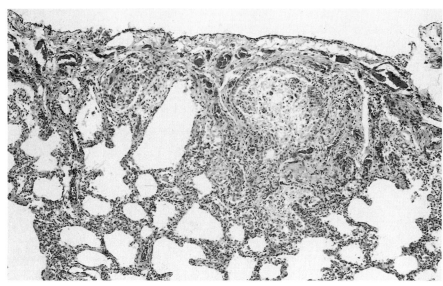

Figure 8–18. Lung, milk granulomas. All four of the following photographs are from the same infant whose clinical history is described above. This infant, even though apparently well at home, clearly had a problem with repeated aspiration of milk. The resultant granulomas again appear in the typical location, just beneath the pleura. In the first three of these pictures, taken at low magnification, the center of the lesion consists of amorphous material; in these photographs it appears gray, but in the original hematoxylin and eosin-stained sections its color was light blue. There are some lymphocytes mingled with the foreign material and the beginning of a fibrous capsule around the periphery.
A (upper): 60x
B (lower): 60x
C (upper, facing page): 60x
D (lower, facing page): In this photograph, at higher magnification, it becomes apparent that the amorphous material bears numerous cholesterol clefts. Macrophages can also be identified in and below the accumulation. 160x

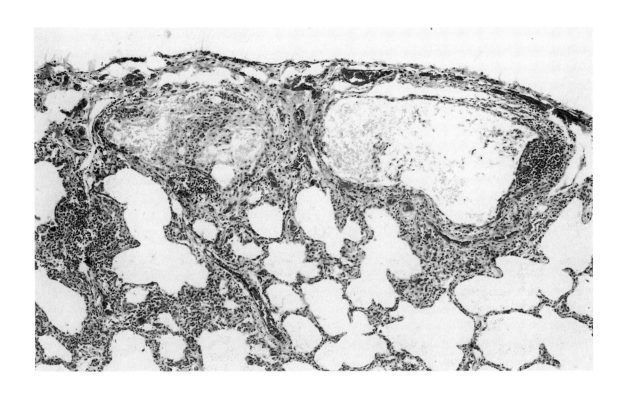

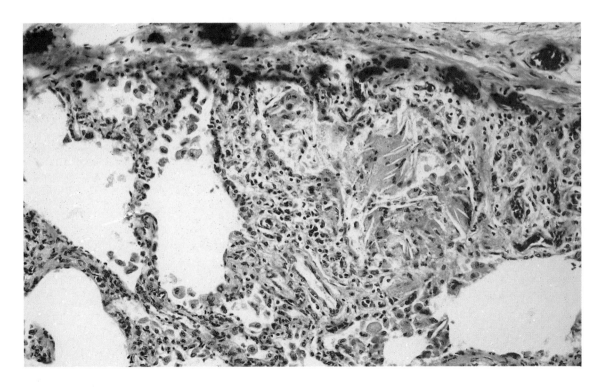

THE "WILSON-MIKITY" PATTERN

Some infants who, as neonates, have been treated with prolonged, intermittent, positive pressure breathing, using high levels of oxygen, in neonatal nurseries experience persistent respiratory distress and develop bronchopulmonary dysplasia. Between 10 and 20 days after the beginning of oxygen therapy, their chest X-rays have a so-called "bubbly lung" appearance. When lungs so affected are examined histologically, patches of alveolar coalescence are seen which appear emphysematous. Surrounding these areas of overexpanded alveoli there are bands of atelectasis. Grossly, the overexpanded areas look pale pink and project prominently from surrounding darker, somewhat depressed pleural surfaces. This pattern corresponds to severe maldistribution of ventilation. Most newborns with persistent X-ray changes of this sort recover by six months to one year of age with about normal pulmonary function. Some, however, require prolonged hospitalization and treatment.[17]

Occasionally, infant lungs at autopsy exhibit this so-called "Wilson-Mikity" appearance. The relationship between this striking histologic pattern and untoward neonatal events cannot always be assessed because neonatal records are frequently not available to the forensic autopsy pathologist. However, based on our experience and some clinical studies, it seems likely that this pattern at necropsy does reflect neonatal respiratory distress treated with oxygen under pressure.[4,12,27]

Case History

This white male infant was born at term weighing 2525 grams. He died at the age of two months. Death was attributed to uremia, the result of congenital cystic hypoplasia of the kidneys. The case was submitted as an autopsy control, not as a SIDS case. Therefore, we do not know with certainty that he had respiratory difficulty as a neonate. It is probable, however, that he had experienced respiratory problems then, which were managed with assisted pulmonary ventilation (Fig. 8–19).

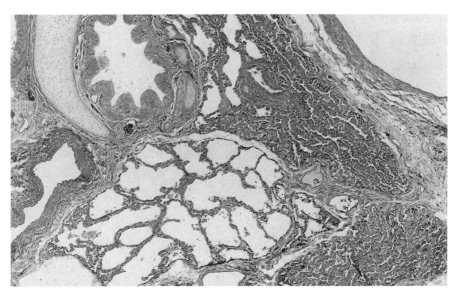

Figure 8–19. Lung, the "Wilson-Mikity" pattern. To the right of the large bronchus in the left upper corner of the photograph is a patch of coalescence of alveoli. The dark, V-shaped atelectatic portion occupies much of the right side of the section. In the center inferiorly is an emphysematous area. This alternating pattern is typical of the "Wilson-Mikity" appearance. 40x

Case History

This white male infant was born very prematurely, about 25 weeks of gestation, with a birth weight of only 681 grams. He experienced severe respiratory distress as a newborn, a fractured femur, and a urinary tract infection. He recovered from all of that and was apparently doing well at home when he was found unresponsive in his crib almost three hours after a feeding. He was four and a half months old when he died. It is not possible to determine in this case, as in the preceding one, whether or not any residual degree of respiratory compromise played a part in the infant's death. Even in the face of this history and the pulmonary pattern observed microscopically, the case was designated a SIDS (Fig. 8–20).

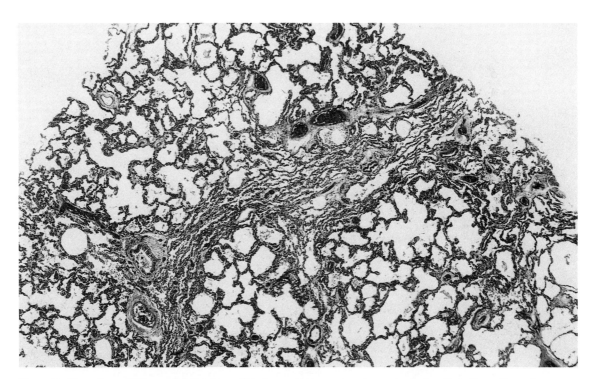

Figure 8–20.   Lung, "Wilson-Mikity" pattern. This figure, at low power, shows clearly the alternating pattern of emphysema and atelectasis; a band of atelectatic lung stretches across the section from lower left to upper right. On both sides of this band, many air spaces are pathologically enlarged. This is not a technical artifact. 25x

Case History

This white male infant was born post-term at 42 weeks of gestation with a birth weight of 4252 grams. He was two and a half months old when he died. Despite the striking histologic appearance of the lungs seen here, this case was designated as a probable SIDS (Fig. 8–21).

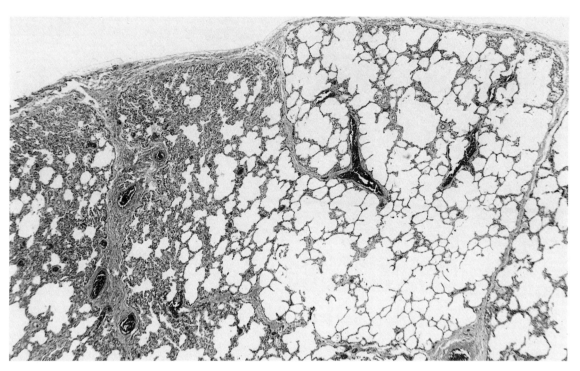

Figure 8–21.   Lung, "Wilson-Mikity" pattern. This is a low-power view of lung, showing what the areas of alveolar coalescence and expansion do to the pleura. The portion of the pleura overriding the patch of emphysema is elevated and the part covering the atelectatic portion, in the left half of the photograph, is depressed. 25x

SEPSIS

It is our opinion that the pathologist is justified in making the diagnosis of sepsis, in the case of a sudden and unexpected infant death, only when at least one postmortem blood culture has yielded a single, potential pathogen. Ideally, the same etiologic agent should be obtained from both the blood and a spleen or lung culture. In our experience no more than 3% of sudden and unexpected infant deaths can be explained by sepsis using this criterion.[33]

There are no morphologic lesions on which to base the diagnosis of sepsis, except perhaps for the presence of many scattered micro-abscesses, and they are found only infrequently.

is impossible to distinguish between them with certainty by means of postmortem examination alone." These deaths must be investigated carefully in other ways.

SUFFOCATION WITH A SOFT OBJECT

Suffocation with a soft object is discussed within the gray zone group, primarily because there is occasionally controversy about it as the cause of death in a specific case and about the criteria that pathologists use to establish it as such.[3,21,29,33,35,38]

In general, experts on the subject agree that it is possible for an adult (and probably for a youth) to suffocate an infant less than a year of age with steady pressure on the nose and mouth for minutes, using a cupped hand or a pillow, without leaving any telltale mark on the body. Furthermore, in many such instances, the autopsy mimics that of SIDS cases in every detail. The most significant evidence for this statement is the occasional confession of a mother or a babysitter.

Not infrequently, the question is raised at meetings of forensic scientists and even of lay people, "How can you tell the difference between the two at necropsy?" The answer is, "It

REFERENCES

1. Beckwith JB. Observations on the pathological anatomy of the sudden infant death syndrome. In: Bergman AB, Beckwith JB, Ray CG, eds. Sudden Infant Death Syndrome, Proceedings of the Second International Conference on Causes of Sudden Death in Infants. Seattle: University of Washington Press, 1970, pp. 83-107.

2. Böhm N. Pediatric autopsy pathology. Philadalphia: Hanley and Belfus, Inc., 1988, p-50.

3. Bowden K. Sudden death or alleged accidental suffocation in babies. Med J Aust 1:65-72, 1950.

4. Coates AL, Bergsteinsson H, Desmond K, Outerbridge EW, Beaudry PH. Long-term pulmonary sequelae of the Wilson-Mikity syndrome. J Pediatr 92:247-52, 1978.

5. Court SDM. The definition of acute respiratory illnesses in children. Postgrad Med J 49:771-6, 1973.

6. Hall CB. Respiratory syncytial virus. In: Feigin RD, Cherry JD, eds. Textbook of Pediatric Infectious Diseases, 2nd ed. Philadelphia: W.B. Saunders Co., 1987, pp. 1653-76.

7. Hall CB. Respiratory syncytial virus and sudden infant death. N Engl J Med (letter) 300:1440-1, 1979.

8. Hall CB, Geiman JM, Biggar R, Kotok DI, Hogan PM, Douglas RG. Respiratory syncytial virus infections within families. N Engl J Med 294:414-9, 1976.

9. Hall CB, Hall WJ, Speers DM. Clinical and physiological manifestations of bronchiolitis and pneumonia. Outcome of respiratory syncytial virus. Am J Dis Child 133:798-802, 1979.

10. Herbst JJ, Minton SD, Book LS. Gastroesophageal reflux causing respiratory distress and apnea in newborn infants. J Pediatr 95:763-8, 1979.

11. Henderson FW, Clyde WA, Collier AM, Denny FW, Senior RJ, Shaeffer CI, Conley WG, Christian RM. The etiologic and epidemiologic spectrum of bronchiolitis in pediatric practice. J Pediatr 95:183-90, 1979.

12. Hodgman JE, Mikity VG, Tatter D, Cleland RS. Chronic respiratory distress in the premature infant; Wilson-Mikity Syndrome. Pediatrics 44:179-95, 1969.

13. Hogg JC, Williams J, Richardson JB, Macklem PT, Thurlbeck WM. Age as a factor in the distribution of lower-airway conductance and in the pathologic anatomy of obstructive lung disease. N Engl J Med 282:1283-7, 1970.

14. Honig PJ, Pasquariello PS Jr, Stool SE. H. influenzae pneumonia in infants and children. J Pediatr 83:215-9, 1973.

15. Hoffman HJ, Hunter JC, Ellish NJ, Janerich DT, Goldberg J. Design of the NICHD SIDS Cooperative Epidemiological Study, in Chapter 11: Adverse reproductive factors and the sudden infant death syndrome. In Harper RM, Hoffman HJ, eds. Sudden Infant Death Syndrome: Risk Factors and Basic Mechanisms. New York: PMA Publishing Corp., 1988, pp. 155-164.

16. Leape LL, Holder TM, Franklin JD, Amoury RA, Ashcraft KW. Respiratory arrest in infants secondary to gastroesophageal reflux. Pediatr 60:924-8, 1977.

17. Kissane JM. Pathology of infancy and childhood, 2nd ed. St. Louis: C.V. Mosby Co., 1975, pp 493-5.

18. Kissane JM. Pathology of infancy and childhood, 2nd ed. St. Louis: C.V. Mosby Co., 1975, pp 495-6.

19. Kissane JM. Pathology of infancy and childhood, 2nd ed. St. Louis: C.V. Mosby Co., 1975, pp 496-9.

20. Kissane JM. Pathology of infancy and childhood, 2nd ed. St. Louis: C.V. Mosby Co., 1975, pp 499-501.

21. Kukull WA, Peterson DR. Sudden infant death and infanticide. Am J Epidemiol 106:485-6, 1977.

22. Norvenius SG. Sudden infant death syndrome in Sweden in 1973-1977 and 1979. Acta Paediatr Scand 1987; Suppl 333:1-138.

23. Paton JY, Macfadyen UM, Simpson H. Sleep phase and gastro-oesophageal reflux in infants at possible risk of SIDS. Arch Dis Child 64:264-9, 1989.

24. Potter EL, Craig JM. Pathology of the fetus and the infant, 3rd ed. Chicago: Yearbook Medical publishers, 1976, pp. 280-2.

25. Rajs J, Hammarquist F. Sudden infant death in Stockholm. A forensic pathology study covering ten years. Acta Paediatr Scand 77:812-20, 1988.

26. Rebban AW, Edward HE. Staphylococcal pneumonia. Review of 329 cases. Can Med Assoc J 82:513-7, 1960.

27. Saunders RA, Milner AD, Hopkin IE. Longitudinal studies of infants with the Wilson-Mikity syndrome. Clinical, radiological and mechanical correlations. Biol Neonate 33:90-9, 1978.

28. Spitzer AR, Boyle JT, Tuchman DN, Fox WW. Awake apnea associated with gastroesophageal reflux: A specific clinical syndrome. J Pediatr 104:200-5, 1984.

29. Smialek JE, Lambros Z. Investigation of sudden infant deaths. Pediatrician 15:191-7, 1988.

30. Stephens BG. Why the autopsy? In: Harper RM, Hoffman HJ, eds. Sudden Infant Death Syndrome: Risk Factors and Basic Mechanisms. New York: PMA Publishing Corp., 1988, pp. 135-41.

31. Stern RC: Bronchiolitis, in Chapter 13: The respiratory system. In: Behrman RH, Vaughan VC, eds. Nelson Textbook of Pediatrics, 13th ed. Philadelphia: W B Saunders Co., 1987, pp 897-8.

32. Stern RC: Bronchiolitis, in Chapter 13: In: The respiratory system. In: Behrman RH, Vaughan VC, eds. Nelson Textbook of Pediatrics, 13th ed. Philadelphia, PA: W B Saunders Co., 1987, pp 898-906.

33. Valdés-Dapena M. The pathologist and the sudden infant death syndrome. Am J Pathol 106:118-31, 1982.

34. Valdés-Dapena M. The morphology of the sudden infant death syndrome—An update, 1984. In: Harper RM, Hoffman HJ, eds. Sudden Infant Death Syndrome: Risk Factors and Basic Mechanisms. New York: PMA Publishing Corp., 1988, pp. 143-50.

35. Werne J, Garrow I. Sudden deaths in infants allegedly due to mechanical suffocation. Am J Publ Health 37:675-87, 1947.

36. Wigglesworth JS. Perinatal pathology, Vol 15. In: Major Problems in Pathology. Philadelphia: W B Saunders Co., 1984, pp. 104-9.

37. Wohl MEB, Chernick V: State of the art: Bronchiolitis. Am Rev Respir Dis 118:759-81, 1978.

38. Wooley PV. Mechanical suffocation during infancy: A comment on its relation to the total problem of sudden death. J Pediatr 26:572-5, 1945.

CHAPTER **9**

ILLUSTRATIVE CASES

INTRODUCTION

This chapter contains the histories and circumstances of death of a selected series of babies, many of whom were *originally* considered to be victims of sudden infant death syndrome (SIDS). These particular cases were chosen either because the microscopic findings are typical of a particular disease entity or because they demonstrate important microscopic abnormalities illustrative of sudden infant deaths in general.

Although only minimal history and investigative information were available in some of the examples, a complete history and thorough scene investigation should be a part of every infant autopsy record. Likewise, growth percentiles are included in the cases presented whenever possible, even when they were not part of the original records. (In those cases they were calculated by the panel and included for the reader's information.) Complete toxicology testing and total body X-rays may be considered part of the forensic infant postmortem examination. Only when pertinent, is that information included in these case studies.

This chapter may be used in two ways. The clinical history, investigative information, and autopsy findings, both gross and microscopic, are presented in such order that the cases may be studied as "unknowns", or diagnostic challenges, or they may simply be read through for the sake of the information they bear.

CASE 1

Clinical History

This black female infant was born at 41 weeks of gestation with a birth weight of 3717 grams. At ten months of age she was brought to the hospital by her mother and grandmother at 4:00 pm on the day of her death. Her mother reported that the baby had been in good health all her life, except for "frequent colds." The infant reportedly had a "very bad cold" for the preceding two weeks, for which her mother had sought medical care three times.

On admission, the infant was lethargic and markedly dehydrated, with sunken eyes, dry mucosal membranes, and leathery lips. She had a faint rapid pulse; her blood pressure was not recorded. Blood gases revealed severe acidosis. The baby was pronounced dead 42 minutes after arrival at the hospital.

Autopsy Findings

At autopsy, the baby's body was clean and well cared for. There were no external or internal signs of trauma. Length and weight were both between the 25th and 50th percentiles for age. Fluid replacement had apparently been satisfactory. Internally, the lungs were described as markedly congested with poor aeration in the dependent regions with blotchy, red foci in nondependent areas. Other organs were normal. Multiple cultures were taken.

The cause of death, reported immediately after the gross autopsy, was bilateral bronchopneumonia and dehydration. Culture results, reported later, included *Klebsiella oxytocia* from the nose, throat, and blood and *Staphylococcus aureus* additionally from the blood. No microscopic examination was recorded.

Microscopic examination by the Pathology Study Panel showed no pneumonia, very mild tracheitis, bronchitis and peribronchitis, and moderate congestion in the lungs. A single section from the left ventricle is shown in Figure 9–1 at low and high magnifications, respectively.

Discussion

Ordinarily, the infiltrate in myocarditis is far less dramatic than this. A small focus of this sort in only one section should arouse suspicion and dictate further sampling of the heart muscle. However, even a single, tiny lesion such as this may be lethal by serving as a focus for arrhythmia.[8]

In this instance, the baby's heart seemed normal grossly, an observation that is typical of gross examination in such cases. The diagnosis is usually established by microscopy.

A similar mistake was made, in reverse, with the lungs. They were thought to show pneumonia grossly when, in fact, none was present microscopically. During this study, panel members were repeatedly impressed that diagnoses based on the gross appearance of the lungs (either positive or negative) were unreliable. Careful microscopic examination of several sections is essential.

Final Diagnosis
Viral Myocarditis

Figure 9–1. Heart, myocarditis. These two photographs demonstrate florid myocarditis with edema, separation of myocardial fibers, and intense infiltration of lymphocytes. A (upper, facing page): Left ventricle of the heart at low power. 60x   B (lower, facing page): The same section at a higher power. 160x

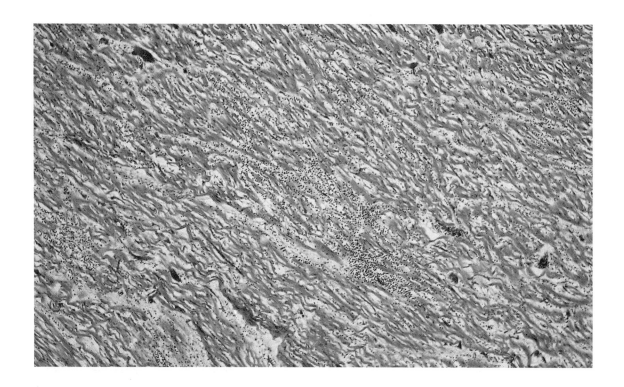

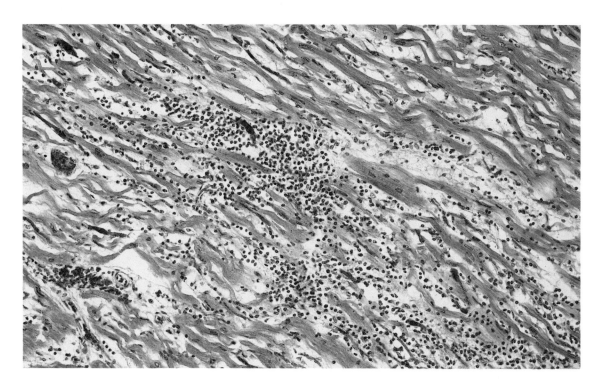

CASE 2

Clinical History

This white female infant was born at term, 40 weeks of gestation, with a birth weight of 3547 grams. At one month of age she was brought to the hospital at 8:45 am by her parents, who said she had a "sore throat" and had previously had a fever, which dissipated after administration of a cool shower. The mother reported that the baby then developed three red spots on her skin. She was pronounced dead 1-½ hours after hospital admission.

The hospital course was unknown as records were not available. The death was reported to the medical examiner because of the short period of hospitalization.

Autopsy Findings

The baby appeared well nourished with a length calculated at the 50th percentile and weight at the 95th percentile for age. Confluent purpura and petechiae covered the entire body, most markedly in the inguinal regions and over the buttocks. Internally, all organs were hyperemic with petechiae and purpura involving the intestines but sparing the thoracic organs. Both adrenals were enlarged and hemorrhagic. Blood and cerebrospinal fluid cultures were taken. No microscopic examination was recorded. The anatomic diagnosis at conclusion of the autopsy was meningococcemia.

Microscopic review by the Pathology Study Panel confirmed generalized congestion, petechiae involving multiple viscera, and adrenal cortical hemorrhage (Fig. 9–2).

Discussion

Although the working diagnosis for this case was Waterhouse-Friderichsen syndrome due to meningococcemia, the autopsy blood culture was positive for *Escherichia coli* only; the spinal fluid culture produced no growth.

Overwhelming sepsis with adrenal hemorrhage (Waterhouse-Friderichsen syndrome) is not specific for meningococcemia but is generally considered a consequence of any endotoxemia and shock.[9,10,14,21,24] *Neisseria meningitidis* (and perhaps *Pseudomonas aeruginosa*) infections may produce the Waterhouse-Friderichsen syndrome relatively more frequently than other organisms. In many geographical areas, however, these two organisms are not the most common cause(s) of *sepsis*. As with bacterial meningitis, the most common organisms, in order of frequency, are *Hemophilus influenzae, Streptococcus pneumoniae,* and *Neisseria meningitidis.*

Another point that should be made is that adrenal glands in infants are often very congested and misinterpreted as being hemorrhagic. In this case, the diagnosis is clearly evident; in others which are less obvious, careful examination may be necessary to confirm true hemorrhage. Sometimes the distinction is impossible.

Final Diagnosis

Escherichia coli *sepsis with Waterhouse-Friderichsen syndrome*

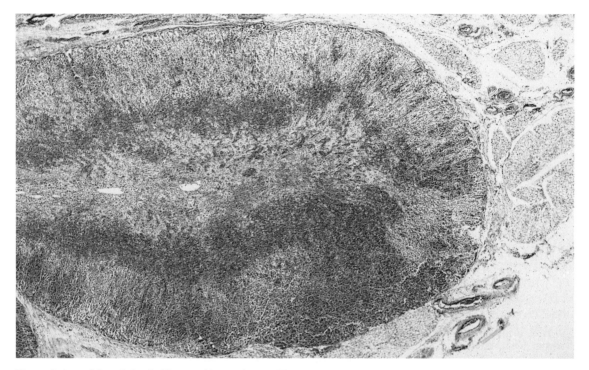

Figure 9–2.   Adrenal gland with central hemorrhage. 25x

CASE 3

Clinical History

This white male infant was born at term, 40 weeks of gestation, with a birth weight of 3630 grams. He had been seen by his pediatrician two days prior to death which occurred when he was 26 days old. At his well-baby check-up, he was thought to be gaining weight and in good health. He was fed and put to sleep at 9:00 pm the night before his death and was found unresponsive in his crib at 7:00 am the following morning. The pregnancy and delivery had been unremarkable. His mother had not taken any medications during the pregnancy and the baby was being fed formula with no problems.

Autopsy Findings

At autopsy, the baby was described as normally developed and well nourished with a length of 20 inches (calculated to be between the 10th and 25th percentile for age) and a weight of 10.3 pounds (75th percentile). The external and internal examinations were entirely normal for the age, showing only petechiae on the heart and over the lungs. Microscopic sections were unremarkable except for an area within the heart described as displaying "prominent myocytolysis" (Fig. 9–3). The original on-site diagnosis after gross and microscopic examination was sudden infant death syndrome.

Discussion

The members of the Pathology Study Panel, each independently, arrived at the diagnosis of rhabdomyomas of the heart (there were several such lesions in the two sections) and questioned whether tuberous sclerosis was also present. When multiple rhabdomyomas are found in the infant heart, the probability of that reflecting tuberous sclerosis is reported to be 50% or higher. If this diagnosis is confirmed, it is a matter of singular importance to the family because the disease is inherited as an autosomal dominant trait.[2, 4, 12, 13, 18, 26]

The clinical history and investigation of the scene for this child were uniformly suggestive of SIDS. The gross autopsy examination was also characteristic (including petechiae on the heart and lungs). It is not surprising that on gross examination of the heart no lesions were perceived. This case emphasizes the importance of careful inspection of these tiny organs and comprehensive microscopic examination, preferably by someone experienced in pediatric pathology. Not only the presence, but also the implication, of multiple cardiac rhabdomyomas may not be apparent to the general pathologist.

Final Diagnosis

Rhabdomyomas of heart; probable tuberous sclerosis

Figure 9–3. Heart, rhabdomyoma.
A (upper, facing page): Rhabdomyoma at low power. 25x   B (lower, facing page): The same section at a higher power. The discrete, pale lesion is the rhabdomyoma. 160x

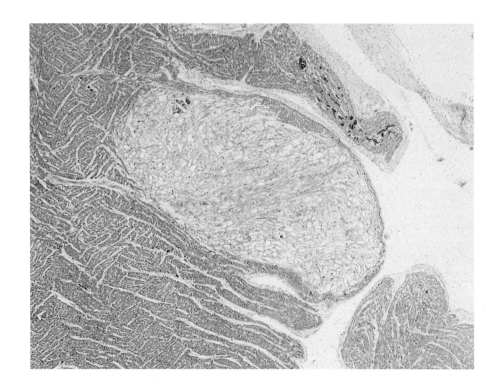

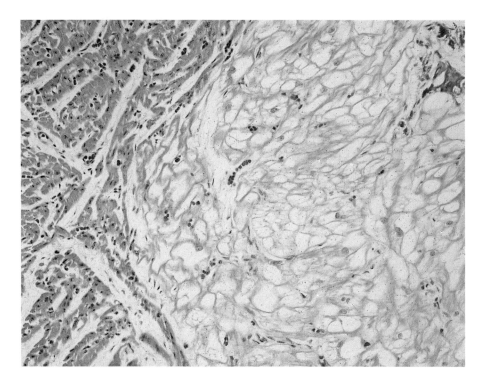

CASE 4

This one month old black male infant was reportedly found by his mother, in the morning, face down in bed, with a small blood stain on the bed sheet beneath his face. The baby had been fed at 11:45 pm the night before and put to bed by an aunt who had been taking care of the infant for the evening. The mother related a normal pregnancy, delivery at 39 weeks of gestation with no problems, and a birth weight of 3005 grams. The baby had been healthy and taking his formula well. His death was reported to the agency responsible for investigating child abuse and neglect because it was felt that the blood in the baby's nose was inconsistent with the history given.

Autopsy Findings

At autopsy, the baby was described as a well-developed, well-nourished, black male infant (calculations of height and weight were between the 10th and 25th percentiles for age). Grossly and microscopically, the lungs showed only congestion and edema. Although no thymic petechiae were described grossly, they were seen microscopically by the Pathology Study Panel (Fig. 9–4).

Discussion

Review by the panel confirmed the fact that there were no significant findings in the microscopic sections; all three reviewers felt that the microscopic findings were consistent with those of SIDS.

Although the child had been dead on arrival at the hospital, an investigator visited the home and spoke with the mother of the child, who reported that she had been out for the evening and that her sister had been taking care of the infant. After feeding the child, the aunt had put the baby in mother's bed and covered him with bed sheets and a blanket. The mother reported that when she arrived home "a little high," she lay down on the bed (with the baby) and went to sleep, unaware of the baby's presence. At some later time, her nine year old son also came to sleep in the bed. When the mother awoke, she found the infant dead in her bed covered over by bedsheets and blankets with a small spot of blood on the bed sheet.

Although the emergency room physician suspected child abuse because of the blood near the baby's nose, this type of bleeding is very common in SIDS and is not necessarily indicative of trauma. It probably derives from blood and edema fluid in pulmonary alveoli, apparently agonal lesions.[29]

Since biblical times, sudden infant deaths have been blamed on "overlaying." In our experience this is uncommon. Even very obese parents tend to be unconsciously "protective" of children with whom they are sleeping, unless they are drugged or drunk. This was one of the few cases we encountered in this study in which such an event was documented. The history of alcohol or drug use (to the extent that the parent's faculties are dulled) is nearly universal in such cases.

The other important issue that this case illustrates (and that the Pathology Study Panel made an inviolable rule) is that no death can be determined to be a sudden infant death syndrome without a comprehensive investigation of the site and circumstances of death. All findings in this instance were absolutely characteristic of SIDS, and that diagnosis was made prior to the scene investigation. It is of the utmost importance that a trained, non-judgmental investigator inspect the scene and question the parents or caretakers.

Final Diagnosis

Probable suffocation/compression asphyxia

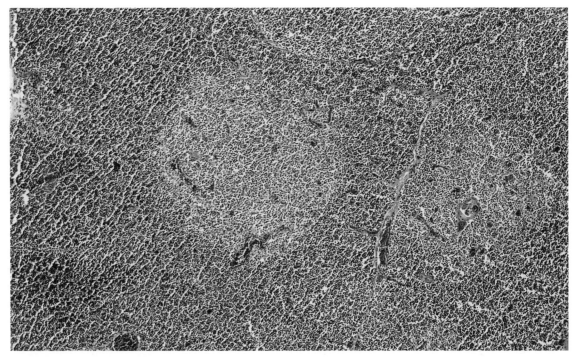

Figure 9–4 . Thymus with petechiae. 60x

CASE 5

Clinical History

This Asian female infant was born at 41 weeks of gestation with a birth weight of 2950 grams. At ten weeks of age she was waiting in the clinic for a routine checkup when her mother noticed that she was having breathing problems and summoned assistance. The infant was cyanotic. Resuscitative efforts, initiated immediately, were unsuccessful. The only other significant medical history was that the child had been born with features suggestive of Down syndrome, although that diagnosis had never been confirmed by chromosomal studies.

Autopsy Findings

At autopsy, the body length was at the 25th percentile for age, weight at the 50th percentile, and head circumference at the 25th percentile. Features of Down syndrome included prominent epicanthal folds, a protruding tongue, and suggestive simian creases. There were no other external abnormalities. Internally, there was an excess of clear fluid in the pleural and peritoneal cavities; petechiae were present. The heart was massively enlarged (calculations revealed it to be three to four times the expected size for the child's size); there was a patent ductus arteriosus, a large (1 cm) interventricular septal defect, and right ventricular hypertrophy.

The microscopic sections as reviewed by the Pathology Study Panel were unremarkable, except for those of the thymus which showed involution indicative of chronic stress (Fig. 9–5).

Discussion

In examining a baby with recognizable abnormalities such as Down syndrome, one might initially consider attributing death to the complex itself. However, in such situations, as in any other case, one is obliged to search for a specific lethal lesion as the cause of death. The fact that a baby has recognizable defects does not necessarily exclude the possibility of death due to SIDS. In this case, however, an obvious cause of death resulting from multiple cardiac malformations was found.[1]

Final Diagnosis

Congenital cardiac anomalies, a large interventricular septal defect, a patent ductus arteriosus, and right ventricular hypertrophy with congestive heart failure (associated with Down syndrome)

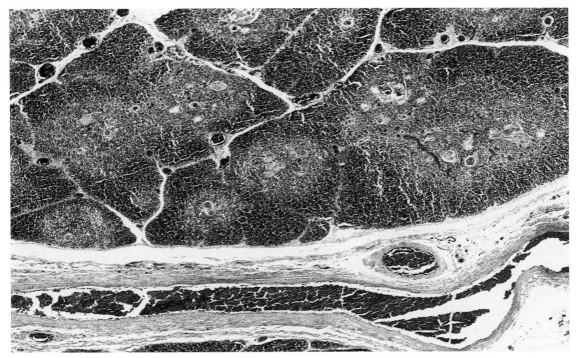

Figure 9–5. Thymus with changes of involution. At low magnification, moderately severe involution can be seen, characterized by thinning of the cortex, generalized loss of cellularity, and numerous prominent Hassall's corpuscles (in contrast to the normal thymus shown in Case 4, Figure 9–4. These findings suggest that the infant had been subjected to chronic stress and are not characteristic of SIDS. In fact, the observation of involution such as this in an infant only two and half months old suggests strongly that the subject has been seriously ill for some time. 25x

CASE 6

Clinical History

This Asian male infant was born at 41 weeks of gestation weighing 3750 grams. At four months of age he was found not breathing, pale, and cold while in the care of a baby-sitter. Initially, resuscitation was successful; however, he later required mechanical ventilation. Approximately five hours after his admission to the hospital no central nervous system function was detectable and life support systems were removed. Although information was difficult to obtain from the parents because of a language barrier, the pediatrician's and hospital's records provided an apparently unremarkable birth history and documentation of routine well-baby care. Investigation of the scene was unremarkable.

Autopsy Findings

Autopsy examination revealed a well-cared for male infant with body length between the 75th and 90th percentile for the age and body weight well above the 90th percentile. Internal examination revealed only petechiae in the thymus and crepitation of the lungs. The original microscopic examiner interpreted a mononuclear infiltrate in the alveolar septa and around the terminal bronchioles as interstitial pneumonitis and bronchiolitis, but considered those lesions to be insufficient to have caused death (Fig. 9–6).[23,29]

Final Diagnosis

Sudden infant death syndrome
(status post-resuscitation attempts)

Figure 9–6. Normal lung. The Pathology Study Panel considered this to be an essentially normal lung for an infant of this age. A (upper, facing page): Connective tissue surrounding this terminal bronchiole contains some mononuclear cells, a normal amount and typical distribution for lymphoid tissue in an infant lung. The thickness of the alveolar septa is characteristic of and normal for an infant. 250x
B (lower, facing page): Focal subpleural emphysema, such as that depicted here, reflects the use of assisted pulmonary ventilation. The affected air spaces are characteristically enlarged, sharply demarcated, and ovoid. 60x

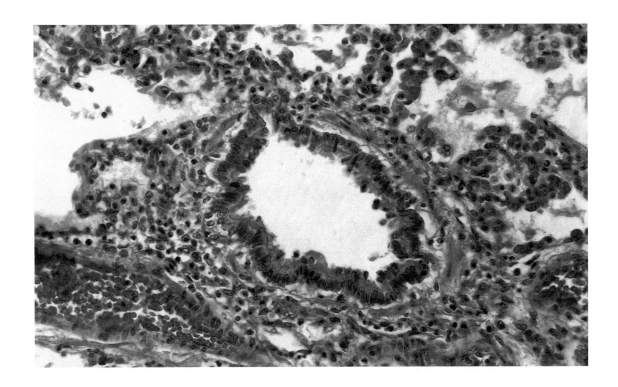

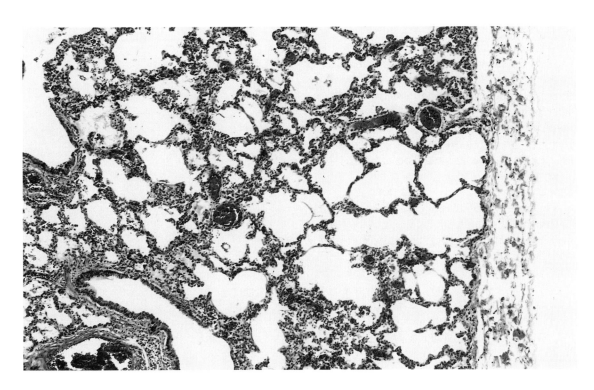

CASE 7

Clinical History

This three and one half month old black female infant was brought into the emergency room by her mother, apparently dead. Froth was bubbling from her left nostril. No other abnormalities were noted. Her mother had fed her and put her to bed at 8:35 pm that evening. When she checked on the baby at 10:50 pm, she found the infant lifeless.

Autopsy Findings

At autopsy, the baby's body weight was between the 25th and 50th percentiles for the age; her head circumference, at the 50th percentile; and her length, between the 75th and 90th percentile. There was no external or internal evidence of injury. Internally, the lungs were described as being deep purple, but no other abnormalities were noted.[20] No microscopic sections were examined by the original pathologist.

The Pathology Study Panel, in their initial review, which was limited to the microscopic sections only, described moderate pulmonary edema without other abnormalities (Fig. 9–7). This feature is characteristic although not diagnostic of SIDS.[30] It may correlate with the clear froth so often found around the nose and/or mouth of babies who have died of SIDS.

Discussion

Following the autopsy, an investigator visited the baby's home and spoke with the family. The baby's mattress had been covered with a thin, plastic, dry cleaner's bag to protect it. The baby had apparently pushed back the lower cotton sheet exposing the thin plastic film which was found adherent to and covering the infant's entire face when she was discovered dead. On the basis of that investigative report, known to them only on their second review, the panel's

diagnosis was changed to accidental suffocation. The microscopic findings had been entirely consistent with SIDS.

Final Diagnosis

Accidental suffocation/asphyxiation by thin, plastic sheet

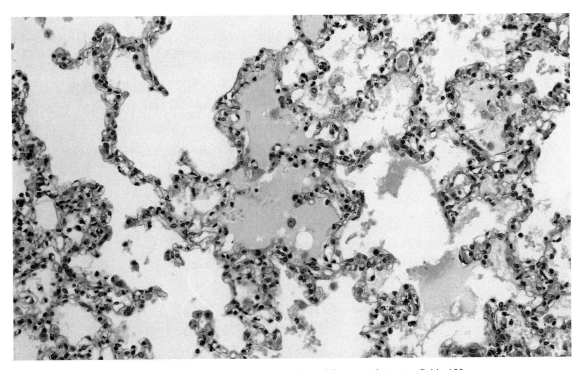

Figure 9–7. Lung with pulmonary edema. Alveoli contain pale-staining, proteinaceous fluid. 160x

CASE 8

Clinical History

This white male infant was born at 39 weeks of gestation weighing 3274 grams. He was 39 days old when he died. He had a slight cough but was not seriously ill before death. He was found unresponsive, wedged between the side rails of his crib and the mattress. He was resuscitated and then taken to a hospital, where he remained on life-support systems for six days before he died.

Autopsy Findings

At autopsy the child was described as well developed and well nourished, with body weight between the 10–25% percentiles for the age; his head circumference, at the 50% percentile; and his length, between the 25–50% percentile. The lungs grossly showed areas of questionable consolidation. The remainder of the prosection was unremarkable.

Microscopic examination by the Pathology Study Panel revealed a patchy pneumonia, involving much of the lung in the five sections submitted, one from each lobe (Fig. 9–8).

Discussion

The cause of death would probably have been simply accidental suffocation had the infant not been resuscitated at the scene. However, he remained alive, but seriously brain damaged, for almost a week, succumbing to secondary pneumonia, probably of bacterial etiology. The Pathology Study Panel considered the underlying cause of death to have been accidental suffocation and the immediate cause, bronchopneumonia.

Final Diagnosis

Accidental suffocation/bronchopneumonia

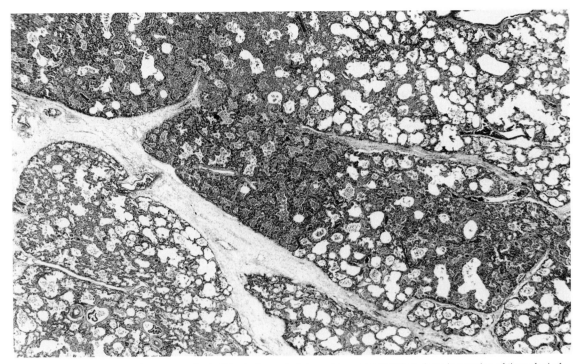

Figure 9–8.   Lung, bronchopneumonia. In this photograph, taken at low magnification, there is a series of three foci of consolidation extending obliquely across the field from the upper left to the lower right corner. In each, all of the air spaces are completely filled with neutrophilic exudate, and the septum, near the center, seems widened by edema. Nodules of florid bronchopneumonia were evident in three of six sections of lung tissue sampled; the remaining three sections showed patchy pneumonia only . 15x

CASE 9

Clinical History

This black female infant was growth retarded at delivery, having been born at 42 weeks gestational age with a birth weight of only 2156 grams. She died at eight months of age. Otherwise, she had been in good health, except for a slight cold and a fractured femur for which her leg had been in a long cast for a few weeks. She was left in the care of her mother's boyfriend. When the mother returned home, she found the child unconscious; the boyfriend was behaving in a peculiar manner and left abruptly. The child died shortly thereafter.

Autopsy Findings

At autopsy, the child was described as well developed and well nourished, although her weight was below the third percentile for her age and her height was between the 10th and 25th percentiles. She had the cast on her leg; her left hip was dislocated and there was a healing fracture of her left humerus (by X-ray). A semicircular, purple contusion involved the left upper eyelid and left cheek bone. Petechiae were discovered in the conjunctivae and the oral mucous membranes. Internally, petechiae were found on the epiglottis and the pleural surfaces of the lungs. The remainder of the examination was unremarkable.

Microscopic examination by the Pathology Study Panel revealed mild laryngitis (Fig. 9–9A), moderate bronchiolitis (Fig. 9–9B), and terminal aspiration of food, with other debris, in the bronchioles (Fig. 9–9C). There was an isolated "starch body" in one bronchiole (Fig. 9–9D).

Discussion

All of these microscopic findings were considered incidental and could well have been found in a typical SIDS autopsy as well. The contusion and the petechiae in the skin, mucous membranes, and internal viscera, however, represent a significant and distinctly abnormal finding.[5,6,20] In contrast to the petechiae found often on the surfaces of the thoracic organs in SIDS, petechiae in other places, e.g., conjunctivae, oral mucous membranes, and epiglottis, suggest suffocation or some other asphyxial mechanism of death. In this case, subsequent questioning of the mother's boyfriend led to his admission of suffocating the baby by holding his hand over the baby's mouth to keep her quiet so that no one would know they were in the apartment. He described swinging her by one leg and one arm "like a plane" causing the dislocation of her leg and, additionally, admitted responsibility for the two fractures. In this case, information derived from the autopsy was so suggestive of child abuse that the investigator was able to conduct an appropriate interrogation of the mother's boyfriend and thus obtain a voluntary confession as to the events leading up to the baby's demise.

Final Diagnosis

Suffocation; child abuse

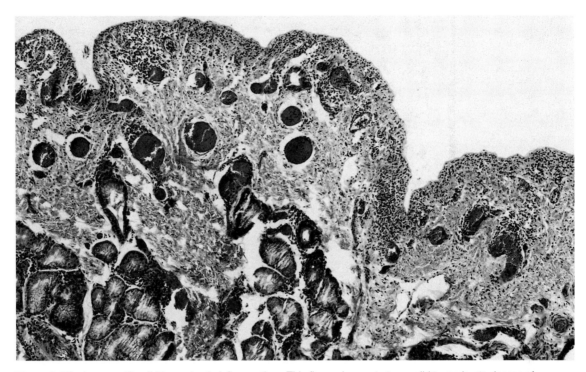

Figure 9–9A. Larynx with mild to moderate inflammation. This figure demonstrates a mild to moderate degree of laryngitis; although it is a significant lesion, it would not be expected to have caused death and is consistent with this child's history of a recent cold. 60x

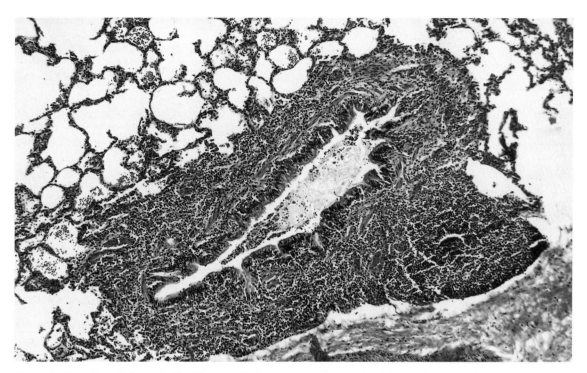

Figure 9–9B. Lung with bronchiolitis. The bronchiolitis demonstrated in this figure was graded as 3+ by the panel. This would have been considered a significant finding, had it been widespread. In this case, however, it was relatively isolated. Note the difference between this inflammatory process (with its circumferential distribution) and the normal lymphoid tissue, in nodules, around bronchioles (Case 6, Fig. 9–6A). 60x

Figure 9–9C (upper, facing page): Lung with aspirated foreign material. The foreign matter within these bronchioles is consistent with aspirated gastric content (food). There is no vital reaction associated with it. Agonal aspiration of gastric material is common in many circumstances, including SIDS, and is not considered a cause or even a mechanism of death, but only a terminal and sometimes artifactual event. 60x **D** (lower, facing page): Lung with "starch body." Demonstration of foreign material, such as this "starch body," is an incidental and relatively common finding at autopsy. 160x

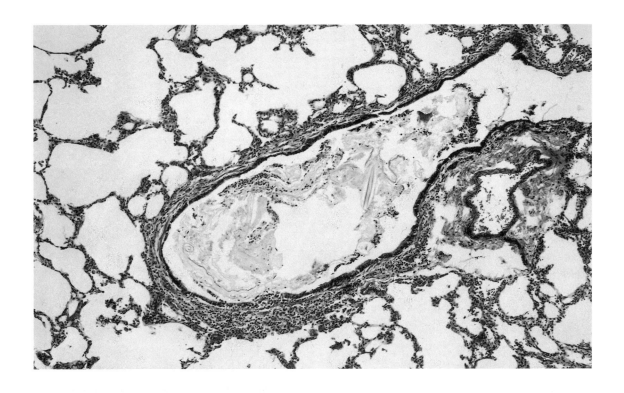

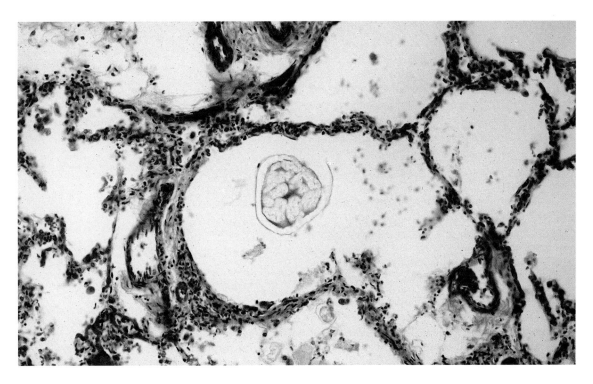

CASE 10

Clinical History

This four month old Hispanic male infant was born by cesarean section at 41 weeks of gestation with a birth weight of 2865 grams. He remained in the hospital for one week following birth. Thereafter, he was in good health, except for occasional bouts of diarrhea, and received regular well-baby care. At four months of age, a few days prior to death, he had a "stuffy nose" and was taken to his doctor. At that time, he was given nose drops and a decongestant. He had no fever. On the day he died, he was last seen alive at 4:00 am but was found unresponsive at 7:00 am. He was taken to a hospital where resuscitation was attempted without success.

Autopsy Findings

At autopsy, the baby was described as "well developed and fairly well nourished." His body length was calculated at the 50th percentile and his weight at the 10th percentile. Other than a "crusty eruption of the scalp," a small amount of serosanguineous fluid in the oral cavity, and evidence of vigorous resuscitation, the external examination was unremarkable. Internal examination demonstrated moderate congestion of all organs and petechiae over the heart, lungs, and thymus. Typical microscopic sections of the lungs are demonstrated in Figure 9–10.

Discussion

These findings are all consistent with SIDS, following vigorous attempts at resuscitation. Congestion may be marked. When septal congestion is severe, there is almost invariably associated alveolar hemorrhage. Intra-alveolar macrophages were numerous (those in Fig. 9–10B are considered few). Although in adults macrophages may be interpreted as indicative of alveolar damage, in numbers such as these, they seem to have little significance in infants.[29]

Final Diagnosis

Sudden infant death syndrome

Figure 9–10. Normal lung. These two photographs show moderate congestion of the alveolar walls and numerous macrophages within alveolar spaces. In other areas, there was intra-alveolar hemorrhage and mild bronchiolitis. A (upper, facing page): Normal lung with congestion. 250x   B (lower, facing page): Normal lung with intra-alveolar macrophages. 250x

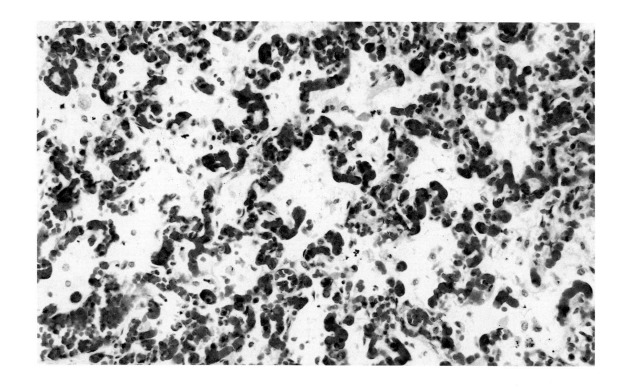

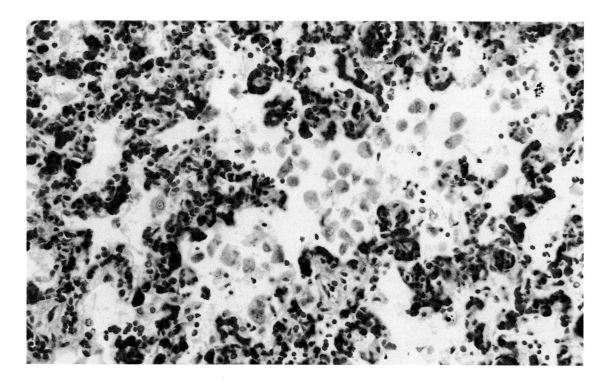

CASE 11

Clinical History

This black female infant was born at term and was severely growth retarded, weighing only 1617 grams. She died at three months of age. Her mother reported that she had been well except for a "cold" for which nose drops had been administered. Also, her mother said the baby was fretful but not "congested" when put to bed. The baby's mother awoke at approximately 4:45 am to find the infant not breathing, with white liquid around her mouth. She rushed the baby to the hospital where she was pronounced dead upon arrival. Two other older siblings were well.

Autopsy Findings

At autopsy, the child was described as "fully developed" for her age. The Pathology Study Panel's comparison with standards, however, revealed her to be below the fifth percentile in weight and height. Her head circumference was just below the second percentile. External examination revealed only a small umbilical hernia and a healing diaper rash. Internal examination showed tan nodules beneath the pleura and throughout the parenchyma of both lungs, diagnosed as diffuse bronchopneumonia. Broad patches of purulent green material involved the leptomeninges over all surfaces of the brain. Microscopic examination was not recorded by the prosector. A microscopic section of the leptomeninges is shown in Figure 9–11.

Discussion

This child had fulminant, purulent bacterial meningitis. The organism responsible for the meningitis in this case was not documented, but the most likely agents at this infant's age, in order of frequency, would be *Hemophilus influenzae, Neisseria meningitidis*, and *Streptococcus pneumoniae.*[3,7,11,15-17,19,22,25,27,28,31]

Noteworthy is the fact that all microscopic sections of the lungs were found to be normal, with no pneumonia. This emphasizes again the difficulty of interpreting gross findings in the infant lung.

This case also demonstrates the fact that a young child may have a significant illness with few, if any, symptoms or signs, and present as do those children who are subsequently found to have died of SIDS. Even a mother who is presumably accustomed to dealing with children's illnesses can be unaware of the severity of such a fulminant illness.

It should be noted additionally that this baby was significantly growth retarded (a critical piece of information that was identified only when autopsy measurements were compared with standards). Growth retardation may be due to a number of factors, e.g., maternal neglect, ignorance, malabsorption states, etc. In any such case, investigation is indicated. The infant who dies of SIDS often has a history of low birth weight and may fall behind ideally matched controls in regard to postnatal weight gain. Some degree of growth retardation is consistent with SIDS but should always alert the pathologist to the possibility of some other underlying problem or disease process which may be recognizable. In this instance the cause of the growth retardation was never identified.

Final Diagnosis

Bacterial meningitis

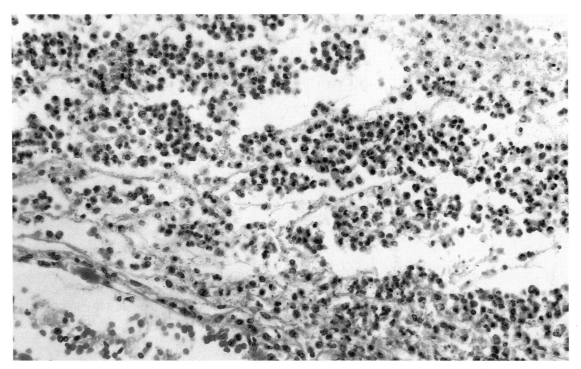

Figure 9–11. Leptomeninges, purulent meningitis. This high power magnification illustrates that the leptomeninges contain large numbers of inflammatory cells that are clearly polymorphonuclear leukocytes. 250x

REFERENCES

1. Arey JB. Chapter 5: Malformations of the ventricular septum. In: Cardiovascular Pathology in Infants and Children. Philadelphia: W.B. Saunders Co., 1984, pp 77-111.

2. Arey JB. Chapter 16: Tumors of the heart and pericardium. In: Cardiovascular Pathology in Infants and Children. Philadelphia: W.B. Saunders Co., 1984, 372-6.

3. Barton LL, Feigin RD, Lins R. Group B beta hemolytic streptococcal meningitis in infants. J Pediatr 82:719-23, 1973.

4. Batchelor TM, Maun ME. Congenital glycogenic tumours of the heart. Arch Pathol 39:67-73, 1945.

5. Beckwith JB. The sudden infant death syndrome. Curr Probl Pediatr 3:1-36, 1973.

6. Beckwith JB. Intrathoracic petechial hemorrhages: A clue to the mechanism of death in sudden infant death syndrome? Ann NY Acad Sci 533:37-47, 1988.

7. Berman PH, Banker BQ. Neonatal meningitis: A clinical and pathological study of 29 cases. Pediatrics 38:6-24, 1966.

8. deSa DJ. Isolated myocarditis as a cause of sudden death in the first year of life. Forensic Sci Int 30:113-7, 1986.

9. deSa DJ, Nicholls S. Haemorrhagic necrosis of the adrenal gland in perinatal infants: A clinico-pathological study. J Pathol 106:133-49, 1972.

10. Devoe IW. The meningococcus and mechanisms of pathogenicity. Microbiol Rev 46:162-90, 1982.

11. Feigen RD: Acute bacterial *meningitis* beyond the neonatal period, in Chapter 11: Infectious diseases. In: Behrman RE, Vaughan VC, eds. Nelson Textbook of Pediatrics, 13th ed. Philadelphia: W.B. Saunders Co., 1987, pp. 569-73.

12. Fenoglio JJ, McAllister HA, Ferrans VJ. Cardiac rhabdomyoma: A clinico-pathological and electron microscopic study. Am J Cardiol 38:241-51, 1976.

13. Fine G. Primary tumors of the pericardium and heart. Cardiovasc Clin 5:207-38, 1973.

14. Greendyke RM. Adrenal hemorrhage. Am J Clin Pathol 43:210-5, 1965.

15. Hand WL, Sanford JP. Post-traumatic bacterial meningitis. Ann Intern Med 72:869-74, 1970.

16. Heerema MS, Ein ME, Musher DM, Bradshaw MW, Williams TW. Anaerobic bacterial meningitis. Am J Med 67:219-27, 1979.

17. Kenny JF, Isburg CD, Michaels RH. Meningitis due to *Haemophilus influenzae* type B resistant to both ampicillin and chloramphenicol. Pediatrics 66:14-6, 1980.

18. Longino LA, Meeker IA. Primary cardiac tumors in infancy. J Pediatr 43:724-31, 1953.

19. Mangi RJ, Quintiliani R, Andriole VT. Gram-negative bacillary meningitis. Am J Med 59:829-36, 1975.

20. Marshall TK. The Northern Ireland Study: Pathology findings. In: Bergman AB, Beckwith JB, Ray CG, eds. Sudden Infant Death Syndrome, Proceedings of the Second International Conference on Causes of Sudden Deaths in Infants. Seattle: University of Washington Press, 1970, pp. 108-17.

21. Martland HS. Fulminating meningococcic infection with bilateral massive adrenal hemorrhage (Waterhouse-Friderichsen syndrome). Arch Pathol 37:147-58, 1944.

22. McGowan JE, Klein JO, Bratton L, Barnes MW, Finland M. Meningitis and bacteremia due to *Hemophilus influenzae*: Occurrence and mortality at Boston City Hospital in 12 selected years, 1935-1972. J Infect Dis 130:119-24, 1974.

23. Cotran RS, Kumar V. Sudden infant death syndrome (SIDS), in Chapter 11: Diseases of infancy and childhood. In: Cotran RS, Kumar V, Robbins SL, eds. Robbins Pathologic Basis of Disease, 4th ed. Philadelphia: W.B. Saunders Co., 1989, pp 415-6.

24. Cotran RS, Kumar V. Waterhouse-Friderichsen syndrome, in Chapter 26: The endocrine system. In: Cotran RS, Kumar V, Robbins SL, eds. Robbins Pathologic Basis of Disease, 4th ed. Philadelphia: W.B. Saunders Co., 1989, pp 1253-4.

25. Schlech WF, Ward JI, Band JD, Hightower A, et al. Bacterial meningitis in the United States, 1978 through 1981. The National Bacterial Meningitis Surveillance Study. JAMA 253:1749-54, 1985.

26. Smith HC, Watson GH, Patel RG, Super M. Cardiac rhabdomyomata in tuberous sclerosis: Their course and diagnostic value. Arch Dis Child 64:196-200, 1989.

27. Spink WW, Su CK. Persistent menace of pneumococcal meningitis. JAMA 173:1545-48, 1960.

28. Symposium on infections of the central nervous system. Med Clin North Am 69:217-435, 1985.

29. Valdés-Dapena M. The pathologist and the sudden infant death syndrome. Am J Pathol 106:118-31, 1982.

30. Valdés-Dapena M. The morphology of the sudden infant death syndrome—An update, 1984. In: Harper RM, Hoffman HJ, eds. Sudden Infant Death Syndrome: Risk Factors and Basic Mechanisms. New York: PMA Publishing Corp., 1988, pp. 143-150.

31. Ward JI, Fraser DW, Baraff LJ, Plikaytis BD. *Hemophilus influenzae* meningitis. A national study of secondary spread in household contacts. N Engl J Med 301:122-6, 1979.

CHAPTER **10**

SUMMARY OF HISTOLOGIC FINDINGS
AND IMPLICATIONS FOR FUTURE SIDS RESEARCH

INTRODUCTION

As described in Chapter 1, the pathology component of the NICHD Cooperative Epidemiological Study of SIDS Risk Factors was designed to ensure that the cases included in the final epidemiological analyses represented definite or probable cases of SIDS. Beginning with the necropsy protocol, which was distributed to each participating medical examiner/coroner's office, standardization of the inherent variability in these complex and diverse systems was attempted. Compliance by field pathologists with requested numbers and types of tissues was outstanding. They provided the materials from which the standard sections were cut and mounted at the Pathology Coordinating Laboratory (PCL) located at the San Francisco Medical Examiner's Office.[1]

In the first stage of the two-tiered review process the three members of the pathology study panel independently and blindly reviewed all histologic sections from each potential case.[23, 25] The only additional information provided was the birth weight, gestational age, and age at death of each infant. During the second review, the panel members, still working independently, examined all accompanying information on each case, including the death investigation report, gross autopsy report, microscopic autopsy report, and any special study reports (toxicology, vitreous humor, chemistry, X-ray, virology, and microbiology), and then assigned a probability of

the case having died of SIDS. After the second review, the Pathology Study Panel met for a final phase of this work to resolve any discrepancies in their individual assessments and to agree on an ultimate designation of each case as being either SIDS (definite or probable), possible SIDS, indeterminate, or explained death.

Based on those proceedings, 757 singleton cases (and 29 multiple birth cases) were classified by the Pathology Study Panel as definite or probable SIDS. If a case that was submitted originally as "SIDS, pending further investigation" was later "turned around" in the field by the responsible medical examiner or coroner, that case was then excluded from the group of eligible SIDS cases. However, the Pathology Study Panel still may have reviewed the case. Although the panel members thought that some "turn around" cases were consistent with the definition of SIDS, those cases were not included in the epidemiological comparisons in accordance with the study protocol.

When the Pathology Study Panel agreed with the pathologists in the field that turn-around cases had died as a result of recognized causes, then those infants were included among the group of explained deaths. At the conclusion of the pathology review process, which included a number of "autopsy control" infants whose deaths were attributable to causes other than SIDS (submitted intentionally by the field pathologists, according to study design, to assure the quality of the work of the Pathology Study Panel), there was a comparison group *altogether* of 65 infants identified as having died from explained causes (nonSIDS).

This final chapter presents a comparison of histopathologic findings in SIDS cases and explained deaths. Findings commonly associated with SIDS, and particularily those in whlch there is still controversy in the literature are given more extensive consideration. The chapter concludes with a discussion of those materials derived from the study which are available for further research and educational endeavors.

COMPARABILITY OF SIDS CASES AND EXPLAINED DEATHS

Before considering the comparison of detailed histopathologic observations in SIDS infants and explained deaths, it is important to examine whether the two groups of infants are similar in relation to such medical and demographic characteristics as, for example, birth weight, gestational age, age at death, race, and sex.[4] Thus, if one of the two groups contained proportionately more very low birth weight and prematurely-born infants, then whatever differences might be discovered could be attributable to that characteristic rather than to the fatal disease processes.

Unlike the two groups of living control infants in the NICHD SIDS Cooperative Epidemiological Study, which were randomly-selected and carefully matched on characteristics such as the infant's age, low birth weight, and race, the "explained death" control infants were not randomly-chosen and no matching had occurred on medical or demographic characteristics. However, the autopsy controls and other explained deaths were all contributed to the study contemporaneously with the SIDS cases by the same

medical examiners and coroners who participated in the geographically-defined, population-based NICHD SIDS Cooperative Epidemiological Study. From the standpoint of pathology, both the SIDS cases and explained deaths were managed in the same way, that is, all of them went through the same two-tiered review by the Pathology Study Panel. In addition, the three panel members had been blinded as to the status of all of the infants at the time of the initial microscopic review.

BIRTH CHARACTERISTICS

The population characteristics for the two groups, SIDS and pathology controls (explained deaths), were similar in several respects (Table 10–1). For example, the proportion of black infants among the SIDS cases and explained deaths was nearly the same, 53.6% and 53.8%, respectively. Similarly, there was an excess of male infants in both groups, 59.7% and 52.3%.

The proportion of preterm infants (<37 weeks) among the SIDS cases and the explained deaths was also similar, 18.2% and 22.2%, respectively. Moreover, the mean gestational ages for the two groups, SIDS and explained deaths, were almost identical, 38.6 weeks versus 38.4 weeks.

The proportion of low birth weight infants (<2500 grams) among the SIDS cases and explained deaths was also similar, 23.6% and 24.2%, respectively. Furthermore, the mean birth weights for the two groups, SIDS and explained deaths, were 2928 grams and 2933 grams. Although there were slightly more explained deaths weighing 3500 grams or more at birth (25.8% versus l9.9%) and a slightly higher proportion of explained deaths with unknown birth weight (4.6% versus 0.3%), neither difference was statistically significant.

Although the explained deaths were not preselected or matched for birth weight, in any way, the agreement between the two birth weight distributions (and gestational age distributions) is important for subsequent analysis. Also, to the extent that pathological differences might derive from such socio-economic or geographic factors as race or sex, the balance between SIDS cases and explained deaths observed for these characteristics is beneficial. Thus, any differences in the results in regard to pathologic lesions described later in this chapter cannot be attributed to differences in race, sex, birth weight or gestational age between the SIDS cases and explained deaths.

AGE AT DEATH

The age distributions for SIDS cases and explained deaths are shown in Table 10–2. The Wilcoxon-Mann-Whitney test is used to test for trends on such data, 2 x k contingency tables with ordered categories.[2,17] In this instance k=5, since there are five age categories. The Wilcoxon-Mann-Whitney test statistic, 0.62, for the two age

Table 10–1. **Number and Percent of Singleton SIDS Cases and Explained Deaths by Race, Sex, Gestational Age, and Birth Weight**

	SIDS Cases No.	SIDS Cases %	Explained Deaths No.	Explained Deaths %
Race				
black	406	53.6	35	53.8
non-black	351	46.4	30	46.2
Sex				
male	452	59.7	34	52.3
female	305	40.3	31	47.7
Gestational Age				
≤ 32 weeks	44	5.8	4	6.2
33-36 weeks	93	12.3	10	15.4
37-41 weeks	549	72.5	44	67.7
≥ 42 weeks	68	9.0	5	7.7
unknown	3	0.4	2	3.1
Birth Weight				
≤ 1499 grams	33	4.4	2	3.1
1500-2499 grams	145	19.2	13	20.0
2500-3499 grams	427	56.4	31	47.7
≥ 3500 grams	150	19.8	16	24.6
unknown	2	0.3	3	4.6
Total	757		65	

distributions is highly significant, p<0.002. This statistic may be interpreted as the probability that an explained death is older than a SIDS case is .62. Alternatively, the difference may be expressed in terms of the median age at death for SIDS cases, which is 77 days (2.5 months), compared to that of explained deaths, which is 111 days (3.6 months). This difference of approximately one month, on average, in postnatal age prompts a further question as to whether gestational age interacts with postnatal age and also needs to be taken into account. The answer is negative. There are no significant differences in the median ages at death for preterm (≤36 weeks gestation) compared to term (≥37 weeks) infants, either among the SIDS cases (2.7 versus 2.5 months) or the explained deaths (3.7 versus 3.1 months). Thus, only the overall difference in median age at death between SIDS cases and explained deaths is significant.

If any of the pathology findings described later in this chapter vary systematically as a function of age at death, the difference in age distributions could be responsible. The analyses of the pathological data, therefore, have been stratified for the categories of age at death shown in Table 10–2. If differences attributable to age at death were found to have influenced the result, they have been incorporated into the following discussion.

CAUSES OF EXPLAINED DEATHS

The comparison group of 65 explained deaths used in this study comprise the following: 15 cases submitted as SIDS from the study centers and later reclassified by the pathology study panel; an additional 11 cases originally submitted as SIDS in which the diagnosis was later changed, or "turned around," at the local study center after toxicology, microscopic results, or other information became available; 39 explained deaths submitted from the study centers as "autopsy controls."

A detailed listing by cause of death is provided in Table 10–3. The 65 explained deaths have been further subdivided into two groups, as due to either: (1) natural causes, those associated with disease processes, or (2) unnatural causes, those attributed to accidents or injuries.

Table 10–2. **Age at Death Distribution of Singleton SIDS Cases and Explained Deaths**

Age at Death	SIDS Cases		Explained Deaths	
	No.	%	No.	%
2–5 weeks	118	15.6	11	16.9
6–11 weeks	311	41.1	15	23.1
12–23 weeks	239	31.6	15	23.1
24–51 weeks	73	9.6	15	23.1
52–103 weeks	16	2.1	9	13.8
Total	757	100.0	65	100.0

Table 10–3. **Specific Causes-of-Death Categories for the Explained Death Infants**

	No.	%
I. NATURAL CAUSES		
Infectious Diseases		
Pneumonia/bronchiolitis	18	
Dehydration/Fluid and electrolyte imbalance	5	
Meningitis	3	
Myocarditis	3	
Adrenal hemorrhage (Waterhouse-Friderichsen)	1	
Cellulitis in the neck	1	
Coronary thrombosis (complication of sepsis)	1	
Febrile seizures	1	
Neonatal hepatitis	1	
Tuberculosis	<u>1</u>	
Subtotal	35	53.9
Congenital Malformations/Inherited Diseases		
Congenital heart disease	8	
Other congenital anomalies	3	
Uremia (due to renal hypoplasia)	1	
Tuberous sclerosis	1	
Sickle Cell disease	<u>1</u>	
Subtotal	14	21.5
II. UNNATURAL CAUSES		
Accidental Deaths		
Suffocation/asphyxia (accident)	4	
Motor vehicle accident	2	
Burns and smoke inhalation (? accident)	1	
Digitalis toxicity (associated with PDA)	1	
Drowning (? accident)	1	
Fall from window (accident)	1	
Subdural hemorrhage (? accident)	<u>1</u>	
Subtotal	11	16.9
Deaths from Child Abuse		
Malnutrition/dehydration	1	
Subdural hemorrhage	1	
Drowning	1	
Suffocation	1	
Liver laceration/trauma (? child abuse)	<u>1</u>	
Subtotal	5	7.7
Total	65	100.0

285

Infectious processes, either directly or by their consequences (including dehydration), were the most common causes of explained death. Overall, 35 (54%) of the explained deaths were attributed to infection. Although all of the infections were difficult for the pathology study panel to assess, the 18 cases of pneumonia, bronchitis, and bronchiolitis, as a group, caused the greatest controversy. In addition, pulmonary infections were both the most overdiagnosed (along with interstitial pneumonitis) in the field, and the most apt to be reclassified by the pathology study panel.

Congenital malformations and inherited diseases accounted for 14 (22%) of the explained deaths. Unnatural deaths comprised 16 (24%) of the cases; suffocation or asphyxia (including drowning) accounted for almost half (seven) of those. The unnatural explained deaths provided an especially interesting group to study since, microscopically, the findings were consistently indistinguishable from those of the SIDS cases, and they were all classified as unexplained during the first (microscopic only) review.

Following subdivision of the 65 explained deaths into these two subgroups, "natural" and "unnatural" deaths, the question arises as to whether they themselves differ from each other in regard to race, sex, gestational age, birth weight, or age at death distributions. If differences were apparent in regard to these characteristics, then there would be an argument for further stratification of the pathology results. However, there were no significant differences between natural and unnatural deaths in relation to male sex (52% versus 53%), black race (54% versus 53%), mean gestational age (38.4 weeks versus 38.5 weeks), or mean birth weight (2919 grams versus 2986 grams). The age at death distribution is slightly different: the median age at death for those with natural causes was 101 days (3.3 months), but for those with unnatural causes was 121 days (4.0 months). Although the variability (and skewness) of the age at death distribution is too large (with the sample size of explained deaths available in this study) for this

result to be statistically significant, fewer of the natural deaths exceeded six months of age (35%) than did to the unnatural death (47%). Since age at death has been recognized already as an important variable for the stratification of results (because the SIDS cases were on average one month younger than the explained deaths), no additional refinement in the pathology analysis was deemed necessary.

APPROPRIATENESS OF AUTOPSY CONTROLS FOR SIDS CASES

In the past, some investigators have questioned the appropriateness of particular sets of control infants for SIDS cases.[4, 19] Some have maintained that only apparently healthy infants of the same gestational and postnatal age, birth weight, race, and even socioeconomic status as the SIDS cases would be acceptable.

In this study, it was found fortuitously that the 65 "explained deaths" constitute an almost ideal match for the 757 SIDS cases. There were no differences between the two groups as regards race, sex, gestational age, or birth weight. As far as age is concerned, since the SIDS cases are, on average, one month younger than the explained deaths, that single factor can be taken into account in any statistical comparison and the two groups contrasted within specific age at death categories.

PREVALENCE OF HISTOLOGIC LESIONS

The primary task of the pathology study panel was not to conduct a research project *per se*, but rather to validate all autopsy cases as being, or *not* being, instances of the sudden infant death syndrome. The advisory and steering committees for the NICHD SIDS Cooperative Epidemiological study decided on this strategy for the pathology component so that the results of the epidemiological investigation would be as generally applicable as possible to the accepted pathologic classification of SIDS cases at centers across the United States, as described in the report of the 1976 conference in Santa Fe, New Mexico.[14, 26]

According to the plan, the pathology panel members did not establish criteria for specific microscopic diagnoses beforehand but, instead, described the presence and severity of all pathologic lesions observed, according to their own independent interpretation and judgment.

The three pathologists selected for this microscopic review (Dr. Russell Fisher, Chief Medical Examiner for the State of Maryland, Dr. Marie Valdés-Dapena, Professor of Pathology and Pediatrics at the University of Miami School of Medicine, and Dr. James Weston, Chief Medical Investigator for the State of New Mexico) each received, in turn, sets of microscopic slides, six cases to a box, from the pathology coordinating laboratory in San Francisco. In addition to the slides for the six cases, each box contained an envelope with six blank forms for the pathologist to use in recording his or her diagnoses for each organ, mailing labels for forwarding the slides, and stamped addressed envelopes for sending the completed microscopic forms back to the pathology coordinating laboratory. The format of the blank forms included subheadings under each organ such as those listed in Table 10–4. For example, for the trachea the subheadings included inflammation, denuded epithelium, neutrophils, etc. For each organ the pathologist was required to check either normal or abnormal and, then, to evaluate the *positive* diagnoses, providing for each an expression of the degree or extent of involvement from minimal (1+) to marked (4+).

It was agreed at the outset that each of the three principal reviewing pathologists, who were located in Maryland, Florida, and New Mexico, could ask their co-workers to read slides from a portion of the cases. For example, one of the pathologists read approximately 60% of all of the cases, while the other 40% were read in conjunction with fellows, co-workers, and residents. At the other extreme, one pathologist took the full responsibility of reviewing and recording all of the desired information. The third pathologist shared the tasks for the microscopic slide review with one colleague only, while referring specific questions to particular experts available on staff. Although this permitted frequent consultations to be sure of consistency in diagnosis locally, there was never, by design, any such communication among the three principal pathologists, either before or during the review of microscopic slides.

From the perspective of the principal pathologists, the single feature of the task which they objected to at the outset, namely, being asked to interpret microscopic sections blindly, upon completion of the study became a unique and valuable aspect of the work.[12] The pathologists knew that their work would be "monitored" during the project. For example, a small proportion (3%) of cases were randomly selected, renumbered, and sent to them a second time to check on their consistency. In addition, "autopsy controls" (for example, deaths attributed to meningitis or tuberous sclerosis), which were known to be explained deaths by the pathologists in the field, were included deliberately among the potential SIDS cases. The pathology study panel members were informed that explained deaths would be inserted and, therefore, realized they had to be alert and as objective as possible in reading every potential case. At the end of the study, the reward for all of their effort was the opportunity to examine the figures shown in Table 10–4, knowing that they were not contaminated by subjectivity since the pathology study panel members never knew what sort of death each case was while the microscopic slides were being read.

The percentages shown in Table 10–4 represent the combined results (normal versus abnormal and positive diagnoses) obtained by averaging across the individual pathologists who reviewed the slides for the 757 SIDS cases and the 65 explained deaths. Differences

Table 10–4.   Histopathological Findings Based on the Pathology Study Panel Review of Microscopic Slides for Singleton SIDS Cases and Explained Deaths [a, b]

	SIDS Cases %	Explained Deaths %
Epiglottis		
Normal	59	49
Inflammation	40	48
Trachea		
Normal	70	55 **
Inflammation	29	45 **
Denuded epithelium	10	13
Neutrophils	<1	<1
Thick basement membrane	<1	<1
Adventitial hemorrhage	<1	<1
Thyroid		
Normal	98	98
Thymus		
Normal	56	64
Petechiae	44	25 **
Lung		
Normal	10	13
Congestion	89	80 **
Alveolar hemorrhage	66	54 *
Edema	63	51 *
Septal hemorrhage	30	13 **
Macrophages	15	18
Emphysema	14	18
Pleural hemorrhage	13	5 *
Bronchiolitis	10	26 **
Poor inflation/atelectasis	7	16 **
Aspiration	10	13
Bronchitis	8	13
Pneumonia	8	34 **
Alveolar collapse	10	12
Postmortem bacterial colonies	5	4
Pneumonitis	4	7
Resuscitative changes	1	2
Granuloma	<1	<1

Table 10–4 *Continued*

	SIDS Cases %	Explained Deaths %
Heart		
Normal	95	92
Endocardial thickening	2	2
Petechiae	3	3
Lymphocytic infiltrate	<1	<1
Interstitial hemorrhage, pericapillary	<1	<1
Diaphragm		
Normal	98	98
Gastroesophageal Junction		
Normal	85	81
Inflammation	12	11
Cellular infiltrate	<1	<1
Liver		
Normal	45	36
Congestion	35	35
Extramedullary hematopoiesis	23	14 *
Fatty change	8	19 **
Triaditis	5	3
Abnormal glycogen	1	2
Hepatitis	1	2
Hepatocellular necrosis	<1	2
Focal inflammation	<1	<1
Portal fibrosis	<1	1
Sinus leukocytes	<1	<1
Foamy vacuolization	<1	<1
Hemangioma	<1	<1
Pancreas		
Normal	88	82
Islet cell hyperplasia	6	10
Cystic fibrosis	<1	<1
Spleen		
Normal	76	63 **
Congestion	18	27 *
Acute splenitis	2	7 **
Hemosiderosis	<1	1
Extramedullary hematopoiesis	<1	1

Table10– 4. *Continued*

	SIDS Cases %	Explained Deaths %
Adrenal		
Normal	59	59
Congestion	40	35
Brown fat present, periadrenal	74	74
Hemorrhage	3	4
Lipid depletion	1	2
Kidney		
Normal	63	58
Congestion	26	30
Relative immaturity	7	7
Calcium deposits	4	8
Pyelonephritis	<1	<1
Vacuolization of proximal tubular epithelium	<1	<1
Ileum		
Normal	95	91
Lymphoid hyperplasia	3	10 **
Eosinophilic infiltrate	<1	1
Lymphoid depletion	<1	<1
Mesenteric Lymph Node		
Normal	93	82 **
Lymphocytic depletion	1	4
Congestion	<1	1
Acute adenitis	<1	3
Blood		
Normal	97	91 **
Sickled cells	<1	3
Brain		
Normal	90	84
Congestion	28	27
Perivascular hemorrhage	17	16
Petechiae	16	17
Calcification	3	6
Hypoxic changes	2	6 **
Relative immaturity	<1	<1

Table10– 4. *Continued*

	SIDS Cases %	Explained Deaths %
Brain		
Encephalitis	1	<1
Meningitis	<1	6 **
Edema	<1	1
Abcess	<1	<1
Inflammation	<1	<1
Excess subependymal neural nests	<1	<1

[a] The findings shown in this table reflect the average percentage, combining the results obtained independently from the reviewing pathologists. Also, the percentages generally do not add to l00% within each organ since the subheadings are not mutually exclusive.

[b] The percentage of SIDS cases and explained deaths, respectively, with missing microscopic slides for this review, by organ, were: epiglottis (20%, 12%), trachea (20%, 16%), thyroid (27%, 23%), thymus (4%, 5%), lung (<1%, 0%), heart (l%, 2%), diaphragm (16%, 5%), gastroesophageal junction (36%, 28%), liver (1%, 0%), pancreas (8%, 8%), spleen (3%, 12%), adrenal (7%, <1%), kidney (2%, <1%), ileum (17%, 15%), mesenteric lymph node (24%, 17%), brain (2%, 4%). The percentages provided in the table were based only on the number of slides reviewed in each organ.

*p<.01

**p<.001

between the two groups which were highly, (p<.01), or very highly, (p<.001), significant statistically are indicated in the table by one or two stars, respectively.

There were ultimately some differences in the individual interpretations by the three pathologists but those were usually not remarkable. This point is exemplified by the diagnoses submitted for pneumonia, as shown in Table 10–5 below.

As might have been expected, there were some items that proved to be of special interest to one or another member of the panel and not to others. One example of that is macrophages in alveoli, about which Pathologist B was particularly concerned. This pathologist made mention of their presence much more frequently than the other two, as shown in Table 10–6.

In the end, such variations in diagnosis proved to be of little consequence as far as the primary outcomes of the study are concerned. The differences reported in Table 10–4 as significant are all robust across the three reviewing pathologists. Conversely, there were no outstanding instances in which one (or two) of the pathologist(s) found a significant difference between the SIDS cases and control infants that was contradicted by the third pathologist.

Table 10–5.   Percentage of SIDS Singleton Cases and Explained Deaths Diagnosed as Having Some Degree of Pneumonia

	Pathologist A	Pathologist B	Pathologist C
SIDS cases	9.7	5.7	9.0
Explained deaths	33.9	32.3	35.5

DISCUSSION OF SELECTED HISTOLOGIC LESIONS

INFLAMMATION OF THE UPPER AIRWAY

Some degree of inflammation in the mucosa of the epiglottis, larynx, and/or trachea is expected in approximately one-third of SIDS autopsies, which is close to what was found in the NICHD study.[22] There was documented inflammation of the epiglottis in 40% of the 757 SIDS cases. Also, it was found in 48% of the 65 explained deaths. The numbers for tracheitis are similar, 29% of SIDS cases and 45% of the explained deaths, which is statistically significant.

The fact that a greater percentage of control infants had upper airway inflammation than did SIDS infants is consistent with the fact that many of the explained deaths were due to lung infections, that is, pneumonia, bronchitis and bronchiolitis.

PULMONARY CONGESTION

Pulmonary congestion is often mentioned as one of the classic findings in a SIDS autopsy and there is a statistically significant difference between cases and controls in this study as well. However, the result cannot be considered to have practical discriminatory value since it was noted to be present in 89% of SIDS infants but, also, in 80% of explained deaths.

PULMONARY EDEMA

Pulmonary edema has also been mentioned as a characteristic feature of the typical SIDS autopsy. It was present in 62% of the SIDS autopsies but, also, in 51% of the explained deaths. Some difference is apparent but it is not marked.

Table 10–6.   Percentage of SIDS Singleton Cases and Explained Deaths with Macrophages in Alveoli

	Pathologist A	Pathologist B	Pathologist C
SIDS cases	2.8	36.5	7.0
Explained deaths	6.4	35.5	11.3

head

LIVER

Extramedullary Hematopoiesis

It is apparent that, in about one fourth of the SIDS cases, some degree of hematopoiesis was evident in microscopic sections of the liver. In fact, it was present in the SIDS cases significantly more frequently than in the explained deaths (23% in SIDS cases versus 14% in explained deaths). This observation confirms earlier research findings on the subject.[7, 18, 21]

Fatty Change

Fatty change in the liver was much more prevalent among the explained deaths (19%) than among the SIDS cases (8%). This is to be expected since many more of the explained death infants were ill and probably had not been eating normally for days. That was not the case for most SIDS Infants.

SPLEEN

Acute Splenitis

The difference seen in the prevalence of acute splenitis, 7% in explained deaths versus 2% in SIDS cases, is not surprising. One should anticipate finding more neutrophils in the red pulp of the spleen in the explained death infants simply because many of them died of acute inflammatory processes. They probably also had higher white blood cell counts in peripheral blood than did the SIDS cases.

ADRENAL

Presence of Periadrenal Brown Fat

In this particular instance, it is not the *amount* of periadrenal brown fat that is being reported but simply its presence or absence. Since the ages of the infants in both the SIDS cases and

explained deaths range from two weeks to two years and since the percent of brown fat in the periadrenal adipose pad normally drops from about 95 percent in the first month of life to approximately 50% at eight months, it is not surprising that in these two "mixed" groups (that vary in regard to both age and mechanism of death), the percentages seen in the two groups are not different from each other.

The morphometric histologic studies which, in the past, demonstrated differences in the *percent* of brown fat in this anatomical location—between cases and controls—were performed by means of painstaking microscopic morphometry and by comparing infants within strictly limited age categories.[18, 20] The data presented here are of a totally different character.

THYMUS

Thymic Petechiae

Thymic petechiae were seen microscopically in 44% of the SIDS cases and in 23% of the explained deaths. They were noted in the gross autopsies of 45% of the SIDS cases and in 22% of the explained deaths. Although these percentages are similar, in some cases petechiae were noted in the gross autopsy but were not seen microscopically and vice versa.

Because thymic petechiae have long been considered one of the "hallmarks" of the typical SIDS autopsy, it is of interest to know how frequently they had been documented either grossly (at autopsy) *or* microscopically in the 757 SIDS cases and in the 65 controls. In fact, they were noted in 526 (69%) of the SIDS cases, slightly more than two-thirds, and in 25 (38%) or slightly more than one third of the explained deaths (p<.001). It is apparent then, that they are not specific nor diagnostic of SIDS *and* that one expects to find them *absent* in about one-third of SIDS autopsies. Nevertheless, these figures confirm the original, long-standing impression that there are thymic petechiae in the majority of infants who succumb to the sudden infant death syndrome. [3, 10, 15]

LUNG

Pleural Petechiae

Much the same can be said of pleural petechiae. If only gross autopsy data are used, these lesions were noted in 408 (54%) of the 757 SIDS infants and in only 23 (35%) of the 65 explained deaths (p<.001).

Microscopically there were, in fact, significantly more hemorrhages in pleura, alveoli and septa in SIDS infants than in explained deaths. The percentages are all listed in Table 10–4. For purposes of the combined analysis, pleural hemorrhages and/or septal hemorrhages were chosen as indicative of lung petechiae microscopically.

Combining the gross and microscopic results, petechiae were noted in 474 (63%) of SIDS cases and in 25 (38%) of explained deaths. The majority were noted during the gross autopsy.

Macrophages in Alveoli

There were no more macrophages in alveoli among SIDS cases than there were among the explained deaths, 15.4% for the former and 17.7% for the latter.

Granulomas in Lung

Similarly, few infants in either the study group or the control group had granulomas in the lung, 0.4% in the former and 0.5% in the latter.

HEART

Epi- and/or Myocardial Petechiae

Petechiae in or on the heart, observed either grossly or microscopically, were documented in 347 (46%) of the 757 SIDS cases and in 15 (23%) of the 65 explained deaths (p<.001). Only about 1% of the petechiae in the heart were noted during the review of microscopic slides;

the vast majority were noted on gross examination.

INTRATHORACIC

Petechiae

In order to compare the percentage of petechiae observed intrathoracically in SIDS cases and explained deaths, the gross and microscopic findings in the heart, lungs, and thymus have been combined. The presence of petechiae in any of the three organs, either on gross examination or microscopic review, has been counted as an occurrence of intrathoracic petechiae. By way of definition, an occurrence of petechiae microscopically was determined to be "yes" if at least two of the three pathologists noted that petechiae were present. Among the SIDS cases, 622 (82%) had intrathoracic petechiae using these definitions compared to 39 (60%) of the explained deaths, which is statistically significant (p<.001). Yet, it is clear that intrathoracic petechiae, by themselves, do not constitute a specific marker for SIDS. They were *not* noted in 18% of the SIDS cases, while they were noted in 60% of the explained deaths.

SUMMARY OF POSITIVE MORPHOLOGIC FINDINGS

The statistically significant *positive* morphologic findings in SIDS infants in this study are the following:

1. Thymic petechiae, grossly and microscopically;
2. Pleural petechiae, grossly and microscopically;
3. Lung congestion and edema, microscopically;
4. Epi- and myocardial petechiae, grossly;
5. Extramedullary hematopoiesis in the liver, microscopically.

SPECIAL STUDIES BASED ON THE NICHD HISTOPATHOLOGY COLLECTION

Two special studies have been conducted with the NICHD histopathology collection that has been stored and maintained by the Armed Forces Institute of Pathology (AFIP). The first of these investigations involved the question of renal glomerulosclerosis and SIDS.[24]   In the past twenty-five years, two different groups of SIDS researchers have indicated that SIDS infants have excess numbers of sclerotic glomeruli in their kidneys.[5, 6] Since two recent retrospective reviews of SIDS autopsies have shown disproportionate numbers of dysmorphic or other minor anomalous lesions in SIDS infants, such a finding would not be surprising.[19, 27]

The NICHD study material was used to conduct a double blind, case-control study to test that assertion. The 99 SIDS cases identified for use in this effort represent a *stratified*, random sample of the total of 757 singleton SIDS cases contained in the NICHD study. A total of 110 SIDS cases were chosen initially, however, because of missing slides, etc., data on only 99 were available for statistical analysis. The stratified sample was deliberately chosen to be balanced on the risk factor of maternal smoking during pregnancy; thus, one-half of the SIDS infants selected had mothers who had smoked during that pregnancy and one-half had mothers who had not smoked. The ages at death for this special study were limited in range from two weeks to one year, and the SIDS cases analyzed had nearly the same age distribution as that occurring in the entire NICHD SIDS population, namely, approximately 80 percent were less than five months of age at death. The control infants were *not* a random sample of any larger set; instead, all available explained deaths (N=65), as finally determined by the Pathology Study Panel, were used. However, because of missing slides, etc., data were available for analysis from only 54 of them.

Relative numbers of sclerotic glomeruli were counted in four fields of renal cortical tissue in two microscopic sections from each infant. Two investigators scored each case independently. Initially, after the two investigators had scored 15 cases, the two sets of determinations were examined and found to be comparable. Thereafter, each investigator proceeded alone. Results did not change when assessed both within and across investigators. No differences were found between SIDS and explained deaths in regard to the percent sclerotic glomeruli.

Data on maternal smoking were available only for the SIDS cases. There were no differences in the relative number of sclerotic glomeruli between SIDS infants whose mothers had smoked cigarettes during pregnancy and those whose mothers had not smoked. Similarly, there were no differences in the percent sclerotic glomeruli between black and non-black infants, among either SIDS or explained deaths. Also, there was no correlation between relative numbers of sclerotic glomeruli and birth weight among either SIDS or explained deaths.

This analysis represents a much larger number of SIDS cases than was examined in the two earlier reports. In addition, relative rather than absolute values were determined. At the outset, it was shown that absolute numbers of sclerotic glomeruli decreased as a function of the infant's age over the first year of life. Thus, the differences in findings between studies are probably due to the fact that the differences in postnatal age between SIDS and control infants were not considered in the two smaller previous studies. By studying the relative occurrence of sclerotic glomeruli rather than absolute value, and by including sufficient numbers of SIDS and explained deaths, and by controlling for infant's age at death in the analysis, no association was found between renal glomerulosclerosis and SIDS.

The other study that has been conducted with the NICHD material examined the relationship of gastroesophageal reflux and SIDS. Results from this study have been reported,[8] but are not yet published. Since reflux cannot be assessed postmortum, esophagitis was used as a marker. Slides from the gastroesophageal junction in 77 SIDS cases and 40 controls (explained deaths) were examined for evidence of esophagitis by three independent teams of pathologists, who did not know which were SIDS cases and which were controls. Each slide was assessed for the maximum number of intraepithelial neutrophils and eosinophils per high-power field, as well as other criteria for reflux esophagitis in infants and children, as proposed by Groben, *et al.*[9] Although interobserver variability was noted, each team's observations led to the same result: there was no statistically significant difference between SIDS cases and controls in regard to the presence of intraepithelial neutrophils or eosinophils. The investigators suggest that analysis of subgroups (for example, SIDS cases in which feeding problems had been noted by the mother) may be worthwhile, but conclude that their data do not add support to the gastroesophageal reflux hypothesis of SIDS.

RESOURCES FROM THE NICHD HISTOPATHOLOGY COLLECTION FOR FUTURE STUDY AND RESEARCH ACTIVITIES

In the course of the NICHD Cooperative Epidemiologic Study of SIDS, several collections of material with significant potential for use in research and education were assembled and saved. They include the following:

1. A set of 386 35mm Kodachromes, the color equivalent of the black and white photographs in this **Atlas**. These slides can be

used in conjunction with the text in the **Atlas** in both teaching exercises and individual study of the subject.

2. A complete set of 30-35 microscopic slides for every autopsy case in the entire study set, that is, all 757 SIDS cases and 65 explained deaths. This collection is housed at the Armed Forces Institute of Pathology (AFIP) and is available for research purposes. Applications for their use will be considered by a special committee of SIDS research investigators designated by NICHD.

3. Paraffin blocks for all (or most) of the slides mentioned in item 2 above are also stored at the AFIP and can be made available to researchers upon request, after appropriate approval of the proposals.

4. Formalin-fixed blocks of wet tissue for the slides mentioned above are also available and stored at the AFIP. Like the slides and paraffin blocks, they can be made available to investigators for their own research, pending approval of research project proposals.

CONCLUSION

The primary purpose of the NICHD SIDS Cooperative Epidemiological Study was the ascertainment of risk factors, with the ultimate goal of developing intervention studies to try to prevent SIDS deaths from occurring.[11, 13] However, early in the study, the pricipal investigators realized that certain benefits in the realm of pediatric pathology might accrue. One of the best features of the pathology component was the insistence by members of the Steering Committee that all of the microscopic sections be read "blindly," to assure that observations of histopathology be as objective and reliable as possible. Although only a few of the microscopic observations have been determined to be significantly different statistically, and fewer still may be significantly different from either a pathological or practical point of view, all of them are important in a fundamental sense because the slides were read blindly without knowledge of which infants died of SIDS and which were pathology controls. For example, we can now assert, on the basis of this well-designed scientific study, that five to ten percent of SIDS infants have some pneumonia when they die.

Other comparisons are equally interesting and important. Thus, 29 percent of SIDS infants have tracheitis, but so do 45 percent of infants whose deaths are explained. Also, SIDS infants were found to have no more macrophages in their alveoli than do infants who die of recognized causes. Neither do SIDS infants have considerably more pulmonary congestion (or pulmonary edema) than controls. Although statistically significant differences were found between frequencies in the last two categories, they were without pathological or practical consequence. Thus, pulmonary congestion was noted in 89 percent of SIDS infants but, also, in 80 percent of explained deaths, which is of no diagnostic value.

Results of this study do confirm prior reports that SIDS infants have hepatic erythropoiesis more often than do explained death controls.[7, 17, 21] Similarly, this study confirms several earlier studies that suggest thymic petechiae occur significantly more often in SIDS infants than in explained deaths.[3, 10, 15] In the NICHD SIDS Cooperative Epidemiological Study, thymic petechiae were observed, grossly and/or microscopically, in slightly more than two-thirds of the SIDS infants, whereas they appeared in only slightly more than one-third of the explained deaths. Yet, these petechiae are neither specific nor diagnostic of SIDS and they are absent in one-third of SIDS autopsies.

Periadrenal brown fat was noted as being present in about three-fourths of SIDS cases and explained death controls. As noted previously, this is an indicator that is highly correlated with the infant's age. In this study, the age distributions of SIDS and control infants are sufficiently similar that no difference in the presence or absence of periadrenal brown fat was found. This result does not contradict earlier reports in this regard, since those studies were based on a painstaking point-counting quantitative approach.[18, 20] For the purposes of discussion, however, it should be pointed out that many of the microscopic findings seen in both SIDS infants and explained death controls represent normal histologic morphology of infants of this age, rather than abnormalities.

Besides a complete and thorough postmortem examination, the diagnosis of SIDS depends upon a careful death scene investigation and case history of the child's health since birth in determining the cause and mode of death. This point is certainly true in regard to correctly classifying the unnatural explained death control infants. In these instances, the morphological findings alone may not clearly distinguish them from SIDS cases.

This Atlas represents the cumulative experience gleaned after several years by pathologists and other scientists reviewing the extensive collection of pathology materials contributed by the study centers participating in the NICHD Cooperative Epidemiological Study of Sudden Infant Death Syndrome Risk Factors. Three different pediatric and/or forensic pathologists reviewed the histopathology of more than 900 potential SIDS infants. They became thoroughly immersed not only in the history of SIDS but, also, with general infant histopathology. It was of great interest to the participants to learn at the end of the two-tiered pathology review process, when the three reviewing pathologists' findings wre compared, nearly identical conclusions had been reached, independently, concerning those findings that were significant and incompatible with SIDS versus those that were incidental to SIDS, or at least sufficiently minor to be compatible with SIDS. These conclusions may provide the most useful guidance to general and forensic pathologists. Many of these pathologists are confronted with the problem of determining whether an infants's death is due to SIDS or to an explained cause. Until now, they have had little recourse other than their own, often limited, experience and informal discussions with colleagues. Hopefully, this Atlas demonstrates that research studies can result in an educational benefit, which is a serviceable contribution to the daily lives of general and forensic pathologists. The authors hope that SIDS research investigators, who are endeavoring to understand the etiology of SIDS or devising interventions that may lead to the prevention of SIDS deaths, will also profit from reading this Atlas.

REFERENCES

1. Allison DJ, Stephens BG. Manual of Operations for the Pathology Coordinating Laboratory of the NICHD Cooperative Epidemiological Study of Sudden Infant Death Syndrome (SIDS) Risk Factors. San Francisco: Office of the Chief Medical Examiner and Coroner of the City and County of San Francisco, 1985.

2. Armitage P. Tests for linear trends on proportions and frequencies. Biometrics 11:375-86, 1955.

3. Beckwith JB. Observations on the pathological anatomy of the sudden infant death syndrome. In Bergman AB, Beckwith JB, Ray CG, eds. Sudden Infant Death Syndrome, Proceedings of the Second International Conference on Causes of Sudden Death in Infants. Seattle, WA: University of Washington Press, 1970, pp. 83-107.

4. Beckwith JB. A pathologist's perspective on SIDS diagnosis and the search for predisposing factors. In Harper RM, Hoffman HJ, eds. Sudden Infant Death Syndrone: Risk Factors and Basic Mechanlsms. Now York, NY: PMA Publishing Corp., 1988, pp. 507-13.

5. de Chadaravian J, Issa-Chergui B. Dlagnostlc relevance of the idiopathic, non-symptomatic, infantile glomerulosclerosis. An autopsy study. Presented at the Interim Meeting of the Society for Pediatric Pathology. Dallas, TX: October 18-19, 1986.

6. Gilbert EF, Suzuki H. Renal changes in the sudden unexpected death syndrome. Presented at the Interim Meeting of the Pediatric Pathology Club. Milwaukee, WI: October 17-18, 1969.

7. Gilbert-Barness EF, Kenison K, Giulian G, Chandra S. Extramedullary hematopoiesis in the liver in the sudden infant death syndrome. Arch Pathol Lab Med, 115:226-9, 1991.

8. Gregg PA, Valdés-Dapena MA, Hoffman HJ, Dahms B, Siegel GP, Askin FB. G-E reflux and SIDS. Presented at the Southern Medical Association annual meeting. Washington, DC: November, 1989.

9. Groben PA, Siegel GP, Shub MD, Ulshen MH, Askin FB. Gastroesophageal reflux and esophagitis in infants and children. Basel, Switzerland: Karger, Perspect Pediatr Pathol 11:124-51, 1987.

10. Handforth CP. Sudden unexpected death in infants. Can Med Assoc J 80:872-3, 1959.

11. Hoffman HJ, Hunter JC, Damus K, Pakter J, Peterson DR, van Belle G, Hasselmeyer EG. Diphtheria-tetanus-pertussis immunization and sudden infant death: Results of the National Institute of Child Health and Human Development Cooperative Study of Sudden Infant Death Syndrome Risk Factors. Pediatrics 79:598-611, 1987.

12. Hoffman HJ, Hunter JC, Ellish NJ, Janerich DT, Goldberg J. Design of the NICHD SIDS Cooperative Epidemiological Study, in Chapter 11: Adverse reproductive factors and the sudden infant death syndrome. In: Harper RM, Hoffman HJ, eds. Sudden Infant Death Syndrome: Risk Factors and Basic Mechanisms. New York: PMA Publishing Corp., 1988, pp. 155-64.

13. Hoffman HJ, Damus K, Hillman L, Krongrad E. Risk factors for SIDS: Results of the National Institute of Child Health and Human Development SIDS Cooperative Study. Ann NY Acad Sci Volume 533, 1988, pp. 13-30.

14. Jones AM, Weston JT. The examination of the sudden infant death syndrome: Investigative and autopsy protocols. J Forens Sci 21:833-41, 1976.

15. Krous HF. The microscopic distribution of intrathoracic petechiae in sudden infant death syndrome. Arch Pathol Lab Med 108:77-9, 1984.

16. Molz G, Hartman H. Dysmorphism, dysplasia and anomaly in sudden infant death (letter). N Engl J Med 311:259, 1984.

17. Moses LE, Emerson JD, Hosseini H. Chapter 11: Analyzing data from ordered categories. In: Bailar JC, Mosteller F, eds. Medical Uses of Statistics. Waltham, Ma: NEJM Books, 1986, pp. 235-58.

18. Naeye RL. Hypoxemia and the sudden infant death syndrome. Science 186:873 8, 1974.

19. Naeye RL. Pathologists' role in SIDS research: The Unfinished Task. In: Tildon JT, Roeder LM, Steinschneider A, eds. New York, N.Y.: Academic Press, 1983, pp. 161-7.

20. Valdés-Dapena M, Gillane MM, Catherman R. Brown fat retention in sudden infant death syndrome. Arch Pathol Lab Med 100:547-9, 1976.

21. Valdés-Dapena M, Gillane MM, Ross D, Catherman R. Extramedullary hematopoiesis in the liver in the sudden infant death syndrome. Arch Pathol Lab Med 103:513-5, 1979.

22. Valdés-Dapena M. The pathologist and the sudden infant death syndrome. Am J Pathol 106:118-31, 1982.

23. Valdés-Dapena M. The morphology of the sudden infant death syndrome—An update, 1984. In Harper RM, Hoffman HJ, eds. Sudden Infant Death Syndrome: Risk Factors and Basic Mechanisms. New York, N.Y.: PMA Publishing Corp., 1988, pp. 143-150.

24. Valdés-Dapena M, Hoffman HJ, Froelich C, Requeira O. Glomerulosclerosis in the sudden infant death syndrome. In: Jaffe R, ed. Festschrift for Ben Landing. Ped Pathol 10:273-279, 1990.

25. Valdés-Dapena M, McFeeley PA, Hoffman HJ, Damus KH, Franciosi RR, Allison DJ, Jones M, Hunter JC. Chapter 1: Study design and protocol for the pathology component of the National Institute of Child Health and Human Development Cooperative Epidemiological Study of Sudden Infant Death Syndrome Risk Factors. Washington, D.C.: Armed Forces Institute of Pathology, this volume.

26. Valdés-Dapena M, McFeeley PA, Hoffman HJ, Damus KH, Franciosi RR, Allison DJ, Jones M, Hunter JC. Chapter 2: Death Investigation and Postmortem Examination. Washington, D.C.: Armed Forces Institute of Pathology, this volume.

27. Vawter GF, Kozakewich HPW. Aspects of morphologic variation amongst SIDS victims. In: Tildon JT, Roeder LM, Steinschneider A, eds. Sudden Infant Death Syndrome. New York, NY: Academic Pregs, 1983, pp. 133-134.

APPENDICES

APPENDIX A

AUTOPSY PROTOCOL

Autopsy # _____

Hospital Chart # _____

Birth Weight: _____

Name: _____

Age: _____

Gestational age: _____

Sex: _____

Color: _____

Date and time of admission: _____

Date and time of death: _____

Date and time of autopsy: _____

Autopsy performed by: _____

PROTOCOL: The body is that of a _____ infant weighing _____ gm.

The crown-rump length is _____ cm; the rump-heel,_____ cm.

The occipito-frontal circumference is _____ cm, that of the chest is _____ cm, and that

of the abdomen is _____ cm. Rigor _____.

Hypostasis _____. Icterus _____.

Cyanosis _____. Edema _____.

_____.

The pupils are _____.

The sclerae are _____.

The ears _____.

The nose _____.

The mouth _____.

There is/are _____ needle puncture mark(s) _____

_____.

The umbilical cord is _____.

The anus is _____.

The external genitalia are _____.

The skin is _____.

_____

_____.

PERITONEAL CAVITY: The peritoneal surfaces are _____

_____

The peritoneal cavity contains _____

_____

The diaphragm arches to the _____ on the right and

to the _____ on the left. The

umbilical vein _____.

There are _____ umbilical arteries.

The measurements of the liver are as follows: _____.

The spleen _____

_____.

The appendix is in the right lower quadrant. The stomach is _____

_____.

The small intestine is _____.

The large intestine is _____.

The mesenteric lymph nodes are _____

_____.

The root of the mesentery _____

_____.

PLEURAL CAVITIES: The pleural surfaces are _____

_____.

The right pleural cavity contains _____

_____.

The left pleural cavity contains _____

_____.

The lungs occupy _____ of their respective pleural cavities.

Each lung has a normal number of lobes.

PERICARDIAL CAVITY: The pericardial surfaces are _____

_____.

The cavity is free from adhesions and contains _____

_____.

CARDIOVASCULAR SYSTEM:

HEART: The heart weighs _____ gm. (Normal is_____ gm)

The foramen ovale is _____.

The ductus arteriosus is _____.

The mural and valvular endocardium is _____.

The myocardium is _____.

The coronary ostia and coronary sinus are in normal position. The great vessels arising from the heart and those arising from the aortic arch do so in normal position.

The measurements of the heart are as follows:

TV _____ , PV _____ , MV _____ , AV _____ , RVM _____ , LVM _____ cm.

The thoracic and abdominal aorta _____

_____ .

RESPIRATORY SYSTEM:

LUNGS: The combined weight of the lungs is _____ gm (Normal is _____ gm)

On section _____

_____ .

The trachea and major bronchi are lined by _____ mucosa, their

lumens contain _____ .

HEMATOPOIETIC SYSTEM:

SPLEEN: The spleen weighs _____ gm (Normal is _____ gm) The capsule is _____ .

On section the parenchyma is _____ .

The malpighian corpuscles are _____ .

The lymph nodes are _____ .

Bone marrow is _____ .

GASTROINTESTINAL SYSTEM:

The mucosa of the esophagus is _____

and its lumen contains _____ .

The mucosa of the stomach is _____

and its lumen contains _____ .

The mucosa of the small intestine is _____

and its lumen contains _____ .

The length of the small bowel is _____ cm; the large bowel _____ cm.

The mucosa of the large intestine is _____

and its lumen contains _____ .

LIVER: The liver weighs _____ gm. (Normal is _____ gm)

The capsule is _____ .

On section the parenchyma is _____

_____ .

The sinus intermedius and ductus venosus are _____

_____ .

The bile, which is, _____ , is freely

expressed from the gallbladder into the duodenum.

PANCREAS: The pancreas is tan and coarsely lobulated. On section _____
_____
_____ .

ENDOCRINE SYSTEM:
ADRENALS: The combined weight of the adrenals is _____ gm. They are _____
_____ .

The cut surfaces reveal _____
peripheral zones and _____ central zones.
GENITO-URINARY SYSTEM:
KIDNEYS: The combined weight of the kidneys is _____ gm. (Normal is _____ gm)
The renal arteries and veins are free from thrombi. The capsules strip easily from
_____ surfaces _____
_____ .

On section the cortex and medulla are _____
_____ demarcated. The renal pelves and ureters are lined
by _____ .
BLADDER: The mucosa of the bladder is _____
_____ .

The relations at the trigone are normal.
  GENITALIA: The prostate is small, firm and reveals no gross abnormalities. The vaginal mucosa
is _____ .
The uterus, tubes and ovaries reveal no gross abnormalities. The uterus and ovaries are of normal
size.
ORGANS OF THE NECK: The thymus weighs_____ gm. The surface is
_____ .
The cut surfaces _____ .
The thyroid and larynx reveal no gross abnormalities. The larynx is lined by _____
_____ mucosa and is empty. The submaxillary glands _____
_____
_____ parathyroids are identified. Positions: _____
_____
_____ .

BRAIN: The soft tissues of the scalp are _____
_____ . The anterior fontanelle measures _____ cm.
The posterior fontanelle is _____ .
The sutures _____ .
The dura mater is _____ .
The falx cerebri and the tentorium cerebelli are intact. The pia arachnoid is _____

_____.
There is no subarachnoid hemorrhage nor exudate. The convolutions and sulci are _____
_____

The brain is fixed in toto. The dural sinuses are free from thrombi.
The middle ears are _____.
A segment of the _____ spinal cord is removed by the anterior
approach and reveals no gross abnormalities.
The pituitary _____.

MUSCULO-SKELETAL SYSTEM:
BONES: The manubrium sternum contains _____ center of ossification.
The _____ , _____ , _____ sternabrae
each contain _____ centers of ossification. There
are _____ pairs of ribs. Two lower costochondral junctions are removed from each
side.

*Reproduced from Valdés-Dapena MA, Huff DS. *Perinatal Autopsy Manual.* Washington, D.C.: Armed Forces Institute of Pathology, 1983, pp 68-71.

APPENDIX B

Letterhead

Date

Mr. and Mrs. _____

_____

_____

Dear Mr. and Mrs. _____ :

We have reviewed the findings of the scientific examinations and these tests indicate that your baby, _____ , died as a result of Sudden Infant Death Syndrome (SIDS). The tests do not indicate any condition which could pose a threat to present or future members of your family.

The pathologist and the medical investigator involved with the autopsy on your child are available for consultation, as are all of our staff. If you have any questions or comments, or if we can be any assistance, please do not hesitate to contact us.

Sincerely,

Letterhead

(When names of parents are different)

Date

Mr. _____

Mrs. _____

_____

_____

Dear Parents:

Please accept the sincere condolences of the staff of the _____ Office of the Medical Investigator on the sudden death of your child, _____ .

The preliminary postmortem examination showed that your child was well formed, appeared well cared for, and had suffered no injuries. Furthermore, no infection of any kind has been found that might be a hazard to present or future members of the family. These findings are consistent with the condition called Sudden Infant Death Syndrome. (SIDS) or "crib death."

Please be assured that no neglect is involved. SIDS cannot, at present, be predicted or prevented. It is the most common cause of death of babies between one month and one year of age and happens to babies of every race, religion, and living circumstance. Its exact cause is still unknown at this time, but a number of laboratories, including ours, are conducting scientific research into the problem. Enclosed are pamphlets which explain some aspects of this condition.

In this moment of sorrow, we do not wish to intrude on your privacy. However, since your child died suddenly and unexpectedly, you may want to know more about this problem. The _____ SIDS Program offers free and accurate information to families and to other interested people. A list of persons specially trained in the problems of SIDS may be found at the end of this letter. When you can, you are urged to contact one of them. They may be able to offer suggestions on how to answer questions from relatives or friends, and about other practical problems unique to the death of a child so young.

Again let me express our condolences. If we can be of any assistance, please do not hesitate to call.

Sincerely,

Letterhead

(Grandparent letter)

Date

Ms. _____
_____
_____

Dear Ms:

Please accept the sincere condolences of the staff of the _____ Office of the Medical Investigator on the sudden death of your grandchild, _____ .

The postmortem examination showed that he/she was well formed, appeared well cared for, and had suffered no injuries. Furthermore, no infection of any kind has been found that might be a hazard to present or future members of the family. These findings are consistent with the condition called Sudden Infant Death Syndrome. (SIDS) or "crib death."

Please be assured that no neglect was involved. SIDS cannot, at present, be predicted or prevented. It is the most common cause of death of babies between one month and one year of age and happens to babies of every race, religion, and living circumstance. Its exact cause is still unknown at this time, but a number of laboratories, including ours, are conducting scientific research into the problem. Enclosed are pamphlets which explain some aspects of this condition.

In this moment of sorrow, we do not wish to intrude on your privacy. However, since your grandchild died suddenly and unexpectedly, you may want to know more about this problem. The _____ SIDS Program offers free and accurate information to families and to other interested people. A list of persons specially trained in the problems of SIDS may be found at the end of this letter. If you wish, you may contact me or one of them. We may be able to offer suggestions on how to answer questions from relatives or friends, and about other practical problems unique to the death of a child so young.

Again let me express our condolences. If we can be of any assistance, please do not hesitate to call.

Sincerely,

Sudden Infant Death Syndrome

APPENDIX C

STUDY PRINCIPAL INVESTIGATORS , CONSULTANTS, AND NICHD STAFF

A large number of individuals contributed to the success of this study. In particular, we wish to acknowledge the principal investigators and project coordinators from each of the study centers, plus other project staff and consultants.

Principal Investigators and Project Managers: Julius Goldberg, Ph.D., and Ronald Hornung, M.S., Loyola University of Chicago; Jess Kraus, Ph.D., and Marilyn Misczynski. M.A., University of California at Davis; Donald Peterson, M.D., and Nina Chinn. R.N., University of Washington; Jean Pakter, M.D., Ehud Krongrad, M.D., and Patricia Hanson, R.N., Medical Health Research Association of New York; Dwight Janerich. D.D.S., Susan Standfast, M.D., and Diane Aliferis, M.A., New York State State Health Department; Laura Hillman, M.D., Barbara Puder, R.R.A., and Sharon Hollander. M.A., Maternal and Child Health Council of St. Louis.

Data CoordinatingCenter: Gerald van Belle. Ph.D. (Director), Marjorie Jones, M.A., Catherine Nanney, M.S., Mary Jane Almes, M.A., and Donald Kunz, B.S., University of Washington.

Pathology Coordinating Laboratory: Boyd G. Stephens, M.D., and Donna J. Allison, Ph.D.. San Francisco Office of the Chief Medical Examiner and Coroner.

Pathology Study Panel Members: Marie A. Valdes-Dapena, M.D., University of Miami School of Medicine; Russell Fisher, M.D., Maryland Office of the Chief Medical Examiner and Johns Hopkins University Medical School; and James Weston, M.D., and Patricia A.

McFeeley, M.D., New Mexico Office of the Chief Medical Examiner and University of New Mexico Medical Center.

Advisory Committee: Henry L. Barnett, M.D. (Chairman), Albert Einstein College of Medicine and Children's Aid Society, New York City, NY; Ralph R. Franciosi, M.D., Children's Health Center Laboratory, Minneapolis, MN; William L. Harkness, Ph.D., Pennsylvania State University, University Park, PA; G. Eric Knox, M.D., Abbott Northwest Hospital, Minneapolis, MN; Richard R. Naeye, MD., Milton S. Hershey Medical Center, Pennsylvania State University, Hersey, PA; James D. Neaton, M.S., University of Minnesota, Minneapolis, MN; and Zena Stein, M.B., New York State Psychiatric Institute, New York, NY.

Consultants: Glen Bartlett, M.D., Ph.D., Milton S. Hershey Medical Center, Pennsylvania State University, Hershey, PA; Theodore Colton, Sc.D., Boston University School of Medicine, Boston, MA; David C. Hoaglin, Ph.D., Harvard University, Cambridge, MA; Lewis P. Lipsitt, Ph.D. Brown University, Providence, RI; William C. Orr, Ph.D., Presbyterian Hospital and University of Oklahoma Health Sciences Center, Oklahoma City, OK; Philip E. Sartwell, M.D., Harvard School of Public Health, Boston, MA; and Harold Morgenstern, Ph.D., Yale University, New Haven, CT.

NICHD Staff: Eileen G. Hasselmeyer, Ph.D., R.N., Howard J. Hoffman, M.A., Charles R. Stark, M.D., D.P.H. (Project Officers); Jehu C. Hunter, B.S. (Study Coordinator); Harvey Shifrin, B.A. (Contracting Officer); and Karla H. Damus, Ph.D. (Epidemiology Consultant).

APPENDIX D

Medical Examiners and Coroners Contributing SIDS Cases to NICHD Cooperative Epidemiological Study of SIDS Risk Factors

LOYOLA UNIVERSITY OF CHICAGO STUDY CENTER

Cook County

Tae Lyong An, M.D.
Lee F. Beamer, M.D.
Eupil Choi, M.D.
Edmund R. Donoghue, M.D.
Mitra Kalelkar, M.D.

Robert H. Kirschner, M.D.
Yuksel Konakci, M.D.
Robert J. Stein, M.D.
Shaku Teas, M.D.

UNIVERSITY OF CALIFORNIA AT DAVIS STUDY CENTER

Contra Costa County

William Bogart, M.D.
Louis Daugherty, M.D.

Merced County

Grant P. Carmichael, M.D.
G. Phillip Mansur, M.D.
Malcolm Murdoch, M.D.
Jack Sjaarda, M.D.

Orange County

Walter R. Fischer, M.D.
Richard I. Fukumoto, M.D.
Robert G. Richards, M.D.
Peter Yatar, M.D.

Sacramento County

Pierce A. Rooney, M.D. and colleagues

San Francisco City and County

Boyd G. Stephens, M.D.

San Joaquin County

Robert Chard, M.D.

San Mateo County

Peter Benson, M.D.
Arthur Lack, M.D.

Yolo County

J. Fred Ransdell, M.D.

UNIVERSITY OF WASHINGTON STUDY CENTER

King County

J. Bruce Beckwith, M.D.
Joseph Seibert, M.D.

MEDICAL HEALTH RESEARCH ASSOCIATION OF NEW YORK

New York City; New York, Bronx, King, Queens, and Richmond Counties

Michael Baden, M.D.
Olive Barlow, M.D.
Jacques Durosier, M.D.
Manual Fernando, M.D.
Millard Hyland, M.D.
Beverly Leffers, M.D.
Josette Montas, M.D.
Geetha Natarajan, M.D.

John O'Connor, M.D,
Jon Pearl, M.D.
Nafees Pervez, M.D.
Phito Pierre-Louis, M.D.
Yong-Myun Rho, M.D.
Monique Ryser, M.D.
Milton Wald, M.D.
Joseph Veress, M.D.

NEW YORK STATE DEPARTMENT OF HEALTH

Albany County
James Cavanaugh
J.N.P. Davies, M.D.
Leon Feltman, M.D.
James Keeher
Aniceto Lomotan, M.D.

Columbia County
Angelo Nero

Dutchess County
Paul Garell, M.D.
Joseph D. Ross, Jr., M.D.
John Supple, M.D.

Fulton County
Milan Kovar, M.D.
Richard Wagner, M.D.
William H. Whipple

Greene County
Covered by Albany County pathologists

Montgomery County
Covered by Fulton County pathologists

Nassau County
M. Araki, M.D.
Orlando Castellon, M.D.
G. Figueroa, M.D.

Daniel Levin, M.D.
Leslie Lukash, M.D.
Daniel P. McCarthy, M.D.

Orange County
Martin B. Grant, M.D.
John Greco
Carlos Greenberg, M.D.
Roy Lippencott, Jr.
Mary McPhillips
Donald Parker

Putnam County
John DelCampo, M.D.

Rensselaer County
James V. Barrett, M.D.

Rockland County
Neil Janis, M.D.
W.J. Redner, M.D.
Edwardo Zappi, M.D.
Frederick Zugibe, M.D.

Saratoga County
Frank Kearney
Jack Paston, M.D.

Schenectady County
Robert Sullivan, M.D.

Henry E. Damm, M.D.

Schoharie County
Jan Platt, M.D.
Jacobus Vrolijk, M.D.

Suffolk County
Howard Adelman, M.D.
Jose P. Fernandez, M.D.
Donald Jason, M.D.
John Grauerholtz, M.D.
Jack Sturiano, M.D.
Carlos Tejo, M.D.
Sidney Weinburg, M.D.

Sullivan County
Covered by Orange County pathologists

Ulster County
Harry C. McNamara, M.D.

Warren County
John Cunningham, M.D.
S. Richard Spitzer, M.D.

Washington County
Covered by Warren County pathologists

Westchester County
Daryl Jeanty, M.D.
Gary Paparo, M.D.
Louis Roh, M.D.

MATERNAL AND CHILD HEALTH COUNCIL OF ST. LOUIS

Franklin County
Stanley Meyer

Jefferson County
James Rehm, M.D.

St. Charles County
Joseph W. Mueller, M.D.

St. Louis City
George E. Gantner, Jr., M.D.

St. Louis County
George E. Gantner, Jr., M.D.

Sudden Infant Death Syndrome

Index

A

Abscesses **251**
Acute interstitial pulmonary emphysema **95**
Adenovirus **226**, **232**
Adipose tissue
   histology **76, 77**
   periadrenal brown fat **73**, **77**
Adrenal **33, 34, 35**
   calcification **205**, **206**
   cysts **75**
   cytomegaly **207**, **208**, **209**
   hematoma **205**, **206**
   hemorrhage **205**, **256**, **257**, **285**, **290**
   histology **73**, **74**, **75**
   histopathology in SIDS **290**, **293**
   neuroblastoma-in-situ **210**
Adrenal hemorrhage **11**
Adrenal hyperplasia **8, 117, 118**
Adrenal hypoplasia **117, 118**
Adrenal rests **207**
Advisory Committee **313**
Age **26**
Age at death **282**, **283**, **284**, **286**
Age at death or maternal interview **5**
Agonal event **175, 272**
Agonal findings **99**
Agonal lesions **105**, **107**, **112**, **260**
AIDS (acquired immune deficiency syndrome) **36**
Alcohol **15**, **17**
Alcohol, drug abuse **24**
Alveolar hemorrhage **11**
Alveoli

histology **48, 49, 50**
Ampulla of Vater **34**
Anorexia **122**
Anoxia **205, 212, 214**
   intrauterine **237**
Anterior fontanelle **32**
Anus **31, 35**
Aorta **29, 33**
   coarctation **29**
Aortic stenosis **23**
Aortic valvular stenosis **117, 145**
Apgar score **15, 16, 237**
Apnea **15, 16, 226**
Arteries
   celiac **33**
   superior mesenteric **33**
Arteriovenous malformation, intracranial **8, 117, 118, 145**
Artery
   splenic **34**
Asphyxia **111, 260, 261, 266, 268, 285, 286**
Aspiration **11, 148, 149, 166, 174, 175, 176, 177, 178, 179, 180, 246**
"Aspiration pneumonia" in newborns **240**
Autopsy **1, 6, 12, 23, 25, 93, 96, 97, 116, 118, 281**
   pathology coordinating laboratory (PCL) **1**
Autopsy protocol **26, 303**

B

Bacterial colonization **167**
Battered child *See also: Child abuse, shaken baby* **8, 118, 144**
Beckwith-Wiedemann syndrome **207**
Bile **34**
Bile duct **35**
Biochemistry **6**
Birth weight **5, 14, 15, 16, 282, 283, 286**
Birth weights and gestational age **14**
Blanched skin **94**
Blankets **144**
Blood
   cultures **27, 29, 36**
   histopathology in SIDS **290**
   sickle cells **218, 225**
   toxicology **36**
Bone
   costochondral junction **7**
   temporal bone **7**

Boric acid poisoning   **8, 118, 139**
  autopsy findings   **138**
Bourneville's disease   **119**
Bradycardia   **15, 16**
Brain   *See also: Central nervous system*   **32, 159**
  abcess   **291**
  basal ganglia   **7, 10**
  calcification   **290**
  cerebellum   **7, 10**
  congestion   **225**
  edema   **225, 291**
  germinal matrix   **291**
  germinal matrix hemorrhage   **225**
  hemorrhage   **11**
  hippocampus   **10**
  histopathology in SIDS   **112, 290, 291**
  inflammation   **291**
  liver, pancreas   **10**
  medulla   **7**
  perivascular hemorrhage   **112, 225, 290**
  petechiae   **290**
  pons   **7**
Brain damage   **175, 236, 242**
Brain stem   **32**
Breast   **35**
Breech   **205**
Bronchi   **33**
Bronchiole
  histology   **46**
Bronchiolitis   **8, 23, 117, 118, 119, 126, 127, 128, 226, 227, 228, 229, 230, 231,
    233, 272, 285, 286, 292**
  in SIDS   **126**
  lesions sufficient to cause death   **126, 223, 226, 229, 286**
Bronchiolitis, minimal   **186, 187**
Bronchitis   **146, 286, 288, 292**
Bronchopneumonia   *See also: Pneumonia*
    116, 117, 118, 122, 129, 130, 131, 132, 133, 146, 232, 233, 234
  incidental or inconsequential   **188**
  lesions sufficient to cause death   **119, 129**
  secondary   **268, 269**

Bronchopneumonia, minimal   **188**
Bronchopulmonary dysplasia   **11**
Bronchus   **7**
  histology   **45**
Brown fat retention   **96**

Burns   **285**

C

Caesarian   **17**
Carbon monoxide   **117, 118**
Cardioesophageal junction   **35, 198**
  histology   **62**
Cardiomyopathy   **117, 118**
Case history   *See also: Death investigation*
Cellulitis   *See also: Cervical cellulitis*   **11**
Central nervous system   *See also: Brain*   **89, 237**
  germinal matrix hemorrhage   **216, 217**
  hemorrhage   **90, 214**
  histology   **89, 90, 91**
  intraventricular hemorrhage   **214**
  pigment-laden macrophages   **216**
  pigment-laden macrophages in the leptomeninges   **214**
  pseudocyst   **216, 217**
  subarachnoid hemorrhage   **212, 213, 214**
  trauma   **214**
Cerebral atrophy   **119**
Cerebral cortex   *See also: Central nervous system*
Cervical cellulitis   **11, 117, 119, 141, 142, 285**
Cervix   **34**
Cesarean   **15**
Chemistry   **281**
Child abuse   *See also: Battered child, shaken baby*
  23, 24, 27, 37, 94, 118, 260, 268, 285
Cholestasis   **11**
Choristoma   **196**
Circumferences
  abdomen   **26**
  chest   **26**
  head   **26**
"Classical" findings   **93, 94, 96, 99**
Clinical history   *See also: Death investigation, medical history*
Clostridium botulinum   **36**
Cold   **18, 19, 126, 186, 226**
Communication with the family   **96, 97**
Congenital adrenal hyperplasia   **8**
Congenital anomalies   **89, 119, 285**
Congenital diseases   **191**
Congenital heart disease   **8, 117, 118, 145, 262, 285**
  anomalous origin of the left coronary artery   **117**
Congenital malformations   **286**

Congestion, **95**
  adrenal **290**
  brain **290**
  kidney **290**
  lymph node **290**
  pulmonary **104, 105, 288, 292**
  spleen **289**
Consultants **313**
Control infants **4, 6, 7, 9, 13, 16, 115, 281, 286**
  living, Control A **5, 15, 282**
  living, Control B **5, 14, 15, 282**
  non-living **6–9**
Contusion **268, 270**
Coronary arteritis **117**
Coronary thrombosis **285**
Costochondral junction **7, 28, 31**
Cough **18, 19, 126, 187, 226**
Counseling **96, 97**
Coxsackie virus **8, 118, 122**
  group B **122**
  B5 **134**
Cranial nerves **32**
Criteria
  cause of death **12**
  lesions insufficient to cause death **11, 12**
  lesions sufficient to cause death **11, 12**
  "without lesions" **11**
Cultures
  bacterial **24, 26, 36**
  blood **27, 29, 36, 251**
  fungal **24, 26**
  lung **27, 29, 36**
  middle ear **33**
  other **26**
  spleen **27, 36**
  viral **24, 26, 36**
Cyanosis **27, 94, 122, 124**
Cystic fibrosis **8, 117, 118, 289**
  autopsy findings **143**
Cytomegalovirus **11, 160, 162, 163, 232**

D

Death investigation **6, 12, 23, 24, 93, 94, 96, 97, 116, 118, 144, 253, 260, 281**
Death scene investigation **297**
Definite SIDS **12, 13, 115**

Dehydration **23, 25, 26, 117,** 118, **119, 126, 146, 226, 285, 286**
Department of Health, Education, and Welfare **96**
Diabetes **207**
Diaphragm **7, 29, 33, 35**
  gross pathology in SIDS **94**
  histology **87**
  histopathology in SIDS **289**
  petechiae **94**
Diarrhea **18, 19, 26, 117, 126, 146**
Differential diagnoses **8**
Digitalis toxicity **285**
Down syndrome **246, 262**
Drowning **118, 285, 286**
Drug abuse **37, 145**
Drug use **15, 17**
Ductus venosus **35**
Duodenum **34**
Dura **31**
Dural sinuses **32**

E

Ears **27**
Eastern equine virus **140**
Echoviruses 4,6,9, and 30 **134**
Economic factors **16**
Ectopic rests **196**
Edema **27**
  pulmonary **11**
Education **15, 17**
Electrolytes **27**
Emphysema **170, 171, 172, 173, 248, 249, 264**
Encephalitis **8,** 117, **118, 122, 140, 291**
Endocardial fibroelastosis **8, 23,** 117, **124, 145**
Endocardial sclerosis **124, 145**
Endocardium
  histology **39, 40**
Endotracheal tube **96**
Enteritis **11, 126**
Enterocolitis **8, 117, 146**
Enterovirus **134, 140, 232**
Epicardium
  gross pathology in SIDS **94, 95**
  histology **39, 40**
  petechiae **94, 95**
Epidemiology **2, 93, 94, 129**

Epiglottis   **164, 288, 292**
  histology   **41**
  histopathology in SIDS   **288**
Epiglottitis   **11**
Erythroblastosis fetalis   **207, 214**
Escherichia coli   **8, 256**
Esophagus   **33, 34, 35, 196**
  ectopic rests of gastric mucosa   **196**
  gastric mucosa   **196**
  histology   **61**
Explained death   **6, 12, 13, 115, 116, 281, 282, 283, 284, 286**
  alveolar hemorrhage   **105**
  alveolar macrophages   **108**
  brain   **116**
  cardiovascular   **119, 120, 124, 145**
  central nervous system   **122, 134, 136, 137, 140, 145**
  gastrointestinal tract   **116, 146**
  histopathological findings (table)   **288, 290, 291**
  histopathology in SIDS   **289**
  liver, fatty change   **110**
  originally submitted as SIDS   **119**
  pancreas   **116**
  perivascular hemorrhage, central nervous system   **112**
  petechiae   **103**
  pulmonary congestion   **104**
  pulmonary edema   **107**
  respiratory   **116, 126, 128, 129, 130, 131, 132, 133**
  specific causes of death   **285**
  systemic   **116, 138, 139, 141, 142, 143**
  thymic petechiae   **111**
Extramedullary hematopoiesis   **11**
  adrenal   **211**
  liver   **189, 200, 211, 289, 293**
  spleen   **189, 211, 289**
  thymus   **189, 211**

F

Failure to thrive   **25, 148**
Fall from window   **285**
Fallopian tube   **34, 35**
Falx cerebri   **32**
Fever   **15, 16, 18, 122**
Follicular cysts
  histology   **72**
Foramen ovale   **30**

G

Gallbladder **34, 143**
Gastric contents **175**
  gross pathology in SIDS **95**
  toxicology **36**
Gastric mucosa
  ectopic **33**
Gastroenteritis **202**
Gastroesophageal junction
  histopathology in SIDS **289**
Gastroesophageal reflux **295, 296**
Gastrointestinal tract *See also: Stomach, intestine* **143**
  Barrett's esophagus **196**
  ectopic rest **196**
  gastroesophageal junction **7**
  ileum **7**
  inflammation **198**
Geographical area **2**
Germinal matrix **90, 91**
Gestational age **14, 282, 283, 286**
Glomeruli
  histology **56, 57, 58, 59**
Glomerulonephritis **11**
Granuloma **224, 242**
Granuloma, milk **176, 182, 246**
Granulomas, aspiration **183, 184**
Gray zone
  defined **223**
Gross pathology **94**
  diaphragm **94**
  epicardium **94**
  explained deaths **118**
  mouth **94**
  mucous membranes **94**
  myocardium **94**
  nose **94**
  petechiae **94**
  pleura **94**
  skin **94**
  thymus **94**
Gross pathology in SIDS **93**
Growth percentiles **253**
Growth retarded **276**

H

Hamartoma **203**
Heart **7**, **28**, **29**, **33**, **35**, **128**
   calcium deposit in a papillary muscle **155**
   calcium deposits **159**
   dissection **29**, **30**
   histology **39**
   histopathology in SIDS **99**, **289**, **294**
   iatrogenic lesions **95**, **156**, **158**
   interstitial fibrosis **153**, **154**
   ischemic necrosis **159**, **224**
   needle track marks **156**, **157**
   papillary muscle **159**, **224**
   petechiae **99**, **128**, **289**, **294**
   rhabdomyoma **258**
Heart's blood
   gross pathology in SIDS **95**
Haemophilus influenzae **164**, **232**, **256**, **276**
   Haemophilus influenzae type b **129**, **134**
Hemorrhage **224**
Hemorrhage, brain **8**
Hepatitis **8**, **118**, **285**, **289**
Hepatosplenomegaly **122**
Herpes virus **140**
Hippocampus **7**
Histology   *See also: Chapter 3*
   normal **39**
Histology sections **7**, **9**, **10**, **12**, **23**, **35**
Histopathology   *See also: Specific processes, i.e., pneumonia*
   explained deaths **118**
Histopathology in SIDS   *See also: Chapter 5*
   central nervous system **112**
   larynx **100**, **101**
   liver **110**
   lung **103**, **104**, **105**, **106**, **108**, **109**
   thymus **111**
   trachea **102**
History   *See also: Death investigation, medical history* **8**
HIV testing **36**
Hyaline membrane disease **96**
Hypertension **15**, **17**
Hypothermia **15**, **16**
Hypoxia **89**, **96**, **159**, **218**, **237**, **290**

I

Iatrogenic lesions   *See also: Resuscitation, and specific organs, (heart, lungs, etc.)*   **99, 169**
   acute   **95**
   airway   **95, 96**
   chronic   **95**
   hyaline membrane disease   **96**
   interstitial pulmonary emphysema   **95**
   intubation   **95**
   lungs   **96**
   needle puncture marks   **95**
Ileum
   histopathology in SIDS   **290**
Illnesses   **18**
Incidence of SIDS   **2, 4, 93**
Incidental or inconsequential lesions   **153**
Indeterminate cases   **10, 12**
Indeterminate cause   **13**
Infection   **205**
Inferior vena cava   **33**
Inflammation
   epiglottis   **11, 164**
   gastrointestinal tract   **198**
   upper respiratory tract   **11, 164**
Inherited diseases   **286**
Instruments
   required for autopsy   **25**
International Classification of Diseases   **93**
Interstitial lung disease   **39, 224, 264**
Interstitial pneumonia   **129**
Interstitial pneumonitis   **286**
Interstitial pulmonary emphysema   **95, 172, 173**
Interventricular septal defect   **145**
Intestine
   histology   **63**
   large   **28, 34, 35**
   small   **28, 34, 35**
Intrauterine growth retardation   **94**
Intubation   **95**
Islets of Langerhans
   histology   **66, 67, 68**
   hyperplasia and hypertrophy   **207, 225**
Ivemark's syndrome   **119**

J

Jaundice   **15, 16, 27, 122**

K

Kawasaki's disease **117**
Kidney **7, 34, 35,** 31, **33, 34**
  calcium **290**
  calcium deposits **192,** 193
  glomerulosclerosis **191, 225, 295**
  histology **56, 57, 58, 59**
  histopathology in SIDS **290**
  "immaturity" of glomeruli **225**
  nephroblastomatosis **225**
  nodular renal blastema **194,** 195
  sclerotic glomeruli **191**
  subcapsular microcysts **191**
  subcapsular scar **190**

L

Langhans giant cell **184**
Laryngitis **42, 101, 271,** 292
Larynx **7, 33, 35, 42**
  fibrinoid necrosis **100**
  histology **42, 80**
  histopathology in SIDS **100, 101**
  iatrogenic lesions **95, 96**
  laryngitis **101**
  ulcers **96**
Law enforcement agencies **96**
Length **26**
Leptomeninges **32**
Leptomeningitis **11**
Lethargy **122**
Letters of condolence **96, 97, 309**
Ligament of Treitz **28, 34**
Lipid storage disease **110**
Listeria monocytogenes **134**
Listless/droopy **18, 19**
Liver **7, 28, 34, 35, 36**
  cholestasis **224**
  extramedullary hematopoiesis **200, 224, 289, 293, 294, 297**
  fatty change **110, 143, 202, 220, 224, 289, 293**
  fibrosis **289**
  glycogen **289**
  hamartoma **224**
  hemangioma **203, 224, 289**

histology **64, 65**
histopathology in SIDS **110, 289, 293**
inflammation **289**
necrosis **289**
sickle cells **220**
triaditis **224, 289**
Liver laceration **285**
Lobar pneumonia **232**
Low birth weight **94**
Ludwig's angina **11, 117, 119, 141, 142, 285**
Lung **7, 29, 33, 35, 39, 226, 227, 228, 229, 230, 231, 264**
alveolar hemorrhage **105, 288**
alveolar macrophages **108, 174, 288, 292**
aspiration **175, 176, 177, 178, 179, 180, 181, 182, 183, 184, 246, 272, 274, 288**
aspiration, chronic **242, 244**
aspiration of amniotic debris **237, 240**
atelectasis **109**
bacterial colonization **166, 167**
bronchiolitis, minimal **186, 187**
bronchopneumonia, minimal **188**
congestion **104, 294, 297**
cultures **27, 29, 36**
edema **95, 107, 267, 288, 292, 297**
emphysema **109, 288**
granuloma **246, 294**
granulomas **182, 183, 184, 185**
gross pathology in SIDS **95**
histology **47-51, 129, 264, 274**
histopathology in SIDS **103, 104, 105, 106, 107, 108, 109, 288, 292, 294**
iatrogenic lesions **168, 169**
interstitial emphysema **106**
interstitial pulmonary emphysema **172**
macrophages in alveoli **236, 294, 297**
patchy overaeration **168, 169**
petechiae **103, 128, 294**
septal hemorrhage **106, 288**
sickle cells **218**
squamous cells in alveoli **237**
subpleural emphysema **170, 171**
"Wilson-Mikity" pattern **248, 249, 250**
Lymph node **7, 28, 35**
gross pathology in SIDS **95**
histology **45, 54, 55**
histopathology in SIDS **290**
inflammation **290**

Lymphocytes
  bronchiolar **51**
  pancreatic **70**
  thymus **79**
Lymphoid aggregates, colonic mucosa
  gross pathology in SIDS **95**
Lymphoid tissues
  gross pathology in SIDS **95**

M

Macrophages
  in alveoli **11, 236**
Malabsorption **147**
Malnutrition **8, 285**
Married **17**
Maternal age **15, 17**
Maternal diabetes **207**
Maternal interview **5**
Measles **140**
Medical Examiners and Coroners Contributing SIDS Cases **315**
Medical history **24, 93**
Meningitis **8, 23, 36, 117, 118, 119, 122, 276, 277, 285, 291**
  aseptic (viral) meningitis **134, 137**
  autopsy findings **134**
  bacterial meningitis **134, 136**
Meningococcemia **8, 256**
Mesenteric lymph nodes **35**
Microbiology **6, 12, 24, 26, 118, 281**
Microcephaly **119**
Middle ears **33**
Milk **175, 176, 177, 178, 179, 242**
Milk granuloma **176, 182, 246**
Morbid lesions **223, 225**
Mortal lesions **223, 224, 225**
Mortality rate
  infant **2**
  neonatal **2**
  postneonatal **2**
  SIDS **2**
Motor cortex **7**
Motor vehicle accident **285**
Mouth
  gross pathology in SIDS **94**
Multiple births **4, 13**
Mumps **140**

Muscle **31**
  histology **87**
  skeletal **35, 88**
Mucous membranes
  gross pathology in SIDS **94**
Mycoplasma **126, 226**
Mycoplasma pneumoniae **140**
Myocarditis **8, 11, 117, 118, 122, 254, 285**
Myocardium
  gross pathology in SIDS **94, 95**
  histology **39, 40**
  petechiae **94, 95**

N

Needle puncture marks **27, 95, 99**
Neglect **148**
Neisseria meningitidis **134, 256, 276**
Nerve **31, 35**
Neuroblastoma **210**
NICHD Cooperative Epidemiologic Study of SIDS Risk Factors **94, 95, 115, 119**
  defined **1–3, 3, 281**
    Pathology Study Panel (PSP) **1, 3, 6, 10, 116, 223, 281, 286**
    purpose **296**
    study centers **1, 4**
NICHD staff **313**
"NonSIDS" **10**
Nose
  gross pathology in SIDS **94**

O

Obstruction, upper airway **117**
Office of Maternal and Child Health **96**
Oral cavity **27**
Ossification centers **28**
Ovaries **34**
Ovary **35**
  follicular cysts **71**
  histology **71**
Overheating **117**
Overlaying **144, 260**

P

Pancreas **7, 34, 35**
  dilatation of acini **225**

ectopic splenic tissue   **204**
histology   **66, 67, 68**
histopathology   **138, 139**
histopathology in SIDS   **289**
hypertrophy of islets   **225**
islet cell hyperplasia   **11, 225, 289**
islet cell hyperplasia and hypertrophy   **207**
Pancreatitis   **8, 118**
Parainfluenza virus   **232**
Parainfluenza 3   **126, 226**
Parathyroid
histology   **33, 43, 82, 83, 84, 85**
Parity   **15**
Pathology Coordinating Laboratory (PCL)   **3, 9, 281, 313**
Pathology Study Panel (PSP)   *See also: NICHD Cooperative Epidemiological Study of SIDS Risk Factors*
Pathology Study Panel members   **313**
Periadrenal adipose tissue
histology   **76**
periadrenal brown fat   **76, 290, 293, 297**
Perinatal Autopsy Manual   **23, 26**
Peripheral nerve   **35**
Peritoneal cavity   **27**
Pertussis   **140**
Petechiae   **158**
brain   **290**
edema   **294**
epicardial   **99, 158, 294**
gross pathology in SIDS   **94, 95**
heart   **103**
intrathoracic   **294**
lung   **294**
myocardial   **99, 294**
pleural   **103, 294**
thymus   **103, 111, 261, 288, 293, 294, 297**
unusual locations   **268, 270**
Peyer's patches
gross pathology in SIDS   **95**
Phakomatosis   **119**
Pharynx   **31, 33**
Photographs   **24**
Pillows   **144**
Pituitary   **32**
histology   **86**
Plastic bags   **144**

Plastic sheets   **266**
Plastron   **28**
Pleura
  gross pathology in SIDS   **94**, **95**
  histology   **52**
  petechiae   **94**
Pleuritis   **129**
Pneumococci   **232**
Pneumonia   *See also: Bronchopneumonia*
      8, **11**, **23**, **36**, **95**, **104**, **109**, **128**, **129**, **159**, **160**, **228**, **231**, **235**, **254**,
      285, **288**, **292**, **297**
  autopsy findings   **129**
  interstitial pneumonia   **129**
  lesions sufficient to cause death   **223**, **231**, **232**, **286**, **292**
  lobar   **129**
Pneumothorax   **28, 106**
Poisoning   **8, 118**
Poisoning (carbon monoxide)   **117, 118**
Possible SIDS   **12**, **13**, **115**
Posterior fontanelle   **32**
Postmortem artifact   **105**, **107**, **175**
Postmortem findings   **99**
Preeclampsia   **15, 17**
Pregnancy
  anemia   **15, 17**
  late prenatal care   **15, 17**
  low weight gain   **15, 17**
Prematurity   **94**, **170**
Preterm   **14**, **15**, **16**, **19**, **282**
Principal investigators   **313**
Probable SIDS   **10, 12**, **13**, **115**
Project managers   **313**
Prostate   **35**
Pseudomonas aeruginosa   **256**
Psoas muscle   **87**
Pulmonary emphysema   **95**
Pulmonary hemosiderosis   **11**
Pulmonary hypertension   **8**
Pupils   **27**
Pyelonephritis   **8, 290**

Q

Quinsy   **11, 285**

R

Race   **2**, **3**, **5**, **14**, **15**, **16**, **19**, **26**, **282**, **283**, **286**
Regurgitated matter   **175**
Regurgitation   **236**
Relative risk   **16**
Renal hypoplasia   **285**
Resources from the NICHD histopathology collection   **296**
Respiratory depression   **237**
Respiratory distress   **122**
Respiratory distress syndrome   **228**, **242**, **244**
Respiratory syncytial virus   **186**, **226, 232**
Resuscitation   **24**, **48**, **50**, **51**, **99**, **106**, **109**, **156**, **168**, **169**, **172**, **173**, **175**, **177**, **180**, **264**, **268**, **274**
Retinal hemorrhage   **27**
Reye's syndrome   **8**
Rhabdomyoma   **117**, **118**, **119**, **120**, **258**
Ribs   **28**, **31, 35**
Rickettsia   **140**
Rigor mortis   **27**
Risk factors
   maternal   **15**, **16**, **17**
   newborn   **15**, **16**
   relative risk   **15**, **16**, **17**
Rokitansky technique   **30**
Rubella   **140**

S

Salivary gland   **35**
Salmonella   **8**
Scalp   **32**
Seasonal occurrence   **129, 226**
Seizure   **18**
Sella turcica   **32**
Sepsis   **8**, **251**, **256**, **285**
Sequestration crisis   **218**, **225**
Sex   **16**, **26**, **282**, **283**, **286**
Sex of the infant   **15**
Shaken baby   *See also: Child abuse, battered child*   **27, 144**
Shigella   **8**
Sickle cell anemia   **8, 11**
Sickle cell disease   **119, 285**
Sickle cells   **218**, **225**, **290**
SIDS
   clinical history   **18**

comparability with explained deaths   **282, 283**
defined   **4, 6, 23, 24, 93, 96**, **287**
definite SIDS   **10, 12, 13, 281**
gastroesophageal reflux   **295, 296**
histopathological findings (table)   **288, 290, 291**
histopathology in SIDS   **289**
incidence   **19**
mortality rate   **2**
Pathology Study Panel   **287**
possible SIDS   **10, 12, 13, 281**
probable SIDS   **10, 12, 13, 281**
relative risk   **16, 17**
Singleton births   **4, 13**
Skin   **31, 35**
gross pathology in SIDS   **94**
Skin turgor   **27**
Smoke inhalation   **285**
Smoking   **15, 17**
Social services   **96**
Soft palate   **31**
Spinal cord   **31, 32**
Spirochete infections   **140**
Spleen   **7, 34, 35**
accessory spleens   **204**
cultures   **27, 36**
extramedullary hematopoiesis   **189, 225, 289**
histology   **53**
histopathology in SIDS   **289, 293**
sickle cells   **218**
Splenitis   **289, 293**
Staphylococci   **232**
Staphylococcus aureus   **129**
Starvation   **148**
Sternum   **28**
Stomach   **33, 34, 35**
gross pathology in SIDS   **95**
Streptococcus pneumoniae   **129, 134, 256, 276**
streptococcus group B   **134**
Stress   **205**
Study centers   **3**
Subarachnoid hemorrhage   **27**
Subdural hematoma   **117**
Subdural hemorrhage   **27, 285**
Submaxillary gland   **35**
Sudden infant death syndrome
histopathology   **274**

Suffocation   **118**, **144**, **260, 261**, **266**, **268**, **285**, **286**

T

Tachycardia   **15**, **16**, **122**
Tachypnea   **15**, **16**, **226**
Temporal bone   **7**
Tentorium   **32**
Testis   **31**
Thoracic cavity   **28**
Thymus   **7**, **28**, **35**
   extramedullary hematopoiesis   **211**
   gross pathology in SIDS   **94, 95**
   histology   **78, 79**
   histopathology in SIDS   **111**, **288**, **293**
   involution   **11, 78**, **79, 95**, **263**
   petechiae   **94**, **95**, **111**, **128**, **261**, **293**, **297**
Thyroglossal duct remnant   **117**, **118**
Thyroid   **7**, **33**
   histology   **43**, **80**, **81**, **82**
   histopathology in SIDS   **288**
Tongue   **30**, **31**, **33**, **35**
Tonsils   **33**
   gross pathology in SIDS   **95**
Total anomalous pulmonary venous return   **145**
Toxemia   **15**, **17**
Toxicology   **6**, **12**, **24**, **26**, **36**, **118**, **253**
Toxin   **110**
Toxoplasma gondii   **122**
Trachea   **7**, **33**, **35**
   histology   **43**, **44**, **80**, **82**
   histopathology in SIDS   **102, 288**
   tracheitis   **102, 165**, **288**, **292**, **297**
Tracheobronchitis   **8**
Tracheoesophageal fistula   **33**
Trauma   **117**, **118**, **212**, **285**
Trauma, brain   **8**
Traumatic delivery   **205**
Triaditis   **11**
Trisomy 18   **194**
Tuberculosis   **185**, **285**
Tuberous sclerosis   **118**, **119**, **120**, **258**, **285**
"Turn arounds"
  defined   **6**
Typical findings   *See also: "Classical"findings*

U

Umbilical arteries   **27, 31**
Umbilical vein   **27, 35**
Umbilicus   **31, 35**
Unmarried mother   **15, 17**
Upper respiratory infection   **186, 187**
Upper respiratory tract
  histopathology in SIDS   **292**
  upper respiratory tract infection   **18, 101, 102, 226, 232**
Urachal remnant   **31, 34**
Urea nitrogen   **27**
Uremia   **285**
Ureter
  histology   **60**
Urethra   **34**
Urinary bladder   **34, 35**
Urinary tract infection   **15, 17**
Urine
  toxicology   **36**
Uterus   **34**
Uterus-cervix-vagina   **35**
Uvula   **31**

V

Vaccines   **140**
Vagina   **31, 34**
Vegetable matter   **180**
Venereal disease   **15**
Ventilation   **248, 264**
Vertebrae   **31, 32, 35**
Viral agent   *See also: Cultures, viral*   **36**
Virall myocarditis   **23**
Virology   **281**
Vitreous humor   **27, 146**
  toxicology   **36**
Vomiting   **18, 19, 146**

W

Wasserhellen cells, parathyroid   **84, 85**
Waterhouse-Friderichsen syndrome   **11, 256, 285**
Weighing scale   **25**
Weight   **25, 26**
Weight, at birth   **14**
Wilms tumor   **194**

"Wilson-Mikity" pattern   **11, 248**, **249**, **250**

X

X-ray   **6, 24, 37, 96, 118, 144, 253, 281**